EROTIC POWER

EROTIC POWER

Exploring the World of BDSM

by
Gini Graham Scott

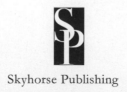

Skyhorse Publishing

Skyhorse Publishing books may be purchased in bulk at special discounts for sales promotion, corporate gifts, fund-raising, or educational purposes. Special editions can also be created to specifications. For details, contact the Special Sales Department, Skyhorse Publishing, 307 West 36th Street, 11th Floor, New York, NY 10018 or info@skyhorsepublishing.com.

Skyhorse® and Skyhorse Publishing® are registered trademarks of Skyhorse Publishing, Inc.®, a Delaware corporation.

Visit our website at www.skyhorsepublishing.com.

10 9 8 7 6 5 4 3 2 1

Library of Congress Cataloging-in-Publication Data is available on file.

ISBN: 978-1-62636-420-2

Printed in the United States of America

Contents

Acknowledgments

I want to thank the many people who helped me in preparing the book. First, many involved in dominance and submission relationships or active in the "scene" gave me information and advice. A dozen of them read the manuscript and made suggestions, although I can't thank most of them publicly. But to those I can, Penny Sunlove and Layne Winklebleck (aka Mistress Kat and Mouse), I offer my deepest thanks. Also, special thank you's to the many members of the Society of Janus, the SM Church, and the Gemini Society, who offered continuing assistance.

In addition, I received much help and encouragement from many sociologists, anthropologists, psychologists, and sexologists. In particular, I would like to thank George DeVos, Marcello Truzzi, and Charles Moser, who offered their comments and support.

Foreword

When I first wrote *Erotic Power* in 1980, the book was something of a breakthrough. The title of the initial hardcover was *Dominant Women, Submissive Men,* and that was quickly changed when the book was brought out in paperback to *Erotic Power,* because it was felt that the description might prove offensive to men who might like be described as "submissive."

At the time, the subject of the book was so controversial that many of the major bookstores wouldn't carry it, even though it was first published by a mainstream publisher of both academic and trade books. However, a launch party at a club that then existed in the Potrero District of San Francisco called The Farm changed everything. Although we publicized the party with flyers passed out mainly in the financial district in San Francisco, in the days before the Internet, Facebook, and cell phones, about two hundred professional and business people showed up for the party, which included demonstrations of S&M, bondage, and discipline techniques performed by Mistress Cat, her submissive partner Mouse, and a half-dozen other members of the then small D&S community, which was then mainly comprised of members of the SM Church, the Society of Janus, and the Gemini Society in San Francisco.

The event was featured in the *San Francisco Chronicle* in a half-page spread on the front page of the local section. And suddenly, that made all the difference. Now the bookstores were willing to cover the book, and now magazine articles appeared on the subject. The book also contributed to the growth of the D&S community, and it even changed the conversation, since the term *D&S* was then unknown.

Then, in 1997, when the book was updated and revised for a new edition by Carol Press, I noted how D&S had become more accepted and openly practiced. As I noted then, about 15 to 75 million American adults participate in "heterosexual erotic activity that includes some form of female dominance—a switch from the usually less assertive female role in heterosexual relationships." I also noted how all there were perhaps ten thousand to twenty thousand people active in publicly exploring female dominance, that there were about one hundred sexually oriented magazines on this theme, that about one hundred thousand to one hundred fifty thousand males each year visit a professional dominatrix, and that the groups I originally wrote about in 1980 had grown and many new groups had emerged.

Well, with this new edition in 2013, the interest in and acceptance of this subject has grown even more. In books like *50 Shades of Grey* and films like *Laura Croft* and *KickAss,* there are powerful women figures, and in music, women from Madonna to Miley Cyrus present themselves as strong and erotic figures. For example, according to recent stats, 2–3 percent of American adults play with dominance and submission in the form of bondage and discipline or S&M: most occasionally, some often, and a few 24/7—about 5 million people. At the same time, about 20 percent of adults report some arousal from D&S images or stories.[1]

In turn, the sales of books and film attendance at films with D&S themes and imagery has zoomed. For instance, the *Fifty Shades of Grey* trilogy has sold more than 65 million copies. And now the Internet and social media has provided even more opportunities for individuals to explore their D&S interest. For instance, the membership of FetLife, a social networking site for D&S enthusiasts interested in B&D or S&M, has grown to nearly 2 million.[2]

So now there is a vast new audience for books and other media featuring D&S, and particularly female dominance and male submission. While it may at the extremes be abused by practitioners who push the boundaries with dangerous activities, the vast majority of enthusiasts use safe words and respect limits in their play, intrigued by the imagery of danger and loss of control evoked in fantasy sessions, but able to control their participation so it remains in the realm of fantasy, much like the books, films, and social media interchanges that push limits in the imagination, but not in reality. This book is dedicated to them—those who are fascinated by this subject and who are committed to using any D&S practice safely and securely while respecting the limits of their partners in D&S play.

Introduction

About 15 to 75 million American adults, depending on the estimates, participate in heterosexual erotic activity that includes some form of female dominance, that is, a switch from the usually less assertive female role in heterosexual relationships.[1] This erotic play—which some characterize as a form of role reversal, others as a form of using power—includes a variety of activities in which the woman is dominant and the man submissive. Indeed, many adults experiment with such activities without considering them a form of dominance and submission (D&S). For example, when a woman playfully orders a man to give her an erotic massage or takes the initiative in commanding the man to bed, the couple's sexual pleasure involves an element of erotic female domination.

This kind of erotic activity, focused on the reversal of power roles, is sometimes referred to as a form of sadism and masochism (S&M) or of bondage and discipline (B&D). Some people use these terms interchangeably to refer to a wide variety of sexual, erotic, and recreational activities that involve a consensual power exchange between partners. In this book, however, I follow those who define S&M and B&D narrowly, reserving S&M to refer to exchanges involving eroticized mental, emotional, or physical pain and B&D to refer to the erotic use of assorted restraints and commands. I use D&S to encompass these and all other forms of consensual power exchange, such as the use of costumes, fetishes, cross-dressing, and infantilism (the erotic return to babyhood). These activities may be used for erotic arousal or for nonsexual fantasy play.

While many people privately and only occasionally explore their interest in D&S, a small but growing number of people—perhaps 10,000 to 20,000 in this country—are involved to some extent in publicly exploring female dominance. They actively seek out partners, meet with other couples, belong to D&S organizations, participate in D&S parties, answer ads in magazines, and purchase and use special equipment. These active participants come primarily from middle- and upper-income occupational groups, and most have a college education or advanced degree. This is not a group of dropouts and losers; they are mainstream Americans. Yet they are involved in an activity that breaks one of the most deeply held social taboos.

Here, then, are two intriguing paradoxes: participants are breaking a serious social taboo, yet they are engaging in behavior and fantasy that, in some forms, are widely prevalent. Second, and perhaps contrary to social stereotypes, the D&S scene attracts people who, except for this interest, seem otherwise to belong to the mainstream.

To explore the public D&S scene, I became an active participant for two years, beginning in January, 1981. I joined the Society of Janus and the Service of Mankind Church, two organizations in the San Francisco Bay Area for persons interested in D&S. I spent several nights each week and a dozen weekends in formal and informal group activities. I went to about two dozen parties, attended a dozen or so social evenings for D&S couples, and dated 10 men who were active in the scene. I also spent a day as a mistress-in-training and two evenings talking to mistresses at two B&D houses.

In writing this book, I adopted the perspective of an outside observer, a journalist or sociologist-anthropologist. I examine the dynamics of the heterosexual D&S scene, using detailed stories and accounts of activities to illustrate how female dominance, the power exchange, and role reversal affect the D&S sexual interaction itself, as well as other areas of the participants' lives.

This book is the first in-depth study of D&S by a participant-observer writing for a general audience. Most of the literature on the topic has been written by a few dozen psychologists and psychiatrists, including Krafft-Ebing, Sigmund Freud, Wilhelm Stekel, Theodore Reik, and Karen Horney. Such individual case studies, however, concern patients involved in S&M or B&D who are psychologically disturbed and therefore seeking treatment. Such patients are but one small segment of the vast D&S population.

Unlike the psychiatrists and psychologists who deal primarily with psychologically troubled individuals who are also interested in D&S, I met a variety of people involved in the D&S scene. I did not find them to be psychologically troubled or socially inept; rather, a spirit of good humor and fun prevailed, and the participants appeared to be mostly attractive, quite ordinary-looking people who had ordinary relationships outside the D&S scene. Most were quite content with their participation, and some saw themselves as special, creative, more exciting people because of their unique interest. Initially, some struggled with guilt feelings, but, once overcoming these, they found D&S a fulfilling form of erotic expression. Through it, they believe they have become more open, better able to understand themselves, and more capable of being intimate with others. They see the power exchange as a creative expression that promotes the development of trust and intimate communication.

So far, this population has been looked at by only a handful of observers and researchers who have written for a primarily scholarly audience. In 1979, Charles Moser, a sexologist at the Institute for the Advanced Study of Human Sexuality in San Francisco, surveyed the interests and backgrounds of about 200 men and women involved in various types of S&M activity, most of them members of two S&M clubs in New York and San Francisco, for his Ph.D dissertation. Andreas Spengler surveyed a West German S&M population of some 250 people who advertised in S&M contact magazines or belonged to S&M clubs and reported the results in a journal article in the *Archives of Sexual Behavior* in 1977. Also, John Alan Lee described his findings from interviews with 35 Canadian gay males who were part of an S&M subculture in *Alternative Lifestyles* in 1979.

Other materials on the D&S scene have been mainly works of fiction, such as the *Story of O*, about a woman's experiences with erotic submission. Or they have been nonfiction descriptions verging on pornography, such as Larry Townsend's *Leatherman's Handbook*, a sexually graphic portrayal of the gay S&M scene, published in 1972.

D&S merits an in-depth study for at least two reasons. First, some form of D&S fantasy and behavior are widespread through the general population, although many people do not identify their activities in these terms. Images of female dominance also appear frequently in the media. Some of these images are explicitly sexual, others are not. But the prevalence of such images suggests that D&S allusions and fantasies are active in the contemporary American psyche. Such images may also reflect the general increase in women's assertiveness in our society. The presence of strong women in traditionally male jobs, for example, provides new images for sexual fantasy. The erotic appeal derives from both the unusualness of women police officers or army sergeants and the reversal of traditional roles.

Second, in the past 10 years, D&S has become more accepted and more openly practiced. The first club was organized in New York in 1971 with a handful of individuals who considered themselves masochists and called themselves the Masochists Liberation Front. Now called the Eulenspiegel Society, the club has several hundred members of all sorts of S&M, B&D, and D&S persuasions. In San Francisco, the Society of Janus, started in 1975, now has about 150 members, as does the Service of Mankind Church, a group specifically oriented toward female domination. Other D&S organizations include the Gemini Society, for dominant males and submissive women; Samois, for gay and bisexual women; and several commercial houses, such as the Chateau and Backdrop, that sponsor D&S parties and activities.

The commercial world of sex likewise shows a growing interest in female dominance. About 100 sexually oriented magazines feature this theme, and each has a circulation of about 10,000 to 20,000. Also, perhaps 100,000 to 150,000 males each year visit a professional dominant or mistress for erotic satisfaction.[2]

In Part I, I discuss how people become involved in female dominance. Some are drawn in because their fantasies and experiences of female domination are so appealing or compelling that they cast aside personal anxieties about breaking social taboos and fears of public discovery. Others become involved when a friend or lover happens to introduce them to D&S while experimenting with a variety of sexual styles.

The psychological and sexual dynamics of the D&S power exchange are discussed in Part II. Typically, D&S sexuality involves a scenario in which an erotic fantasy is played out. The experience is an exaggeration of the usual sexual encounter, and its excitement derives from its uniqueness. The participants are erotically aroused or psychologically satisfied because each enjoys enacting a role: the dominant finds pleasure in exercising power, and the submissive enjoys freedom from responsibility or control and the act of submission itself. The partners are also excited by the unusualness of the role reversal as well as the mental, emotional, or physical stimulation offered by the erotic activity.

Parts III through V are devoted to the activities and behavior of people for whom D&S is more than an occasional and private diversion. Part III focuses on men and women who are beginning to explore D&S seriously and publicly through workshops and social clubs, and who are extending their D&S play beyond a couple relationship. Part IV describes those who are very active in a D&S community, their behavior with those outside the community, and the etiquette and conventions within the community. Finally, Part V explores the commercial side of D&S: professional mistresses and their clients, fantasy tapes and letters, and the market for D&S magazines, books, art, and pornography.

NOTES

1. Kinsey reports that about 50 percent of the 567 men and 2200 women from whom he collected sexual histories had at least some erotic response to being bitten. About two-thirds of the fantasies reported by Nancy Friday in *Men's Sexual Fantasies* have elements of male submission. A *Playboy* survey of college students in 1976 found that about 8 percent of the women sampled had fantasies about inflicting pain.

2. No reported figures on the number of professional mistresses and clients are available. I estimated the size of the clientele by using the advertisements placed by dominants in city newspapers and national publications. I estimate that there are about 2500 professional mistresses in this country at any given time—an average of 20 in each of the 100 major cities, and outside these cities another 500 who advertise nationally. Since most work either part time or occasionally, I estimate that each might serve two or three men a day, five days a week, for a total of about 1½ million visits a year. Assuming that the average client visits once a month, I estimate that 100,000 to 150,000 men visit mistresses in a given year.

PART I

DISCOVERING DOMINANCE AND SUBMISSION

1

The Attractions of Female Dominance

W hy, outsiders usually ask, would anyone want to get involved in any form of D&S and in female dominance in particular? Why would a woman want to hit a man, humiliate him, treat him like a slave? How can a man enjoy being hit, humiliated, or treated like an object? What motivates some people to behave in a way that outsiders generally consider not only perverse, but crazy or sick? And why do some brave social taboos and the risks of disclosure by "coming out" into the public scene instead of participating privately, as millions do?

To find out, I spoke with about 50 males and 25 females active in the San Francisco D&S scene and 25 additional males who had a long-lasting interest in female dominance but had so far mostly cultivated this interest alone or with a partner. In this chapter I discuss what attracted participants to D&S and whether any special social or personal characteristics distinguish these people from others.

The central reason that men and women become involved in female dominance, or in any other form of D&S, is that they find it erotic. They describe it as a profound, exciting, exhilarating experience that enables them to feel a greater sensation of ecstasy or sexual satisfaction than they ever achieved in normal "straight" or "vanilla" sex, as they call it. Also, they claim that it satisfies certain fundamental psychological needs, which may include the experience of power and control for the woman and the experience of giving up power and release for the man. Then, too, many D&Sers find through the sexual interchange a profound closeness, intimacy, and sense of communication and trust with one partner, particularly when they are involved in a long-term D&S relationship, coupled with a greater awareness of self, and an experience of self-expansion, as they explore new realms of creative sexual expression.

Why do some find D&S erotic? Are they different from other people? These questions are not easy ones to answer, since D&Sers are by no means a homogeneous group. D&Sers differ greatly in their levels of interest in female dominance and other forms of D&S; in their orientations to being occasionally-to-exclusively dominant or submissive; in their gender preferences—heterosexual, bisexual, or gay; and, of course, in their

3

engagement in different kinds of erotic activities. However, I did discover certain patterns that suggest some of the major attractions of D&S and the types of persons who seem especially likely to find it appealing.

The erotic attraction of D&S derives primarily from its intensity, which D&Sers claim is at times even greater than that of ordinary sex, and participants find that this intensity can carry over into nonsexual aspects of their relationships. In the casual D&S encounter, sexual intensity is heightened as participants enact deeply held fantasies, experiment with role reversal, exercise and exchange power, and explore and challenge their abilities to experience pain, pleasure, and other sensations.

For some D&Sers, this intensity yields an extremely profound, extremely intimate, and sometimes even spiritual experience in which they come into touch with their own deep feelings and those of their partner. D&S offers them not only immediate sexual satisfaction but a lingering spiritual or psychic fulfillment. They speak of a blissful surrender in which they communicate with their partner in an unmediated mental or physical fusion in which the pleasure the dominant gives and the submissive receives becomes intermingled.

Others characterize the D&S experience as one of becoming aware of their own limits and then bypassing those limits to attain another level of endurance, acceptance, or personal growth. Much as the solo adventurer confronting the wilderness discovers new capacities in themselves, they experience D&S as a frontier of self-exploration and intimacy, and, much more than a physical release, they see D&S as an arena for mental and psychic discovery. By working on the edge of the erotic and exploring the power exchange in other aspects of their lives, they feel they are delving more deeply into themselves and into others, through the use of fantasy, power, pleasure, pain, humiliation, role reversal, and other elements of D&S.

To an outsider, who observes the trappings of D&S—the whippings, the ropes, the ritualized insults, and so forth—this kind of inner experience may be hard to imagine. Yet D&Sers testify that an inner transformation occurs through the combination of intense physical, mental, or emotional stimulation. Some describe profound personal changes that result from their D&S activity: the discovery of new qualities in themselves, a heightened awareness of their own power or ability to submit, and the experiencing of a deep sense of communion with another person. For some the experience is almost a mystical or spiritual transformation.

Though D&Sers may feel this in a casual encounter, more typically, they do so in an ongoing relationship that encompasses far more than D&S activity. In such a relationship, they explain, the D&S play helps to bring the partners closer together, as they share their most intimate fantasies. To make their D&S activity more pleasurable, they must communicate well, and not only about sexual matters. But this sexual openness enhances their trust and thus their ability to share intimate nonsexual parts of themselves, too. In turn, the process of communicating their feelings helps them to look more deeply within themselves so they can understand themselves better and conceptualize and verbalize these feelings.

A social worker involved in D&S for two years explained that her participation had freed her to explore a wide range of inner thoughts and emotions, previously unexpressed, and integrate them with her outer, more public face. A lawyer who had earlier struggled with and suppressed his submissive feelings for many years found an emotional intensity in his D&S relationships that he had never experienced before, and this intensity became an integral part of his life.

For these reasons, as peculiar as it sounds to outsiders who see only the external trappings, some D&Sers describe their erotic exploration as a form of inner growth. As one woman teacher who enjoys being both dominant and submissive explains: "We're unusual people. We are looking for life, intensity, growth, expansion, and fulfillment. So we play with pain where it meets pleasure, because it meets the edge there. But we're seeking growth."

Of course, this ideal of intense intimacy, communication, and growth through D&S remains only an ideal for many, and not all D&Sers have such high expectations. D&Sers also engage in a great deal of light erotic play, seeking fun and erotic excitement, not spiritual illumination or profound awareness. Yet even so, many who engage in light play fantasize about such profound experiences and hope eventually to attain them in a session or, ideally, in an ongoing relationship. For some men who have had long-standing D&S fantasies, this desire for spiritual or psychic intensity drives them continually to seek out submissive experiences or a relationship in which they can be submissive. Although they may share society's view that D&S is wrong, this search for intensity propels them, in spite of themselves, to realize their nonsexual ideals through D&S play.

And some women, though they may come to the D&S experience late, report that same compelling attraction. As one administrator puts it: "Now that I've experienced D&S sex, I can't experience anything else."

In short, the attractions D&S offers range from the light and playful eroticism of a D&S session, which can occur between complete strangers as well as close intimates, to a transforming discovery that affects all aspects of the D&Ser's life. D&S activity can be conceived of as a pyramid—with light, casual experiences at the bottom and the most intense experiences at the top. Most participants are at the bottom, viewing D&S activity as an extension of traditional sex play, a casual experimentation with exchanges of power. D&S is an occasional part of their lives, confined to the casual, though intense, D&S session. It is pleasurable and adds to their sexual repertoire. At times they may crave it, particularly in the case of men with long-standing fantasies, but, in general, they can take it or leave it.

At the middle levels of the pyramid are those who regularly engage in D&S sexual activity, though they may participate in straight sex as well. Though they consider D&S essential, it is still confined to a small segment of their lives. Finally, at the pyramid's apex are those—perhaps 10 to 20 percent of those involved in D&S—for whom D&S is part of their everyday lifestyle. They participate in D&S sexual sessions frequently, at least several times a week or more with a single partner, or more generally with several partners, though they may have a primary relationship with one of them. And, typically, they play with the power exchange outside the D&S session. Some of the women work as professional mistresses; and both the males and females are active in various commercial or organizational aspects of the scene—running groups, writing articles, selling products, offering D&S workshops, or putting out D&S publications. Others choose a more private D&S lifestyle, confined to having a close D&S relationship or interacting with small groups of people involved in D&S.

SOCIAL CHARACTERISTICS OF D&SERS

Although interest in all types of D&S and in female dominance cuts across socioeconomic, religious, and ethnic lines, D&Sers tend to be better educated and from higher income and occupational brackets than the average American. National studies on the incidence of S&M behavior, reported by Dr. Charles Moser[1] and referred to in the 1980 KQED–San Franciso documentary *One Foot Out of the Closet*,[2] support this finding.

One explanation of this upscale pattern is that such individuals have more leisure to explore recreational sexual activity and tend to be more accepting of variety in sexual behavior. Thus, when they have fantasies or opportunities to explore erotic dominance and role reversal, they feel freer to act. Also, more affluent people are more likely to join any sort of organization. A similar predominance of upper-status participants is found in swinging, the largely middle-class sport of swapping partners.

This upscale pattern may, in turn, partially explain why relatively few members of minority groups are involved in the scene, though cultural strictures may also account for the relative scarcity of participants from certain racial or ethnic groups. For example, the black subculture places a high value on male toughness, and black women tend to play a strong, assertive role within the family. Possibly, the kind of role playing involved in female dominance may conflict too strongly with the black male image or may too closely resemble the black woman's usual role to be erotic for either. Or maybe minority group members just confine their D&S activities to private encounters and so don't appear in a mostly white upscale scene.

Although I observed these class, educational, and ethnic differences, I found no preponderance of individuals from any particular religious group. In general, D&Sers are not religious. In fact, most of the ones I met view traditional religion as a kind of moralistic straightjacket that constrains members' erotic nature and sexual expression; most came from a nonreligious background or had abandoned their religious beliefs before or while entering the D&S scene.

Finally, these D&Sers came from a wide diversity of social arrangements and affiliations. For example, some were in traditionally monogamous marriages; some in open marriages; some were living with other people in either monogamous or open arrangements. Some dated extensively in ordinary heterosexual relationships; some were involved in a fairly serious monogamous relationship; some were very shy and didn't date at all. Others had a mixture of gay and straight experience. A few discovered D&S as a result of being involved in swinging and other freewheeling sexual activity. Some had been involved in various growth and human potential movements; many had not.

PERSONALITY CHARACTERISTICS OF D&SERS

Although all types of individuals may enjoy the eroticism and power exchange of female dominance, the more specific attractions of D&S reflect a participant's personality. Also, the attractions for men and for women differ, as might be expected, since the men are drawn to submission, and the women to dominance. We can begin to look at the relationship between personality and attraction to D&S by distinguishing between the individual's basic orientation to assertiveness or passivity in everyday life and his or her interest in dominance or submission in a relationship or erotic encounter.

Using gender and everyday orientation to power, we can sketch four very broad categories of individuals: assertive men, passive men, assertive women, and passive women. Members of all four categories can be found in D&S relationships, but the attractions of D&S vary by category. For example, males who are generally assertive in everyday life may find submission an erotic release or counterbalance to their everyday behavior. Conversely, males with a generally passive nature may be attracted to submission as a complement to their personal style. Similarly, passive women may experience sexual dominance as erotic and fulfilling because it allows them to release their suppressed power, while assertive women may find sexual dominance a natural extension of their nature. Let us call those passive men and assertive women who carry over their everyday orientation into their D&S activities *natural submissives* and *natural dominants*, respectively. Those whose everyday orientation is the opposite of their D&S role, we will call *balancers*.

Quite obviously, these four categories constitute a vastly simplified model, since people's personalities range over a spectrum of dominance and submissiveness in their everyday lives, and their expression of assertiveness or passivity varies with time and circumstance. In addition, a person's work style may differ from his or her recreation style; for instance, after a difficult day at work, some assertive people like to relax by being passive, while others work off their residual aggression by being active. Likewise, an individual's enjoyment of erotic dominance or submissiveness varies with given circumstances. Nevertheless, our four categories enable us to make some useful and valid generalizations about the attractions of D&S.

Let us examine each of these groups.

THE MALE BALANCER

Most males involved in the D&S scene are balancers. In their everyday lives, they project the image of the typical, well-socialized American male—outwardly strong, outgoing, and assertive, and frequently quite successful in a responsible, high-level job. Yet these generally assertive males enjoy sexual submission, finding the unusualness of assuming the passive role in the power exchange to be erotic. Some of these males want to be socially as well as sexually submissive to a woman, but most combine sexual submissiveness with the traditional male role in their relationships with women. Thus they clearly distinguish between occasional sexual submission and other parts of their relationships and lives.

Some male balancers visit a professional mistress, which allows them to express the submissive part of themselves in a situation fully separate from the rest of their lives. Such arrangements protect them from exposure and disapproval for their erotic tastes—a particularly important consideration for males in high-level positions. Most male balancers, however, prefer to experience submission as part of a noncommercial and more or less ongoing relationship, though they may visit a mistress at times, particularly when they are not in an ongoing relationship.

Male balancers enjoy submission for any number of reasons. For some, being submissive offers release from daily responsibilities and restrictions. Others find submission a way to compensate for their usual aggressive or manipulative behavior: the symbolic punishment becomes a form of penance for their everyday aggression, and, having done this penance, they feel comfortable in then resuming their aggressive role. Or they consider the punishment as atonement for their feelings of guilt at having hurt others; the humiliation of D&S atones for the times they have humiliated others.

Then, too, an assertive male can find in submission an exciting catharsis that results from surrendering control. Instead of controlling others, someone else is controlling him, and he can lie back, relax, let go of the male preoccupation with being strong, and abandon himself to his feelings. American males are taught to suppress or rationalize their feelings, and, for some, submission allows them to become more aware of their emotions and sensory responses. For example, one male observed: "When I'm treated rough physically by a woman, I feel overcome by a flow of loving, tender, submissive energy. Surrendering to that energy and to the dominant woman on top of me is one of the most joyous experiences in my life."

Submission also enables the male balancer to relinquish responsibility for his behavior to another person. He can then do what he wants to do without feeling he has initiated an activity that he otherwise might consider taboo, sinful, or a little wicked. By claiming that a woman made him do it, he can shift the burden of accountability to her and thereby release his inner impulses. For example, Lester, a computer programmer who likes to cross-dress, appeared at an SM Church Halloween party with a wardrobe of skimpy women's dresses, nightgowns, and bathing suits. At the beginning of the party, he asked one of the women to take control of him for the evening and instruct him when to change outfits. Lester could then enjoy cross-dressing while feeling that the woman, and not he, was accountable for his costume.

Other balancers simply like the physical sensations and intense stimulation D&S offers, and some may initially act quite aggressively or coerce a woman into playing the dominant role with them. For instance, Teddy— one of the most experimental, exploratory, outgoing people I met—was a professional comedian in his 20s trying to break into the theater. Although he looked almost clerkish with his slight build, short stature, and glasses, he was actively involved in exploring virtually every type of sexual activity imaginable—including all forms of D&S. He explained that he enjoyed giving people pleasure, and, when he met a new woman, he often offered himself to her almost immediately as her masseur and pleasure slave. Also he would spend hours calling friends all over the country to treat them to erotic phone fantasies in which he described at length how he was pleasing them. In contrast, Davis used a very different, though also aggressive, style in seeking out erotic stimulation from women. He would approach a dominant woman at a D&S party, suddenly touch her aggressively, usually on the breasts, buttocks, or genitals, and then, when she inevitably turned around to slap or whip him, he would have an orgasm.

Other male balancers find still other sources of satisfaction in occasional submission, such as reexperiencing childhood cravings by being mothered, protected, or nurtured by a beautiful, sexually appealing woman; acting like a little boy again; or expressing worshipful feelings to a woman, as they did when boys. Some like the chance to express the normally repressed feminine side of their nature.

In short, male balancers find many different sexual and psychic pleasures in being submissive, and there are many ways in which being submissive balances their otherwise aggressive nature. Yet, even as they seek this submission, they do not give up their power or will completely, for they may have a specific agenda for being submissive in a certain way or may only fantasize being submissive. To achieve this end, they may more or less surreptitiously manipulate a dominant woman into enabling them to be submissive in the way they wish.

THE NATURAL MALE SUBMISSIVE

In contrast to the male balancers, who are submissive only sporadically, some men feel they are passive by nature and want to be submissive in all aspects of their lives. They seek relationships in which their submissiveness extends beyond the bedroom. Some of these natural submissives pretend to be assertive in their jobs or with other males, while others are passive or submissive in their everyday lives. In contrast to the balancers, these men are submissive both to women and to people generally, because of their shyness or social ineptness. Often, such men have feelings of uncertainty or inferiority because they are aware that they are not conforming to the traditional male role.

Some natural submissives choose D&S because they have difficulty in relating to women or because they lack social skills. They feel it will be easier for them to succeed with women if they let women take the lead. The strategy does not always work, because their lack of social skills may lead dominant women to reject them, too. But such men believe they will be more successful if they don't have to take the traditional male initiative, find the D&S scene erotic and occasionally gain some attention; so they persevere. Other natural submissives seek out strong, powerful women as a way of compensating for their own feelings of uncertainty and inferiority. By looking up to dominant women or identifying with them, they feel more personally worthwhile.

For example, Winston, a computer systems analyst in his 30s, was one of the shyest males I met. Slightly built, very thin, and a little owlish looking, he had quit a legal career because he found it too competitive to suit his passive, retiring nature. He explained that he was drawn to strong, dominant women, although his shyness made it difficult for him to initiate contact with such women. When he encountered someone new, he never seemed to know what to say. Although he had enjoyed a relationship with a dominant woman who had picked him up at a department store and wanted another D&S relationship, his shyness seemed to relegate him to waiting for a dominant woman to initiate a relationship with him.

In a similar case, Travis, a biology student in his late 20s, had been very shy and withdrawn in high school, though very good looking, because he never felt good enough. He felt he didn't measure up to his professional parents' standards of excellence, so he withdrew from his parents and classmates and never dated. At 15 he began fantasizing about being with the popular girls in school and having them dominate him. Once he passed three of the most popular girls who were sitting in a car talking, and he imagined what it would be like to be trapped between them, ordered around, and finally beaten up. For several years he tied himself to his bed or fantasized about being overpowered by a dominant woman while he masturbated. Then he began to go to mistresses occasionally and participate in D&S groups, although his shyness, lack of confidence, and uncertain social skills made these encounters less than satisfying. He was never sure the woman liked him or if he was doing the right thing, even as he tried fervently to please. As a result, he began seeing a therapist occasionally to deal with his social problems and insecurities.

Thus passive males seek out submissive experiences for very different reasons than assertive males. Yet, even so, they may enjoy the same sort of experiences submission offers, such as feeling out of control, feeling nurtured and protected, becoming more aware of their bodies, experiencing punishment, and so forth. However, passive men seem to have more problems in integrating their submissiveness into a successful and satisfying lifestyle, in part because of their shyness, low self-esteem, or social ineptitude. Then, too, compared to the assertive males, these men tend to have much more powerful, deep-seated fantasies that surpass erotic submission and entail a desire to submit their total being to a woman in all aspects of life.

For men this kind of thinking can be quite threatening, for it challenges the traditional concept of male identity. The naturally submissive male usually has difficulty in accepting his self-image and incorporating his submissive identity into his life. In contrast, the assertive male who only occasionally plays at being submissive generally does not have to confront this identity issue so profoundly, and it may not be an issue at all, though he may initially feel uneasy with that part of himself that wants to be submissive at a given time.

THE FEMALE BALANCER

The female balancers represent a counterpart to the male balancers in that
their everyday personalities generally meet society's expectations for
their gender. These women have a soft, gracious, feminine manner; and
typically, in their everyday lives they play the traditional feminine role. For
example, they are often teachers, secretaries, nurses, lower-level adminis-
trators, or hold other jobs frequently performed by women.

In turn, much as male balancers at times enjoy being submissive,
female balancers occasionally like being dominant sexually or being assertive in other areas of the male-female relationship. Some female balancers
are sexually dominant but otherwise passive in their relationships; others
are dominant in nonsexual spheres as well, with the particular arrangements usually based on negotiated agreements with their partners. Dominance gives these women a sense of power, authority, and control that
compensates for their feelings of powerlessness or, in some instances,
oppression in daily life, and these feelings are a source of erotic pleasure.
Also, dominance gives them a chance to explore their own potential,
exercise their creativity, take initiative, be assertive, and assume leadership. Thus dominance offers psychological ballast for their everyday passivity. As one woman put it, "Why should I want to be submissive in a
relationship? I'm that way normally in everyday life." For some, erotic
dominance is also a symbolic enactment of their general hostility or anger
at men for oppressing women, though in a redirected, stylized, safe, and
mutually enjoyable form.

Indeed, female balancers frequently seek D&S activity after a trying
day that leaves them feeling tense, upset, frustrated, or angry. For example,
Sharon, an administrative assistant in her 30s who was primarily socially
passive in her relationship but sexually dominant most of the time, told me:
"Whenever someone gets me angry, I 'take it out' on my love." By this, she
meant that she would symbolically transform her anger into a creative
expression of dominance over him. "It's a way of letting out the angry
energy in my soul in a constructive way." In turn, her lover, Lance, a real
estate contractor with whom she lived, enjoyed being directed by a powerful woman who was acting firm and mean. For instance, one evening at a
small dinner party, Lance opened a bottle of champagne and it sprayed all
over the living room. Though Lance apologized profusely, the thought of
the clean-up task ahead made Sharon feel angry and frustrated. Rather than
yelling or arguing, she sought to even the score symbolically in a way that
would both release her anger and give her and Lance pleasure. She went
into the bedroom, got a rug beater, and slapped it against Lance's buttocks.
Since the guests were also involved in D&S, they understood her response
and cheered her on. And Lance experienced a pleasurable, though painful,

feeling of release, through the combination of the erotic stimulation and the symbolic punishment and penance imposed by her act.

THE NATURAL FEMALE DOMINANT

Other women attracted to erotic dominance are highly assertive in daily life and see themselves as having a dominant personality. Their interest in sexual dominance represents an extension of their usual way of being. As such, their attraction to dominance is much like the naturally passive male's interest in submission. However, unlike naturally submissive males, who may encounter social difficulties and feelings of low self-esteem when they are submissive in the everyday world, natural female dominants typically have a healthy level of self-respect because American society looks favorably on the qualities associated with dominance and power. The naturally dominant woman generally experiences success in daily life and thus, though she doesn't conform to feminine stereotypes, she usually feels good about herself.

When an assertive woman encounters dominance and finds it erotic, she tends to feel that she has discovered a natural mode of sexual expression and fairly easily integrates this conception into her own identity as a strong, successful woman. As one woman who managed a small business told me: "When my lover suggested I be dominant, I took to it like a duck takes to water. I already had a strong personality. I was successful in managing all sorts of projects. So this was something I felt really comfortable doing. I was just exercising my dominance in another part of my life." And although the naturally dominant woman's motivations may differ from the female balancer's, she too finds in dominance a way to exert control, exercise her power and authority, explore her creativity, and expand her self-awareness.

NOTES

1. Charles Allen Moser, "An Exploratory-Descriptive Study of a Self-Defined S/M (Sadomasochistic) Sample," Ph.D. Dissertation. The Institute for Advanced Study of Human Sexuality. August 1979.

2. *One Foot Out of the Closet*, KQED–San Francisco Documentary, February, 1980.

2

Becoming Involved

As we saw in Chapter 1, participants find female dominance to be erotically stimulating and psychologically satisfying. But these attractions and benefits do not explain why they were first drawn to female dominance or other forms of D&S. Why does a man choose D&S rather than socially more acceptable ways to relax and be passive? And why does a woman choose to express her desire for power through sexual dominance in the bedroom rather than through assertiveness in the workplace or community? Are there common themes in the backgrounds and personalities of those attracted to female dominance?

Neither social nor personality factors seem to explain the broad appeal of D&S. Rather, the erotic appeal of female dominance seems to develop from either predispositional or situational circumstances, sometimes dating back to childhood. For example, most people who find female dominance or other D&S activity to be arousing and pleasurable discover this when they happen upon an experience that involves dominance. Sometimes the incident is implicitly sexual, as when a woman takes the initiative in a sexual scene and her partner finds this exciting. Although very often the experience is not a sexual one, the person becomes sexually aroused, as a young boy might when he is paddled by a teacher or tied up while playing cowboys and Indians. If the pull of this eroticism is strong enough or if situational factors are favorable, or both, the individual will continue to seek out such experiences.

In short, regardless of their reasons for being presently involved in female dominance, D&Sers generally go through a coming-out process, during which they discover that D&S can be erotic. They then begin, more or less easily, to express and fulfill their desires to dominate or submit.

For some, coming out is a long and relatively difficult process, for they must overcome prevailing social taboos about D&S, S&M, and B&D. Males, especially, tend to have a difficult time, since they must also overcome the societal attitude that male submissiveness is unmanly. Also, many males have to resolve their guilt about their fantasies of submission, guilt that may date back to childhood fantasies.

By contrast, women who feel comfortable taking the initiative and playing an assertive role tend to find coming out easier. Society regards the qualities associated with dominance—strength and power—positive, and in the 1980s these qualities are considered appropriate for women to have. Then, too, women usually do not have the long-standing sexual fantasies and the guilt men do, since women tend to come to dominance late, usually introduced by a male who encourages them to be dominant. And those who do come to dominance on their own initiative tend not to feel guilty about it, because society considers strength an admirable quality or because these women tend to feel an exhilarating sense of liberation as they discover and use their power.

Since there are so many more males than women involved in the D&S scene, let's examine their coming-out process first and then turn to the women.

THE COMING-OUT PROCESS FOR MEN

When men explain how they became interested in submission, three major themes recur. Most had submissive fantasies as children; their current style of submission is often related to their first erotic submissive experience; and men coming to the scene late experience the sudden emergence of powerful, though undiscovered, desires to be submissive.

The Role of Early Fantasies

Again and again, the men I spoke to cited their childhood submissive fantasies as the reason they became actively involved in female dominance. As adults they continued to feel a compelling need to express this submission, which they found extremely erotic or psychologically satisfying, and this need had become an integral, essential part of the self.

These men typically reported spending many years privately—and guiltily—experiencing submissive fantasies. They felt their interest to be wrong or forbidden, because in American society, males are supposed to be aggressive and independent. Being submissive is considered weak, unmanly, and feminine.

Many of them also felt guilty when someone, usually a parent, discovered or nearly discovered them acting out a submissive fantasy, such as dressing up as a woman or tying themselves up. After a discovery or a near miss, most continued to fantasize; some even more so, excited by the drama of being found out. Though some stopped acting out their fantasies because they feared being discovered again, most simply became more secretive. And some found their feelings of guilt and the threat of discovery and humiliation erotically arousing, too. The minority who put aside or repressed both the fantasies and the activities found that the fantasies resurfaced when later experience retriggered their earlier feelings.

Thus, eventually, these men began to respond to their recurring feelings and fantasies—some acting earlier than others, some more openly, and some with less guilt. Typically, they first acted privately: masturbating to climax while fantasizing, reading pornographic magazines, or manipulating themselves into a submissive role by provoking a teacher or parent to discipline them. Others explored different ways of enacting their fantasies alone—for example, by dressing up and photographing themselves, tying themselves up, whipping themselves, holding themselves for a long time in an awkward posture, or depriving their senses for an extended period. Most tried a combination of techniques.

For instance, Alex, now a pediatrician in his 30s, had his first experience in cross-dressing at age 11, when his mother and sister thought it would be "cute" if he went to a church costume party as a girl. He found it exciting, and to recapture that experience occasionally continued to cross-dress in his mother's clothes, until she discovered him a few times. So he tried to put this interest aside, but, in his teens the feelings returned, and he began to acquire magazines on cross-dressing, fantasize about being dressed up, and take photographs of himself dressed. Since he still felt guilty about having these desires, he began to fantasize that a woman forced him to dress by tying him up and making him follow her orders. To symbolize her power, he tied himself up and soon found the bondage as exciting as the cross-dressing. In a short time, he was doing both.

Once these men began to act on their fantasies they usually did so secretly for many years because they felt their fantasies too private and too unacceptable to share. But then, typically, they did want to share them as they reached their 20s and 30s, though a minority waited until their middle years; one even held back until he was 70. Usually these men proceeded to act on their fantasies by going to a professional mistress or trying to share their desires with a date, girlfriend, or wife.

Those going to a professional did so because they felt she would understand or they felt freer to express their taboo desires with someone they didn't know. In many cases, an experience with a mistress represented a man's first open encounter with his submissive side—it was a kind of initiation. Others went to a mistress only after their girlfriends or wives refused to share their fantasy. While some visited a professional only once or twice and then sought to confine their submissiveness to an ongoing relationship, others continued to go to a mistress occasionally or even regularly, depending on how well their other relationships satisfied their continuing need for submission and on their ability to afford the fees.

Those who tried to get a date, girlfriend, or wife involved often used an indirect approach, first hinting around at their interest, rather than expressing themselves openly, to protect themselves against rejection. By introducing the subject gradually, they felt they would be less likely to shock their partner and be refused, and, if they encountered resistance, they could back down gracefully and even deny their interest—they were only kidding. A few reversed their fantasies and initially asked the woman to be submissive, hoping she would be more receptive to D&S in general if she played the submissive role first; then they encouraged her to be dominant. For example, some men kidded about what it would be like to be tied up, or experimented with spanking their partner or holding her arms back to see how she would react. Or they casually suggested the woman try something, like instructing her partner to perform some action or slapping him with a slipper. Then, if she responded, they experimented a little bit further or gradually shared a little bit more. But if she didn't, they backed off. Others were more direct in describing their interests.

Most of these efforts to share with girlfriends or wives were unsuccessful, regardless of the tactfulness or gentleness of the man's approach. Often the women were completely unreceptive and thought the request weird, strange, or sick. Then the men usually dropped the topic to preserve the relationship, though they continued to practice privately, go to mistresses, or seek out others with similar interests. For example, when Lester, the computer programmer who liked dressing up, being whipped, and being forced to do things, asked his wife if she might like to try some of these activities, she told him that such play was sick. So he got a post office box number, kept a box of clothes in his car, answered some ads, joined some D&S organizations, and participated in female dominance activities in these groups or in short-term relationships about once a week. For him, the only solution was a double life.

Some women refused because the men were inept in presenting their interest and were too direct or revealed their own ambivalence about participating in D&S and thus turned off their partner. Or the male was too demanding in wanting the woman to respond to his desires right away, before developing a solid, secure, loving, and caring relationship. Had these women been more gradually introduced, some might have ultimately been receptive.

In many cases, women refused because they found it difficult to play the dominant role. One common reason is that many women by nature or socialization learn to be submissive—and few have the strong sexual fantasies males have to express another side of their nature. Thus, frequently, women were willing to experiment when asked by their partner, but they weren't very good at being dominant. Typically, they performed as the men requested, but did not enjoy the dominant role. As a result, their efforts to please or humor their partner were unsuccessful, since the males could enjoy their submissiveness only if the woman was being truly dominant and liking it. If a woman couldn't really "get into it," neither could her partner.

For example, after years of experimenting in private, Alex finally decided to share his fantasy of cross-dressing and bondage with several women. Although his diplomatic approach convinced his partners to experiment, he felt they were merely going through the motions of tying him up or telling him to dress up like a woman, because he asked them to do so. Since the women he was attracted to were by nature submissive, they couldn't effectively perform the dominant role. They couldn't exercise real power or express the firmness, forcefulness, or meanness he wanted to experience from a woman. So, eventually, he lost interest in dating them.

Many men like Alex who gradually opened up their submissive side to others experienced a continuing problem of coming to terms with their own identities. In addition, many encountered assorted frustrations in their quest for fulfillment with others, because professional mistresses did not satisfy their emotional needs, because their girlfriends or wives rejected their overtures or could not play the dominant role, or because no activity was as satisfying as their fantasies. Thus, for various reasons, most put their desires for submissiveness aside for a time.

But the desire continued to return, and so, sometimes reluctantly or ambivalently, still concerned about breaking social taboos or uncertain of their chance for success, they again sought to express their submissiveness. They found the eroticism of submission so pleasurable, the pull of it so compelling, that despite all the difficulties they encountered, despite any lingering reservations about being perceived as deviant or unmanly, they resumed their quest for a satisfying relationship involving female dominance. Thus the men commonly went through a series of cycles, first denying or dismissing their desires for submission, then resuming their search.

For example, Marvin, a 40-year-old internist, was normally dominant at work and in his social relationships. He described his desire for submission as a compelling inner drive that he could not diffuse. He began fantasizing about being submissive in his late teenage years and initially tried to repress these feelings. He later briefly expressed them with a few mistresses and with his second wife, who complied a few times, but indicated she wasn't interested. After his second marriage dissolved, in part because of this issue, he began to attend meetings of D&S organizations, though his guilt precluded him from speaking to other members. But gradually, as he discovered that the others seemed like "nice, respectable, normal people," who enjoyed D&S without feeling guilty, his guilt dissipated and he began to fully enjoy the submissive experience.

Like Marvin, many men come to terms with their submissive needs only after years of frustration, guilt, and confusion. A few seek some therapeutic help; most work out their conflicts on their own. However, almost all gradually come to accept and enjoy their submissive side after gaining support from reading magazines, joining D&S organizations, visiting mistresses, or meeting supportive women who are already dominant or willing to become so. Other men, who find the social taboos too strong or were unable to find a receptive woman, finally, though with difficulty, reject their submissive desires.

The case histories of Alvin and Hal illustrate this long process of men coming to terms with their early fantasies. Alvin finally became happily involved in the scene; Hal, ridden with conflicts over his behavior, dropped out.

Alvin, now an attorney in his late 40s, had some powerful experiences with cross-dressing and bondage as a child. When he was eight, he and a little girl played at cross-dressing. As he put on the clothes, he felt a surge of submissiveness and femininity. Soon after, he played hide-and-seek with another girl, and he liked the experience of being blindfolded while she hid. He enjoyed feeling helpless and thinking of her as more powerful, and he pretended to have difficulty finding her to prolong the game. Then, at 13, when he was at camp, he saw a boy beaten up in a fight by a girl. Along with the other boys, he jeered the hapless victim, but secretly he wished he had been that boy.

Throughout his teenage years, Alvin continued to have fantasies of being bound, whipped, dressed up as a woman, and forced to orally serve a woman. But like most men with these fantasies, he was ambivalent about submissive feelings and did not act on them. He married in his early 20s and played the traditional dominant male role. But his fantasies continued, and, afraid to confide in his wife, he secretly purchased some women's clothing and a wig. When he put them on, he felt a rush of relief and fulfillment. He drove around in this costume for several minutes, and in a "fit of daring," as he described it, picked up a male hitchhiker. However, when the hitchhiker asked him if he was going to a party, he felt embarrassed and said yes. Once alone, he pulled into a gas station, threw out the clothing, and did not cross-dress again for many years.

After Alvin's first marriage broke up, mainly because he was dissatisfied with the dominant role, he moved from the East Coast to Southern California, where he again sought to repress his submissive feelings. He dated several women, told none of them his fantasies, and finally, after an est workshop, decided to marry a secretary he had dated. The workshop helped to convince him that he should accept his present situation and stop fantasizing.

However, his second marriage also proved unsatisfying. Although he shared some of his fantasies with his wife and she briefly tried to be dominant, she was uncomfortable with that role. As this second marriage began to break apart, Alvin first began to visit professional mistresses. He found the experience largely pleasurable, although, like many men visiting mistresses, he felt the encounter lacked emotional feeling and was limited by the clock. What he really wanted, he concluded, was an enduring relationship with a caring, dominant woman. This decision was reinforced by two visits to a therapist who helped Alvin recognize and accept his true submissive nature. No wonder his marriages hadn't worked, the therapist pointed out, because he had chosen unassertive women.

Alvin divorced his wife and actively began to look for a dominant woman. He placed and answered ads and resumed cross-dressing in private. Also, he continued to see the therapist from time to time to get additional personal support for what he was doing. Through an ad, he discovered two local D&S organizations and became active in the scene. Although he has not yet found the relationship he wants, he now feels certain he is doing the right thing in trying to realize his long-repressed inner fantasies.

Like Alvin, Hal had submissive fantasies as a child, but his ambivalence and inner conflict led him to drop out of the scene. Now 35 and a law student, formerly in construction. Hal first became interested in being submissive when he was seven. He remembers lying on the floor while his older sister sat around with her friends drinking coffee or wine, and he found gazing at their legs to be very stimulating. At times, his sister playfully put her foot on his back and kiddingly teased, "You little twerp." And once, he spent an hour locked in a dark closet with her shoes and was highly excited.

In his teens, Hal began collecting magazines on foot fetishism, and he read extensively on the psychology of fetishism, hoping to understand his feelings. While he was drawn to submission, at times he tried to deny the feeling, and for long periods he unsuccessfully tried to put aside his interest.

Until he was 25, he explored submission privately and intermittently. Then, for the first time, he expressed his feelings to a woman he had been dating for almost a year in a traditional relationship. He persuaded her to act out some of his fantasies involving foot worship, being stepped on by a woman, and satisfying her orally. She acceded a few times, but she never felt comfortable doing so and thought Hal's requests were weird. As a result, their relationship gradually deteriorated, and, when he dated other women, he refrained from mentioning his fantasies.

Later, he visited a few mistresses, but didn't find this satisfying because the mistresses seemed mainly interested in making money. In his early 30s he told his fantasies to another girlfriend, whose reaction was much like the first. So, once again, he dismissed his fantasy and played the traditional male role in dating, which he did quite successfully.

Yet, Hal's drive to be submissive persisted, and he briefly explored a few Bay Area D&S organizations—the Society of Janus, the SM Church, and Backdrop. But since he wanted an ongoing exclusive relationship and didn't find the right woman at these meetings, he dropped out.

A few months later he answered an ad placed by Katrina, a 30-year-old woman interested in exploring D&S. Enthusiastically, he wrote to her: "I have been waiting for a woman to run an ad like yours for a long time....I now fully accept that part of me that yearns for a dominant woman....I'm looking for a woman that I can really develop a good and lasting relationship with. There is a submissive part of me that is just waiting for the right woman to take and mold me to her."

But, when he met Katrina, his ambivalence about submission resurfaced. They talked intensely for about an hour about his interests, and he asked Katrina to call him if she was eager for a "slave" to please her. Yet when she did call he was strangely cold and distant. "No, I've thought about all this since we met," he said. "But now I've decided to put it all aside. I'm just going to drop it all completely." Hal still seemed to fear the emotions that might be released by realizing his long-held fantasies. He wanted to explore his fantasies and yet was afraid, and his persistent fear was stronger than his recurring desire.

The stories of Alvin and Hal are classic examples of a common pattern experienced by men interested in submission: early fantasies accompanied by feelings of guilt, efforts to repress their submissive interests, dissatisfaction in traditional male-female relationships, and a decision to either accept and express his inner feelings or to deny or repress them.

THE IMPORTANCE OF THE FIRST SUBMISSIVE EXPERIENCE

A second recurring theme among men is the relationship between their first erotic fantasy or experience and their later style of submission. Though most of these first-time fantasies or experiences dated from childhood or the early teens, others came later. But almost always the content of this first erotic experience became an important part of their later sexual repertoire.

It is not easily determined whether this first experience caused their later interest or whether they had a predisposition toward being submissive which this initial experience triggered. Or perhaps they just wanted to repeat what they found to be an enjoyable experience. But, whatever the reason, they seemed to develop a connection between being submissive in a certain way and experiencing erotic pleasure. Then they found similar experiences or fantasies erotically arousing.

Typically, the men's initial submissive experiences were ordinary everyday events that provoked an erotic response. For example, males who like bondage remember that they enjoyed being captured or tied up when they played cowboys and Indians as children or that they first discovered a submissive thrill when a lover playfully tied them up with scarves. Males who like cross-dressing report having dressed up in their mothers' or sisters' clothing as children or having been dressed up for fun by their families. Males who like spanking or whipping describe early incidents of being punished by someone, usually a teacher, and finding this erotic. Males who are excited by particular objects, like shoes, recall early triggering events, such as being stepped on by an attractive woman. And males who like being mothered or babied say they felt this need as children because they did not have enough love or mothering or because they found a disciplinary action involving babying, such as being put in diapers as a teenager, both embarrassing and erotic.

In short, there seems to be a continuity between early erotic associations and later erotic experiences and fantasies, even for males who are extremely active in the scene and experiment with all sorts of D&S activity. For example, Bertrand, a 75-year-old retired accountant, had his first erotic experience at the hands of his second-grade teacher. She whipped him in front of the class for throwing spit-balls and then required him to sit under her desk. He felt humiliated, yet sexually aroused. As an adult he had recurrent fantasies of being hit and spanked, particularly by a teacher, although he didn't act on these until his early 70s, when he enacted his fantasy with a mistress, and thereafter joined the scene.

Lance, a 35-year-old real estate contractor, who likes bondage and chains, recalls a childhood game of cowboys and Indians when a neighbor girl tricked him into letting her tie him up. Then, as a teenager, he became fascinated with chains when reading about black slavery in America; being black, he identified with the slaves.

Likewise, Warren, a student in his 20s, cites his first erotic experience, which involved "golden showers"—the D&Ser's term for urination. He was about 13 and playing around in the bathroom with a girl of 12. They undressed, and he was aroused when she suddenly urinated on him. Though suprised, he remained sexually excited. Thus the act of urination acquired erotic connotations for him, and, since then, though he came to like spanking, bondage, humiliation, piercing, and other D&S activities as a dominant and submissive with both males and females, his favorite activity is still being a woman's "toilet slave."

As for Mark, a 50-year-old factory worker who expecially likes dressing as a baby, his first erotic experience occurred when his mother disciplined and humiliated him by forcing him to wear diapers to school because he wet his bed. When he took off his trousers in the locker room, his fellow students teased him. But he found their humiliating taunts sexually exciting, and thereafter he continued to replay the essence of that early experience by finding dominant women, usually mistresses, to check his

diapers for stains, make him write sentences promising never to wet his
pants again, and paddle him when he made the inevitable faux pax in his
diaper or underwear.

DISCOVERING SUBMISSIVENESS AS AN ADULT

Although most men in the D&S scene report having had early fantasies, a
sizable minority—perhaps a quarter of the men I spoke with—discovered
their submissive side as adults. They remembered no early fantasies or
experiences about being submissive, but encountered D&S in adulthood
and enjoyed it. Most often, they were playing around with a girlfriend with
whom they had been traditionally dominant when they discovered something she did aggressively to be exciting, or they suggested she try something involving a role reversal and liked it. For instance, when Alan, a
31-year-old scientist, and his girlfriend, Nikki, a 30-year-old legal assistant,
were rolling around on the bed, Nikki grabbed a scarf from the dresser and
began to tease him with it, threatening to tie him up. When she did, he had
an intense erection and afterwards wanted to further explore sexual role
reversal.

Other males discovered submission while experimenting with swinging or bisexuality and, by chance, encountering a sexual scene in which they
were submissive. Then they added submission to their repertoire as
another form of enjoyable sexual activity. As an example, Bart, a writer and
former professor in his late 30s, had had an active sex life since he was 15,
mostly with older women, since he skipped a few years in school. His early
and occasional fantasies about being required to serve a woman were not
important to him at the time, and, through his college years and early 20s,
he had traditionally male-dominant sexual relationships. However, soon
after he married a woman psychologist, he and his wife starting doing
research on swinging couples and participated in numerous swing sessions.
On two occasions the couples they met enjoyed D&S and they introduced
Bart and his wife to female dominance. In the first case, the husband asked
Bart to orally satisfy his wife, and afterwards she urinated on him in the
shower and they tied him down. In the second instance, the wife ordered
Bart around and called him names. He found both experiences exhilarating
and sporadically continued to experiment at swing sessions; but his wife
was not interested in being dominant in their relationship.

Still others, not so sexually active, had unexpected chance encounters
in which they discovered that being submissive was erotic, in part because
its novelty and forbidden quality seemed exciting. For example, Terry, a
35-year-old attorney, lived an ordinary, monogamous life with his wife
until he was 34. Very conservative in outlook, he had never had any

submissive fantasies. Then, on a business trip, he started talking to a couple sitting across from him at the bar at his motel. After about an hour, the woman whispered to him: "I'd really like to suck your cock." He recalls that her remark "practically blew me away." However, her husband reassured him: "Yes, she would."

They led him upstairs to their room, where the husband tied up his wife, slapped her around to stimulate her, and then she orally brought him to orgasm. Terry says he experienced "an exhilaration and thrill that was just incredible. I felt myself come alive in ways I never knew existed."

Back home, he answered a half-dozen ads from couples and women involved in D&S, and through these encounters he learned to play the submissive role. He tried to involve his wife, but she firmly said she wasn't interested, so he quickly dropped the topic. But he continued to participate in occasional D&S sessions, sometimes involving female dominance. As he did, he developed more elaborate fantasies, centered primarily around light bondage and orally satisfying a woman.

Most men who discover submission as adults typically enjoy it in an occasional, playful, experimental way. And perhaps because they are only dabbling with it, or perhaps because they discovered submissiveness after their concept of their own masculinity was already developed, they don't find being submissive at times a threat to their masculine self-image. In contrast, many men who had submissive fantasies or experiences before their sense of self was formed do feel threatened by this impulse to behave in a way not normally considered male. These latecomers, already sure of their own sexuality and identity, consider submission as one more way to experience sex, and they approach it in this uncomplicated, open, experimental spirit. Some have an occasional twinge of concern about how their submissiveness might affect other areas of life, but such concern is usually brief, and most appraise any effects as positive. For example, Bart initially wondered how being submissive might psychologically affect him. But as he continued to explore it occasionally in swinging, he decided, "I've become a better person as a result. I'm more gentle now, more relaxed, all around a better lover."

For a few latecomers, however, the experience had a deep, powerful, life-altering effect, since it brought to the surface certain submissive needs they had repressed and had not acknowledged. This was the case for Jesse, a 27-year-old credit investigator, whose sexual experience prior to his D&S involvement was limited by his shyness with women. Also, Jesse's parents had brought him up to be a strong, tough leader who must never show weakness. Through his early 20s, he had largely repressed his needs for tenderness and love.

At age 24, Jesse was flipping through a sexually oriented publication and saw a large ad for a B&D house picturing a beautiful woman who offered "a fantastic experience." Not knowing exactly what this meant, but intrigued, he went to see her. He was immediately struck by her large size—about six feet—and her beauty. She ordered him to undress, but he only stripped down to his underwear. In moments she tackled him, held him around his shoulders with a heavy grip, twisted his arms behind his back, and snapped him into handcuffs. He hadn't obeyed her first order to undress, she explained, so now she would teach him a lesson. She flourished a paddle and began striking his buttocks and back so hard that soon he had tears in his eyes; he didn't find the experience erotic. Next, she tied him up and left him sitting on the floor for half an hour, while she sat across from him in a chair, watching. For most of this time, he screamed, hoping someone would come, until he realized it was fruitless—no one responds to the cries of a man in a female dominance session, only to those of a woman. When he stopped screaming, she took his clothes, put them in a pile on the floor in front of him, and released him.

"You can crawl over to me now," she told him, "or you can put on your clothes and leave."

He didn't understand why he did it, but he crawled over to her, and she held him in her arms, mothering him for an hour—an experience he found emotionally satisfying and erotic. No one had ever mothered him like this before, he realized. It was the first time he had been able to express this long-repressed need.

He continued to seek out further experiences of being babied, and, as he met other mistresses and people in the scene, he discovered he liked other aspects of D&S, including being both dominant and submissive and participating in sessions with both men and women. He felt no guilt or inner conflicts about expressing this part of his nature; rather he felt he had touched a deep, inner part of himself, that his D&S experience had opened a new world of sexuality to him.

Unlike Jesse, some men who in their 20s and 30s discover their interest in being submissive are frightened to see this part of themself emerge. They are initially intrigued by the new-found eroticism but then become ambivalent about acknowledging the submissive side of their character, feeling it unmanly or fearing they will be unable to control their desires and will thereby disrupt their established masculine role pattern. They pull back not only because the newness of the situation is scary but also they fear that further involvement will threaten their view of what it means to be a man.

This was the case with Alan, a personnel manager in his late 30s. He had long thought of himself as a dominant male, and he enjoyed "putting women through their paces" by treating them like slaves or pieces of furniture and ordering them about in play sessions. But then he enjoyed a few fleeting experiences of submission with two of his usually submissive girlfriends. One playfully raked her long fingernails along his back; the other teasingly played with his nipples. He enjoyed the sensation and felt a strange thrill at having the woman take the initiative and briefly dominate him. He began fantasizing about a dominant woman and asked some of the women he usually dominated to try the role. But they felt uncomfortable, and so he answered a few ads by dominant women and attended a few meetings of D&S organizations. Yet as soon as he was attracted to a dominant woman who encouraged him to initiate an ongoing relationship with her, he pulled back and dropped out of the scene, afraid he could not handle the reality of the submissive role he fantasized about. As he explained: "I'm ambivalent. So far, everything has worked for me, and I'm in a job where I have to be strong and dominant. But I'm afraid if I start releasing the submissive qualities in myself, it may carry over into my work. And I'm concerned about that."

STAYING INVOLVED

Once men do decide to come out and openly express their interest in female dominance, they typically try out a wide smorgasbord of D&S activities, either with a particular person or a series of partners. Some remain active on a fairly intense, ongoing basis; others drop in and out of private D&S activity and the D&S scene. Some alternate private one-on-one relationships with a dominant woman and group activities, depending on their relationship with a particular partner and their partner's interest in organized D&S activities.

Most generally, these men are interested in exploring female dominance with a number of partners, and the scene is characterized by a spirit of creativity and experimentation that encourages this exploration. They enjoy interacting with numerous women, and most prefer playing with nonprofessionals, with whom they feel a more emotional and less business-like connection. Some, though, go to mistresses occasionally, usually when they want to play more than they can with the nonprofessional women they know. Fewer want to explore female dominance with a steady partner.

While some men are very successful in finding women to explore with, many others have difficulty. Some of the men having difficulties are older, less attractive, or less adept socially, and would have difficulty attracting women in any social context. But often men who are quite personable experience similar difficulties, simply because there are so many more men who want to be submissive than women who are dominant—at many D&S group meetings, men outnumber women two or three to one. Unable to find a female partner, some men express their submissiveness in private fantasy or go to a professional mistress. Others only fantasize, finding mistresses too expensive or impersonal, and wait until they meet a nonprofessional dominant woman they like.

The younger single men in their 20s and 30s are usually more interested than the older males in having a series of shifting relationships to experiment with a variety of people. They have relatively good success in doing so, much as they might in the straight heterosexual scene. For example, Andrew, a 30-year-old stock-broker who liked to dress up, went out with a half-dozen nonprofessional women he met at D&S parties and group activities over a period of several months and simultaneously dated several straight women he met at singles bars and at work.

However, as men enter their 40s and 50s, they tend to become more interested in settling down to a more serious, ongoing, even exclusive relationship and exploring D&S within this more secure, personal context. This urge is similar to that of older men seeking any type of relationship. A good example of this stage of life is Arnold, a surgeon in his 50s and a very meek, mild-mannered man who had to force himself to be assertive at work. After his 20-year conventional marriage dissolved, Arnold became determined to express his long-standing desires to explore his submissive, feminine qualities. Soon after his marriage ended, he moved to California, since he felt it would be a freer place to express these needs. He visited a few mistresses, but decided it was "silly" to share his fantasies with a woman who did not want to enter into a relationship. "What I want eventually is a monogamous relationship," he told me. "I'm not interested in one-night stands or short-term experiences. The close emotional connection and understanding—that's what's important to me."

HOW WOMEN BECOME DOMINANT

Woman are drawn into dominance in a very different way from that of men who are attracted to submission. First, most women who are involved do not report the early D&S fantasies that men do, in part because women generally think much less about sexual matters than men. Second, most do not go through the agonizing struggle to recognize and accept the dominant aspect of themselves, for American society praises and rewards assertive, independent behavior. However, some do have a difficult time accepting their aggressive feelings and playing a more assertive, initiatory role with a male. Then, too, it is easier to be dominant than submissive in a D&S session, since the dominant is in control and need not fear physical danger, as a submissive might. Third, women who want to remain active in the scene don't have the trouble meeting partners that men do, since there are so many available men who want to be submissive.

Rather, most women—excluding any commercial dominants strictly interested in the money—are initially drawn into dominance by a male they are close to who is interested in it and encourages them to experiment in their sex play. In some instances, the male asks the woman to be dominant from the start, but in many cases she plays the submissive before she tries dominance, typically with the same man. Only a few women I spoke with had their first experience of submission with one male and subsequently wanted to try out their dominant side with someone else.

To be sure, many women introduced to dominance or submission by a male rejected the idea. Of those who agreed, some were amenable because they wanted to learn more; some were adventuresome and curious by nature; others truly cared for the male and wanted to follow his interests. Then, as these women began to experiment with dominance, they began to like the feeling of being dominant and found it erotic.

Thus most women are initially drawn into dominance in the course of an emotional relationship, rather than because they initially find it erotic. Those who do not come to find it erotic generally lose interest in being dominant and sometimes in the relationship as well.

Melody's case is a classic example of a woman who learned to like dominance after she was introduced to it by her lover. Until her early 30s, she was a conventional housewife, married to a doctor. She had a strong Baptist upbringing, never explored any kind of extramarital sexual activity, and played the traditional passive feminine role. Her husband suddenly announced that he wanted a more open relationship in which they would both be free to date other people. This change led her to meet Marvin, a friend of her husband, whose own marriage was breaking up.

At first, her relationship with Marvin, a 40-year-old internist, was quite conventional, though Melody remained contentedly married. Gradually, Marvin began sharing his fantasies with her, but he put no pressure on her to play them out, so she wouldn't feel threatened. Also, he told her his dominant male fantasies first, so she would experience less conflict with her usual female role. His strategy, which he used successfully with other women, was one of gradual revelation to gain acceptance.

Melody soon became curious, and Marvin encouraged her to play out some of her lighter fantasy ideas, such as his fantasy of tying her up. Marvin then started sharing his fantasies about being submissive, and Melody agreed to try these out, too. She had already broken the first barrier by getting involved in D&S, so it was easier to proceed to the next step: switching roles.

Once she did, she found she liked it, and soon Marvin began introducing her to people in the D&S community who offered her additional training and support. Within a few weeks, she was eagerly trying out new techniques with Marvin, and she began to enjoy activities that he once thought were beyond his own limit, such as piercing his backside with a needle to draw a small heart. When she did it, even though he wasn't sure at first he would like it, he found it erotic and wanted her to do even more. After several months of playing exclusively with Marvin, she began to playfully try out her dominance on other men in the scene.

In short, through her close emotional relationship with Marvin she discovered that she liked dominance. Dozens of other dominant women report similar experiences. They had no previous fantasies of dominance and were in conventional relationships when introduced to D&S. Less commonly, some women did have early dominance fantasies or experiences as children. But they usually set these aside and never acted upon them until they met someone who introduced them to D&S.

For instance, Sharon, an office administrator in her 30s from a conservative Episcopalian East Coast background had childhood fantasies of herself as Nancy Drew, the teenage detective sleuth who was forever encountering difficulties in which she was tied up, locked up, blindfolded, gagged, kidnapped, or otherwise tormented by evil foes. However, Sharon never enacted these fantasies until shortly after she graduated from college and met a couple, Jim and Judy, who offered to act out her fantasy with her. She moved in with them to form a triad in which both she and Judy were submissive to Jim, and Judy was dominant over her. After a year and a half of feeling increasingly oppressed by their domination, she was eager to find a relationship in which she could be dominant. When she met Lance, who was looking for such a woman for an ongoing relationship, she left the triad and began learning to be dominant.

Likewise, Danielle, a real estate salesperson from a conservative Southern Baptist background, had had some dominance fantasies as a child and played out many of them with other children. In a nurse game, she examined a dozen little girls in the neighborhood, and, in a wicked witch game, she gleefully captured other girls and held them prisoner in her "dungeon"—an appropriately dim and musty room in the basement. As a teenager, she participated in a variety of playful fantasy activities in which she somehow bested or humiliated a male, such as when she and another woman wrapped toilet paper around a popular boy's car before he went out on a date. When he told her he arrived at his date's home with strands of toilet paper still streaming down, since he didn't have time to remove them, Danielle was heartily amused. But otherwise, she was extremely conventional and active in numerous church functions, including teaching Sunday school, cooking at church suppers, and hostessing church events.

Then, at a party, she met Fred, a traveling salesman, who was interested in being dominant. Fred fasincated her, and though she was engaged to marry another man at the time, she soon moved in with Fred, leaving behind her fiancé, church, and former lifestyle. A few months later, she followed Fred to the West Coast and married him. Meanwhile, he taught her how to be properly submissive.

At first, she complied willingly with all his requests, including working at a nearby B&D house as a mistress to earn money. There she discovered that she liked being dominant and lost interest in being submissive. She began to feel oppressed by her relationship with a dominant male—a common complaint of submissive women who later turn dominant. Their marriage became increasingly difficult and dissolved during its seventh year. Danielle then became strictly dominant and remained so in several dozen ongoing and casual relationships over the next five years.

Of the few women who discover dominance on their own initiative, most have fairly unusual backgrounds or training in psychology or the social sciences that leads them to be more open to sexuality than most women or to want to better understand unusual sorts of sexual behavior.

For instance, Laura, a tax consultant in her 40s, had previously worked as a sex therapist for several years. She had been actively interested in sexuality since her teenage years and had had numerous relationships, ranging from one-night stands to serious, committed relationships, though none had involved D&S. However, she was curious about D&S as an aspect of sexuality she hadn't yet explored. When she decided to pursue a business career, she sought to fulfill her twin interests in being more assertive at work and in her sexual life. She knew she needed to become more assertive to succeed in business; but she felt that assertiveness training programs were of limited use, since they emphasized assertiveness in impersonal relationships. When she saw an advertisement for a workshop on dominance for women, she decided to sign up. As a result, she began to learn techniques of dominance, discovered the D&S community, answered ads from male submissives, developed some close relationships with D&Sers, and, like Danielle, enjoyed playing around with a number of men.

Another woman with an unusual background, Vickie, was studying for her graduate degree at a sex-training institute while working part time as a sex therapist. She wanted to learn about D&S because she had some submissive male clients. At a demonstration on dominance sponsored by the Society of Janus, she volunteered to be a submissive subject. She later explored female dominance, too, and occasionally went to D&S group meetings.

Regina, a sociology and psychology student in her late 20s, was an ardent feminist, whose political beliefs led her to explore dominance. She reasoned that dominance represented the logical extension of assertive feminism, and she wanted to learn more about it because of its ideological possibilities. She turned up at the offices of the SM Church one day and went to several church meetings. However, as noted earlier, Regina, Vickie, and Laura are atypical, for most women are drawn into dominance by a male who is looking for a woman to fulfill his submissive fantasies.

In either case, once women discover female dominance, some find that it becomes more than an occasional pleasure and instead turns into a driving force or need, as powerful as the need for submission that drives some males. As Sharon describes it: "Now that I've discovered dominance, I'll never go back. I can't. Now I find vanilla sex so tame and ordinary. But dominance gives me a special rush. It's something I've come to truly need. It makes me feel super-charged, alive."

Generally, these dominant women experience far less psychic conflict than submissive men. Once women overcome any initial hesitancy to experiment, most women do not experience the kind of soul-searching torment men often do in recognizing and accepting this new side of their personality. Since American society values assertiveness and independence, these women feel good when exercising the authority, responsibility, and control associated with being dominant. Further, dominance does not threaten their femininity; rather, it seems to enhance their sense of self as they feel more powerful, self-aware, and self-confident. Also, the symbols of the dominant woman highlight women's sexual allure, further enhancing their femininity.

Indeed, some newly dominant women positively glory in discovering their capacities. For example, Catherine, a married woman in her 40s who worked as an administrative assistant, took the dominant role in virtually all aspects of her relationship with Carl, a real estate contractor who liked dominant women. She was delighted to "call the shots" most of the time. As a girl, her family insisted she be properly polite, passive, well behaved, and obedient. As she explains: "I've had all that up to here. And now I'm the one who's in charge." Meanwhile, Carl, burdened by a heavy high-responsibility schedule at work, was delighted that she took command.

A minority of women who become dominant initially experience dominance as a challenge to their conception of the feminine role. As they explore dominance they see themselves expressing qualities that they feel are inappropriate to a woman, such as being mean or expressing strong anger.

For example, one newly dominant woman became concerned when she began releasing feelings she didn't know she had or had not been able to express before. She was startled when she saw she could be "mean," after being such a "nicey nice" for most of her life. But she finally concluded that it was legitimate occasionally to have hostile, dark feelings, particularly if she expressed them in a controlled, positive, constructive way; thus she continued to explore her interest in dominance.

Another woman realized that in controlling and humiliating men in sessions she was releasing some of her general hostility and resentment toward men's power and financial and social advantages over women. At first, she was disturbed by this realization, but she concluded that it was "okay" to express her hostility with males who liked being recipients of her anger, which was then transformed into erotic energy during a session.

Since many women are originally drawn into dominance by a male, many drop out when the relationship breaks up, for their desire for D&S is only a reflection of their emotional ties to the male. Yet women like Sharon and Danielle stay because they learn to like D&S in itself and develop sufficient supporting ties with others in the scene. Such support is readily available, since there are so many submissive males seeking dominant women.

To be sure, many women in the scene actively play with many partners, as do the men. Yet, because a relationship is important to them, most dominant women are involved in primary or ongoing relationships. In fact, some seem to form a relatively stable core to which a number of submissive males attach themselves, as they drift in and out of the scene. This pattern is like that characterizing most kinship networks—the women form the core while the males are more outwardly oriented toward their friends and work associates.

Still, women's involvement in D&S assumes many different forms. Some women remain in primary relationships, sometimes with the male who introduced them to the scene, while others date many males. Some participate in D&S organizations and parties on a more-or-less regular basis. Others mostly participate privately. A few answer or place ads to meet submissive males. Some occasionally act as professional mistresses, or more rarely, do it full time. Most typically, women stay in the scene because of a relationship with a submissive male or because they develop strong ties with other women in the scene. Unlike men, women's fantasies and the erotic intensity of D&S are usually not enough to keep them in the scene. They also need emotional fulfillment based on a relationship with others.

PART II

D&S RELATIONSHIPS

3

Types of D&S Relationships

Although the D&S scene—comprising organized groups, D&S parties, commercial sessions, and other activities—is growing, at the heart of dominance and submission is the D&S relationship, confined to a couple and occasionally involving a triad. Many couples engage in D&S activity without any contact with the scene, and some couples do not view their sexuality as including D&S, although their relationship involves consensual dominance and submission. They think of themselves as "straight" but they occasionally perform characteristic D&S activities. For example, a woman might playfully slap her partner, kiddingly tie his hands together with a scarf, tease him by threatening to do something he doesn't like to humiliate him, or forcefully ask him to do something to her. Or he might perform some action that makes her seem superior, such as kissing her feet and legs like a humble servant.

Unlike couples who engage in such activities sporadically and spontaneously, D&S partners not only share a power exchange that has erotic overtones but also consciously define their activities as D&S. The male is aware that he wants the woman to take over at times, and she is aware that she enjoys taking the initiative. With this awareness, their relationship evolves as an exploration of her dominance and his submission. For some couples such exploration is a casual part of a mostly straight relationship; other couples more regularly experiment with female dominance in both sexual and nonsexual situations. For instance, if a couple goes out to dinner, the woman may demand that he wait to eat, beg her for the privilege of eating, serve food to her, or eat his food as instructed. To an outsider, such demands might seem quite foolish, but they serve to highlight the exchange of power in the relationship and overturn social conventions of role behavior, thus making trivial everyday interactions more exciting for D&Sers.

Play with dominance occurs in relationships of a wide range of duration and intensity, from fleeting encounters with a mistress and one-night stands to long-standing marriages. Some D&Sers have committed, long-term monogamous or nonmonogamous relationships; others engage in a series of short-term monogamous relationships; still others have several partners to whom they have varying levels of commitment. Some D&Sers enjoy frequent one-night stands and short-term relationships.

Like any group of adults, D&Sers differ extensively in their sexual predilections and in the type of person they find sexually appealing. For example, some males claim to be strictly submissive, while others are occasionally so. Conversely, some women describe themselves as exclusively or mostly dominant, some as primarily submissive but dominant at times. While most D&Sers I met were strictly heterosexual, a hefty minority—perhaps 15 to 20 percent—described themselves as bisexual. A few dominant women described themselves as primarily lesbians, though they dominated men occasionally, sometimes in professional sessions.

Furthermore, like other adults, D&Sers' sexuality changes over time. Within an ongoing relationship, for example, there are changes in the relative amount of female dominance during sexual play and in everyday interactions, the importance of D&S activity, and the extent to which each partner wants to assume the dominant or submissive role.

Most of the couples I met viewed D&S as an occasional experiment that enlivened their sex play; in all other aspects, their relationship was based on more or less traditional male-female roles. However, I also spoke to couples in which both partners, and most especially the male, at times felt a compelling need to experience female domination to feel sexually fulfilled; in other couples the woman's dominance extended far beyond the sexual sphere. Some couples experimented with D&S and developed a need for it; other couples found their desire for female domination fulfilled after they experimented briefly, and then they became less involved.

Although some couples were primarily monogamous and went to D&S clubs or parties for support or to socialize with others with similar interests, most couples in the scene wanted to experiment with others in various forms of nonmonogamous erotic play. Each partner was free to engage in D&S or other sexual activity with others, and some couples participated in triads. While most engaged in sexual intercourse as well as erotic play, some reserved the intimacy of intercourse for their partners. Most took turns being dominant, even though the female usually assumed this role.

Besides having a high level of interest in sex, the D&S couples whom I met generally felt a strong closeness and intimacy, based on openness, honesty, and trust. In part, these qualities derive from the exploration of D&S, which requires partners to share their intimate erotic desires, so they understand that "what turns each other on." Couples explained that such sharing extended to other aspects of the relationship. Again and again, they told me: "We have a very strong relationship," "We're very close," and "We tell each other everything." D&S activity also requires a high degree of trust, since some play is potentially dangerous if partners aren't careful. In addition, the submissive partner is psychologically vulnerable, placing himself in the hands of another, and to do so comfortably—or at all—he must trust her. Finally, couples who participate in nonmonogamous play typically tell each other what they are doing—so there is nothing to hide. This openness and honesty helps to bring the couples even closer together. At times, nonmonogamous activities do evoke jealousy, although most couples are nonpossessive and tolerant and feel, according to D&S scene values, that they should be. As a result, a jealous partner will usually try to rationalize his or her feelings or seek a short-term affair—just as many straight partners do.

Short-term D&S relationships, whether one-night stands or relationships lasting a few weeks or months, are usually erotically intense. While both males and females often have casual encounters, generally, as in the straight world, women tend to be somewhat more interested than men in having enduring relationships, and commonly they once had or still have a committed relationship with the male who first introduced them to D&S. In contrast, men are much more interested in having a wide variety of partners or in keeping their D&S relationships casual and external to an ongoing relationship or marriage that does not involve D&S.

One cannot accurately estimate the numbers or percentages of people involved in these different relationships, for individuals and couples move in and out of the scene, change from one type of relationship to another, alter their orientation toward D&S, and try new types of activities and partners. The nature of D&S, which is based on exchanging power through creative sexual expression, often leads people to want to explore, and their experimentation defies a census.

Despite the variety and flux, certain common patterns occur. Perhaps a third of the people I met in the D&S scene are involved in strong, enduring relationships. About half of these couples are married, and most of the rest live together. A few are exclusively monogamous, but most are not. Typically, these couples play with D&S—both in the bedroom and outside—on an occasional basis, but a few couples have experimented with living female dominance on a full-time basis for at least several months.

Another third have enduring relationships with a few regular partners, often concurrently. Some of their regular partners know or have intimate relationships with each other, forming a network of close, interlocking relationships.

The final third are free-floating individuals, primarily males, involved in a number of relatively short-term or casual relationships with a variety of people. Many in this category don't want a committed relationship because they like to play around. Others are married men, living double lives, who don't want their D&S relationships to interfere with their primary commitment to their marriages. While some of their wives know about their husbands' involvement, they aren't interested in participating. Other men don't tell their wives, feeling they won't understand. Some men in this third category visit a mistress occasionally to satisfy their desire for submission, though most continue to seek a more enduring D&S relationship with a nonprofessional.

As in the straight world, some relationships work and others do not; some people are satisfied with their relationships and others are not; some prefer enduring relationships and others like to play around. Thus there is no typical D&S relationship. But there are common threads, such as the desire for exploration and variety and the closeness, trust, and intimacy that occur in good relationships. Also, certain issues commonly arise at different stages of these relationships. Issues focused on power and the assumption of the dominant and submissive roles appear in various forms as a relationship develops from a short-term encounter into an ongoing relationship and a committed long-term relationship. These issues are the subject of the next three chapters.

4

Casual D&S Relationships

L ike most sexual relationships, many D&S encounters last only briefly. These include the classic one-night stand, the one- or two-date affair, and the D&S session that lasts from a half-hour to a few hours. As in the straight world, relationships last a short time for various reasons: those involved want a brief encounter; they meet in passing and have a fleeting attraction; they have other commitments and can't get involved; they talk and find they don't have much in common; the chemistry or "spark" isn't there. Or the individuals have social difficulties in sustaining a long-lasting relationship. There is no difference between the two worlds here.

However, in D&S, four other dynamics contribute to the brevity of many relationships. First, the desire to experiment leads some D&Sers frequently to seek new partners. Second, many males exploring female dominance are initially ambivalent about their involvement: they find it difficult to accept their own submissiveness, have reservations about being identified with D&S, or fear others may look down on them, since D&S is socially taboo. Third, many men find that their fantasy or the forbiddenness of the initial encounter is their primary source of excitement; they are fulfilled by the initial contact with a dominant woman by phone or letter or by a single session. Fourth, many relationships last a short time because they fail to satisfy the fantasies, needs, or expectations of either or both participants. Let us examine each of these dynamics in turn.

EXPERIMENTATION

Because D&Sers like to experiment, many brief encounters are intended to be intense and erotic D&S sessions in which the participants can play out their fantasies, learn new techniques, and simply enjoy the experience. These experiments may lead to a relationship if the participants enjoy them, have no other commitments, and find they have enough in common; but, if not, D&Sers regard these encounters as essentially complete in themselves. Experimentation includes sessions with a professional mistress and the frequent spontaneous play sessions D&Sers engage in when they meet someone who appeals to them.

41

A classic example of this kind of one-time encounter occurred when Natasha, a 30-year-old graphics artist, was first getting involved in the D&S scene. She had participated in a few informal evening demonstrations on female dominance, led by Kat, a woman active in conducting workshops and programs on D&S. Natasha asked Kat if she knew any submissive males interested in experimenting. Kat mentioned Daniel, an office worker and aspiring poet, who had written in response to her column on female dominance in the *Spectator*, a Bay Area sexually oriented weekly, saying he would like to be her lifelong slave. Since Daniel had a wife whom he loved, this "slavery" was limited, but he had performed assorted chores for Kat, such as office work and gardening, and occasionally went out with her to the movies or dinner and participated in sessions. Kat decided to give Daniel to Natasha for a few hours as a kind of male prostitute. Daniel agreed, for the "uninhibited, abandoned, and decadent" plan pleased him, and his intermingled feelings of excitement, anxiety, and fear highly aroused him. Kat laid down the ground rules: he would see Natasha only once; his ongoing D&S relationship would be with Kat.

When Kat brought Daniel over to Natasha's house one Saturday morning in February, he was wearing a slave collar—a symbol of his servitude for the next three hours. Kat left him outside in the car while she and Natasha worked out an overall scenario for the encounter. Kat urged Natasha to have Daniel do "only what will please you. Don't consider what will please him." Then Kat led Daniel into the living room by a chain, handed Natasha a bag of D&S toys, and left.

Natasha began the session by telling Daniel to call her Mistress Gwyneth, to keep his eyes down, and to ask permission for whatever he did. As she instructed, he carried the bag to the car, and she drove to a nearby wooded park, where she asked him to climb a scaffolding by a merry-go-round, rub up against a tree like a dog, and fetch a stick she threw. Without any question or hesitation, he bounded off to do as she asked, and Natasha, fairly new to dominance, felt a surge of power. Someone was actually obeying and enjoying her commands.

She asked him to lead her down a path where she blindfolded him, and for several minutes he crawled at her feet, playing the role of her Egyptian slave who was moving boulders and building a pyramid for her. Then she tied him to a tree and asked him to imagine his humiliation if anyone found him. Visualizing that, he felt a mingling of mortification and excitement. She untied him but kept him blindfolded and drove him to an open field. She asked him what he imagined would happen there. "You'll tie me up, take off my shirt, whip me, and I'll kiss your feet. Then, I'll perform cunnilingus on you, till you have an orgasm." When they arrived, she enacted most of this fantasy, except for the cunnilingus, which she felt too overtly sexual for their first meeting. Afterwards, she tied him up as a hostage in the back of her car, placed him under a plastic ground cloth so no one would see him, and left him on a downtown street for a few minutes, telling him she would be gone for an hour. Fearful, yet excited at the prospect of discovery, he remained nearly motionless, savoring the experience. Finally, Natasha returned him to Kat as a hostage, and Kat approvingly untied him and led him from the car.

When later discussing the experience with Kat, both Daniel and Natasha said they enjoyed the adventure. Daniel especially liked the exhilaration of being blindfolded and not knowing what would happen next, while Natasha liked the rush of power and control. But both knew this was a one-time encounter, and neither expected anything more.

In some encounters, the participants enter the session with few preliminaries other than perhaps a brief discussion of what each would like. But often the participants first spend a short time getting acquainted over coffee, drinks, or dinner and have a longer talk about their fantasies, ideas for a session, and, most crucially, their limits regarding pain, bondage, or humiliation, or the types of activities they don't want to engage in. Then, if they share mutual interests and the chemistry or energy is there, they'll do the session. The session may or may not conclude with sexual intercourse, but it is intended to be sensually and sexually stimulating in either case.

For example, Lester, a computer programmer in his 40s who liked cross-dressing and pain, met Tanya, a stockbroker, at a meeting of the Society of Janus and learned she liked to be dominant. He explained that he was married, but since his wife didn't understand his interests, he sought out people to experiment with once a week. He suggested dinner, and Tanya agreed, indicating that afterwards, if she were so inclined, they would have a session. At their meeting, both dressed in the spirit of the occasion— Tanya in an outfit styled to look dominant: black heels, tight black slacks, flashy red sweater, and studded leather belt; Lester in a seemingly ordinary yellow T-shirt and levis—except that they were women's clothes.

After dinner they went to Tanya's. In her large carpeted playroom she kept several baskets of toys, including crops, whips, ropes, scarves, handcuffs, and belts. Lester brought in his suitcase, containing about a dozen costumes. To give Tanya an idea of what he liked, he described some favorite experiences, when a dominant woman or man required him to dress up as Jane, his alternate persona. In one case, he had to ride the subway wearing a short, blue-denim jumpsuit with pompoms; another time he had to wear a white women's tennis dress and boots on a walk through the financial district at midnight. Now it was up to Tanya to dress him up and order him about as she liked.

Tanya dimmed the lights, put on some music, shone a flashlight on him as if he were on stage, and described a fantasy as he donned each costume—a fantasy about a baby when he put on pink, frilly shorty pajamas; about a little girl in a playground when he put on a tight white dress; about a girl on a beach when he put on a bikini; and about a cheerleader when he put on a short skirt and ribbed sweater with a college letter. Since Lester had said he liked pain—"But not too hard. You can't leave any marks"—Tanya whipped him. As he bounced up and down as a cheerleader, she struck him in time to the beat of each jump. And when he was a little girl in the playground, she played a mean little boy who tied her up and slapped her on the buttocks. Once again, the encounter was brief and mutually fulfilling: Lester played out his desires to be forced to dress up and experience pain; Tanya experimented with fantasy and power.

Some participants, mostly males, use such brief encounters to act out fantasies that they have nurtured for a long time but felt unable to realize in their primary relationships. Even when the encounter turns out to be extremely fulfilling and exciting, the participants usually do not continue meeting because they have commitments to other relationships. For example, Katrina, a teacher in her 30s, met Rick, a musician and student in his late 20s, at a dinner she and three other dominant women organized for four of the submissive men who answered an ad. At dinner, Rick described a fantasy he had had since high school when he read *The Odyssey* and identified with Odysseus' dangerous adventures: being tied to a mast, trapped in a cave, sucked into a whirlpool, turned into a pig, and humiliated by losing the winds he needed to blow his ship back home. However, Rick had not acted out this recurring fantasy, since the women he dated thought the idea to be weird. But Katrina was intrigued, and a week later, they met to play it out. Rick had told Katrina that he had a steady girlfriend, and both agreed to a one-time encounter.

After they talked in more detail about Odysseus' adventures, Katrina placed incense and candles around the room, asked Rick to undress, blindfolded him, and gave him a serape to wear. With a meditation record that sounded like a swirling storm playing in the background, she treated him like the long-suffering Odysseus, deftly moving him from one adventure to another: "Now, kneel down.... Imagine you are on a boat beset by the elements." When he did, she alternately hit him and stroked him with feathers and a glove. "And now, you're going through a whirlpool. You have to struggle to keep from going down." He lurched back and forth on his knees, swept his arms about in the air, and breathed heavily, as if gasping for air. "Now you can see the Sirens in your mind's eye. They are calling to you, and you want to go to them. But you know you must not, for you will never return to Penelope. So you ask your men to tie you to the mast." She wrapped several belts and scarves around his shoulders, torso, and legs. He moaned for her to release him and writhed on the floor. "But you can't get free," she told him, moaning occasionally in Siren's voice, "Oh, Odysseus...Odysseus, come to us."

Then Katrina took Rick to the land of the goddess Circe, who offered Odysseus some wine and turned him into a pig. After she handed Rick a wooden goblet with wine, he sipped some, then threw himself on the floor, groveling at her feet and oinking like a pig. Similarly, Katrina led him through Odysseus' misadventure with the winds and through his capture by the Cyclops and his escape. Afterwards, she told him he was back in the real world again and could open his eyes. Rick described for her the intensity of the experience and the release he felt having acted out his long-held fantasy. There their encounter ended, mutually satisfying and complete.

Although the woman is ostensibly dominant and the man submissive, at times he directs the scenario in order to obtain the kind of submissive experience he wants or to guide the woman if she is new to dominance and doesn't seize the power offered her. Such sessions enable a more experienced male to teach a woman new techniques, which she can later use with other men. Katrina received such a lesson from Pat, a communications specialist in his mid-30s who answered her ad. Pat had been actively involved in bondage for three years. He had played numerous bondage games with his lovers and he had been to professional mistresses who tied him up. He had even designed and built some of his own bondage equipment, which included leather cuffs, poles with eye hooks, harnesses, and a massage table with hooks for tying.

Thus, when Pat met Katrina, he had a clear picture of what he wanted. They discussed their likes and limits over coffee, agreed to do a session, and he directed most of the action. After they returned to her living room—playroom, he arranged the pillows in a pile on the floor, while she put on a slinky red dress. Next, he demonstrated his leather leg restraints, fur-lined wrist cuffs, and long wooden bar. Then, after undressing, he lay down on the floor, his legs apart, and showed her how to tie him to the bar in a spread-eagle position, with his legs stretched and secured to either end of the bar and his penis tied tightly to the center. At his direction, she fastened his arms and legs to the legs of two nearby couches. He then advised her with some irony: "And now that I'm completely helpless, you can do with me what you want."

In a sense Katrina could, for she proceeded to tease him with scarves and sashes, rubbed him with ice, rough sponges, and a horse-cleaning brush and informed him sternly that he was now in her power and she could do whatever she wanted. Yet he had directed the play and had granted her power in the ways he chose. Having engineered his own helplessness, in effect he was still in control.

Similarly, Katrina received other lessons from Bart, a travel agent in his late 20s. He had experimented with B&D for about six months, mostly with professional mistresses, and before their session, he described his experiences and likes at some length: nipple and cock torture, tight harnesses, dildoes, and butt plugs; having hot wax dripped on him, being ordered to please, and performing cunnilingus. The equipment he brought for their session included several "butt plugs," "cock rings," a blindfold, and a gag. He showed her how to put on his "cock cage," a small harnesslike device for his penis, and he demonstrated how to attach several nipple clamps: "You pull out the nipple gently, and put it on." After showing her how to insert a butt plug—"It's painful, yet stimulating to have your ass stretched"—and how to use a vibrator to massage his clamped nipples and the tip of his harnessed cock, he told her to take over and "beat my ass good, so I'll have the proper respect."

The sessions just described were largely inspired or directed by the man and didn't end in sexual intercourse. But in many other one-time sessions, the woman takes over immediately after a brief discussion of likes and limits. Then the man feels he is in her power and experiences the loss of control that some men find intensely pleasurable. He isn't sure what will happen; he doesn't know what she will do. So she whips him, binds him, forces him to crawl, kneel, beg, kiss her feet, or whatever, at her pleasure. And many brief encounters do become highly sexual, since explicitly sexual activities are a central part of many sessions. Partners touch, suck, and lick all parts of the body; use vibrators and other devices for stimulation; orally or manually manipulate the penis or clitoris to orgasm; and, at times, have intercourse. These activities are variously combined with the use of assorted D&S equipment and with fantasies that heighten the intensity of the stimulation.

Though brief, such sessions may be as intense and exciting, sometimes even more so, as an experience within an ongoing relationship. Some sessions lead to further meetings and long-enduring relationships, but many do not, and the participants do not always expect or want a relationship. Rather, they see the session as part of their experimental play. If an encounter is mutually enjoyable and satisfying on its own terms, it need not lead to anything else.

MALE FANTASY AND AMBIVIALENCE

In contrast to the mutual experimentation that leads to intense, mutually enjoyable one-time encounters, many potential relationships end up being short term or even terminate without personal contact, because the male is satisfied by merely fantasizing about the encounter or because he is ambivalent about participating. For example, professional mistresses report that many males who call for appointments do not show up, while others pledge their undying devotion during a session but do not make a return visit.

These dynamics repeatedly occur in social relationships as well. Males describe the intensity of their feelings or repeatedly affirm their desire for a long-term commitment, but they break off the relationship. For some, declaring such commitment is part of the fantasy that excites them. Others mean what they say, or think they mean it at the time, but after a phone call, a letter, or the first or second encounter, their ambivalence about being submissive or about acknowledging their submissiveness causes them to back off.

Several of the men who replied to Katrina's ad showed these patterns. Fulfilled by fantasizing about a prospective session or ambivalent about having one, they backed off after initially claiming sincere interest. In a typical case, a male who described himself as a good-looking, tall professional excitedly wrote in his first letter to her: "I would love to explore submitting myself to the dominance of a woman like you.... I'm interested in being your plaything." His letter concluded with his private phone number and a pseudonym he used to protect his identity. She called, they arranged a meeting, and he sent another letter detailing some of his fantasies about what would occur: "We completely change roles. I put on your clothes; you put on mine. Then, we do something congenial like chat. However, you are out to seduce me.... I'll try to resist. But eventually you'll win, and I'll begin to give in. You'll get me stripped down to my panties, and coax me into your bedroom.... Then, when you have me spread out naked, I'll lose my resistance and let you have your way with me.... I'd like to wrestle with you nude. I'll lose consistently, and eventually you can completely overpower me and kill me by strangling me to death. You can abuse my naked cadaver, and for the finale, castrate me!" He enclosed a picture of himself in the nude and told her when he would call her; but he never did.

Rip, a 28-year-old pilot, who had had infantalism fantasies for years, similarly backed off, because, as he subsequently explained in a letter of apology, he got cold feet. Rip sent a letter to Mistress Kat's column on female dominance in the *Spectator,* asking if she knew some women who could help him explore his long-standing desire to be mothered by a dominant woman. Kat included his letter in her column, and Natasha responded, asking him to call. He did and described himself and his fantasies at length, explaining that he had had this desire since he was a teenager, possibly because he came from a very conservative, work-oriented family that stressed ambition, and he never felt he had been loved or babied enough. He went to a professional twice, once tried dressing up as a baby, and even visited a psychiatrist a few times to dispel his fantasy, which he felt he could share with no one. But still he wanted to be babied by a woman who would understand, though not a pro.

When Natasha agreed, he said he would call as soon as he returned from his next flight and they would get together. About a week later, he sent a letter apologizing and explaining why he was backing off. "Dear Natasha," he wrote. "How delightful it was to talk to someone with your refreshing approach to life. However, I have been deeply saddened since our talk. I pride myself in my forthrightness, but feel as though I betrayed your open willingness to seek out the new by withholding all there was to tell. I am married to a woman who loves me....I withheld this truth from you, out of desperation to explore this fantasy which has captured my interest for so many years.... I could not engage myself in an experience with you, for to do so would result in a tarnishing of our exploration; tarnished by projecting onto you the need for secrecy. To involve you in this would be contrary to your free spirit and openness to self-examination. You are not an object, a thing to be used, or a professional dominant, but a warm, inquisitive woman, and deserve to be treated with the dignity accorded to such a person. Therefore...I am sorry and humbly yours. Rip."

An even more dramatic instance of male ambivalence occurred when Tanya briefly met a male actor, Frank, who responded to her ad by writing: "I am a handsome, 40-year-old professional male, healthy, physically active, aggressive, and ambitious with a compulsion for the physical, emotional, and sexual dominance of an intelligent, creative, and sensitive woman....Oh, dear Mistress, bind me, gag me...use my mouth, my cock, my mind...make me do what you wish done! Make me do what you need to be done to you, for you...beneath you. Force me to tell you what I would not tell God. Then laugh at my foolish needs and use my tongue not for words, but to bathe your cunt! Coffee? Or lunch? Then, perhaps an hour in your power? I'm afraid...but I want you to find me....I want you to have me....Please....Don't hurt me....Not too much.

Tanya went to the play in which Frank was acting. Ironically he played the role of a very tough army sergeant, and she was impressed by his apparent sincerity when she heard two stagehands moving furniture link their names together in a line he later told her he had inserted in the play. "Did you hear," one said to the other, "Tanya and Frank are a swinging couple, too."

After the play Frank took her to a nearby bar, where he spoke revealingly about himself—in fact so revealingly, he said, that he told her things he had never told anyone else. As he explained, he had had submissive desires since he was about seven, when he played cowboys and Indians and a little girl tied him up. Then, on his eleventh birthday, he dressed up in his sister's clothes, and found this exciting, too. But, apart from a few brief experiments with an actress, who played dominant to indulge him, he never discussed this aspect of himself with anyone. He felt he could never tell his wife, a conservative woman who saw him as a very masculine male. "It might destroy our entire relationship to reveal myself," he said.

But now, finally, he wanted to, felt he had to, act on his fantasies. Could she, he implored, explore dominance with him? When Tanya said she could, he seemed relieved, and they talked of what she might do when they next met. She could tie him up as her hostage, show him off to her friends, dress him up in her clothes. Simply thinking about what would happen was exciting, he told her, adding a little wistfully that he wished he hadn't waited so long.

When they left the bar, he asked her to wait for an empty elevator, and as soon as the door closed behind them, he knelt down at her feet. "Oh, mistress, how may I serve you?" he begged, while she stroked his head. As she drove him to his car, he continued to play the role of the abject, submissive male. Could he touch the fur of her coat, he pleaded. As he stroked it, he spoke of how much he would like to touch her thigh and have her treat him as her slave. "I'd like it if you could bind my cock and pull me towards you by it. I wish I could be licking you. I'd like to be able to suck and fuck you. But of course, that's for you to decide." He also offered to bring ropes to their meeting the following week. "Whatever you want. You only have to ask." Finally, at his car, he talked about how much he looked forward to their meeting when she would do with him as she liked. As he closed her car door, he said breathlessly: "God, you don't know how much this has excited me. I'm all wet."

But Frank did not appear for the next meeting. When Tanya called him to find out what happened, he was distant and abrupt. No, he wasn't coming, he told her. "You mean we're supposed to forget everything we said to each other last week?" Tanya asked. "Yes, that's right," he said coolly and hung up. Perhaps Frank was ambivalent about expressing his submissiveness or felt he had shared too much. Or perhaps he merely played out his fantasy for that night and as an actor gave an excellent performance. There is no way to tell.

SHORT-TERM RELATIONSHIPS THAT FAIL TO FULFILL FANTASY NEEDS

Some relationships last only briefly, although both partners are seeking an ongoing relationship, because the relationship doesn't satisfy one or both parties. In many respects, this situation parallels any new relationship in which the partners find they have little in common or that the chemistry isn't right. What is unique to the D&S relationship is the importance of fantasy and role playing, apart from the issue of common interests or sexual attraction. Regardless of whether these latter elements are present, once the fantasy or role playing is disrupted, or once the partners find their fantasies aren't fulfilled, the relationship ends, for these D&S components are essential.

A dramatic example of this occurred when Katrina met Sidney, an extremely shy computer programmer of 35, who was relatively new to the scene. He had briefly explored being submissive with a girlfriend after she slapped him playfully with a slipper, and he found that to be erotic. For the next few months, she occasionally tied him up with scarves or teased him with a variety of household items, such as toothpicks, spatulas, and a hairbrush. They broke up, and for the next two years he only fantasized about finding another woman to whom he could be submissive. Over time, Sidney's fantasies of servitude became more important and intense.

He responded to Katrina's ad by enthusiastically outlining the slave-master relationship he wanted. He lowercased his *I*'s and capitalized his *You*'s to emphasize his humble submissiveness: "As a relative novice, my experience is somewhat limited. i have known the leash, the harness, the stretch, the squeeze. You are the sole source of discipline. Through Your discipline, i will learn better to pleasure, to cook, to clean, to serve You (and if You desire Your friends).... i'm trainable.... Dreaming of the remote possibility of being at Your feet, kneeling respectfully, and tenderly kissing Your ankles. Sidney."

A week later, after Katrina called him and they arranged to meet, he sent another letter, describing more fully his fantasy of complete service: "Most esteemed Lady Katrina: From the depths of the core of me, i offer You many thanks for the kindness and consideration of Your call. i take heart and hope that i may prove to be of value to You.... i'm completely at Your service.... If our acquaintance blossoms into a friendship which contributes something to Your happiness, Your pleasure, Your prosperity in life, then i will know my own rewards.... Now i am yearning to learn to serve You wine, to share Your rituals, to evolve into an obedient thrall.... Will call Friday. Just hoping that i will be capable of speech. Thank You for existing Katrina. Respectfully...Sidney."

When they met over coffee, he continued to play the role of a humble, possibly unworthy, servant. After briefly talking about his work and Katrina's, he turned quickly to the matter at hand. Yes, he truly wanted to be dominated by a powerful woman. But he wondered if he would be worthy. Since the idea of a docile, eager-to-please "slave" appealed to Katrina, they returned to her house for a session. She dressed up as an army officer and ordered him to undress, crawl around, do push-ups, and kiss her ankles. Then she hit him with a whip to discipline him as her lowly, stupid, largely incompetent private, who had gone AWOL and was generally a disgrace to the army.

At the end, Sidney groveled on his knees at her feet, and told her he loved his punishment and was so thankful, because he really needed to be treated like that. He would eagerly await their next meeting. In another letter a few days later, he continued the fantasy: "Most Esteemed Mistress

Katrina," he wrote: "Kneeling, trembling, i salute you. Through the guidance of Your discipline, may my rear bloom red....i pray to kiss again the crop that stings me....i want to be a good recruit for deeper introduction into Your army....Until we meet again, i am happy imagining myself tethered to a post in your stable....Sidney."

A week later, Sidney took Katrina out for Sunday brunch and began the day with a special request: Could he put on a "cock cage" with two chains dangling from it to remind him throughout the day of his worship of her? It would pull and slap against him anytime he crossed his legs or walked and would thus be a constant reminder. She agreed, and he put it on. Over brunch, carrying the fantasy further, he enthusiastically praised women as naturally superior to men, for they were more successful rulers and more honest than men, who were sneaky, manipulative creatures, lacking self-control. Perhaps he believed this; perhaps not. But these ideas fueled the fantasy.

In addition, he asked her permission from time to time to do such ordinary things as taking off his coat, having a cup of coffee, and going to the bathroom. He even reminded her that she might forbid him to have things, and when the waitress asked if he wanted more coffee, he was delighted when Katrina told her no, immediately after he told the waitress yes. "But he just asked for it," the waitress said confused. "Well," Katrinia advised her, "he's changed his mind." "That was wonderful," Sidney complimented her when the waitress went away baffled. He was also pleased when Katrina laid her crop across the table as another symbol of her power.

In turn, Katrina enjoyed playing this superior queenly role. After brunch, she took Sidney to a park, where she demanded that he perform various demeaning actions in public: kissing her crop as she waved it behind her and he crawled after her on his knees, performing a series of exercises for her, and bending over an exercise bar with his pants down while she cropped him.

But a week later, this mutual fantasy came to a crashing end—and with it the relationship. Katrina wanted to run in the highly publicized Bay-to-Breakers race through San Francisco dressed in her army uniform and chase after Sidney with a crop. Others ran the race in costume, so they would not attract any unusual attention. To complete the fantasy, she asked Sidney to wear a white T-shirt that said "Property of the U.S. Army." The shirt would make her feel she was chasing after someone she owned—an extension of Sidney's fantasy of being a total slave. Sidney immediately liked the idea and agreed to obtain such a shirt.

However, when he appeared to meet Katrina near the start of the race, he was wearing a dark blue T-shirt with a symbol of an anchor and the words "U.S. Navy." He couldn't find the appropriate T-shirt, he explained, and he didn't have the time to have one made. Katrina was disappointed and angry, because now she felt foolish about running after Sidney with a crop. His costume didn't fit. She would no longer be running after a slave she owned, as in her fantasy, but after an ordinary person in a T-shirt. So, for her, the fantasy was ruined. When she told Sidney she wouldn't run after him in costume, he felt his own fantasy was crumbling and tried desperately to salvage the scene.

"No, wait," he said. "I brought another T-shirt. I have a magic marker. I can write on the words with that." He laid the plain white shirt over the side of his car and quickly started to write. But after a few scratches, the point broke, and that was enough for Katrina. She whipped off her army jacket and put on a pair of yellow shorts and shirt she had brought along just in case. She invited Sidney to run with her if he wished.

For awhile they did run together, but the original excitement was gone. They were no longer playing out the fantasy. So soon Sidney dropped out of the race and went home, and Katrina was glad he did. For her, as for him, the fantasy was over. Once she took off her uniform, she was no longer his all-powerful mistress, and he could no longer play the game of looking up to her and worshipping her. Furthermore, once the fantasy was over, there was no reason to continue the relationship. The relationship had been based on sharing a mutual fantasy, and once that fantasy was destroyed, the relationship was, too.

In other cases, early in the relationship, one or both partners develop expectations of the relationship that go far beyond what is possible or what the person truly wants. When reality inevitably intervenes, disillusion results, and the relationship built on this fantasy breaks up. Most commonly, this unrealizable expectation involves a long, enduring commitment based on a fantasized but unrealistic D&S relationship. Such a fantasy took hold of Danny, a long-distance bus driver in his 40s, when he met Danielle, a real estate saleswoman in her early 30s who was teaching classes on sexual fantasies for the SM Church. Danny had been having submissive fantasies for a long time and, like many men, had been unable to enact them with his girlfriends. He saw an ad for the SM Church and came to one of Danielle's fantasy classes. Immediately, he was taken by her, and he began fantasizing about a long-term relationship: here finally was a woman who could understand him and control him. She was everything he wanted, he imagined, and within a day, he told her he wanted to marry her.

Danielle had before seen men build up elaborate fantasies but then retreat when the fantasy started becoming real. She treated Danny's protestations of undying devotion with a wait-and-see attitude: possibly the relationship might develop, possibly not. In the meantime, she would see how submissive he really was. If he meant what he claimed, fine. If not, she wasn't interested. Thus she told him she wasn't ready for marriage yet, but if he was truly serious about being submissive to her, he could buy a house for them and put it in her name. That way, if she were to live with him she would be in charge. "Yes, anything, anything," he submissively agreed. He attended two of her fantasy classes and clung closely to her, often sitting at her feet, to show that he truly did want to be servile to her.

However, very soon, it became clear that he enjoyed only the fantasy of being a full-time slave to a wife. For once Danielle began making demands, he balked. He didn't want to do the chores she requested, and he would massage her feet only when it pleased him to do so. Also, he preferred the missionary position, though she desired cunnilingus. Although Danny fantasized about being her humble forever-devoted slave, in reality, he wanted to control when, how, and if he would be submissive.

The next week, Danny told Danielle he would continue attending her classes after he returned from a week long cross-country drive. But he neither showed up nor called. Danielle, in turn, was blasé about the whole matter. She had met many men who had pledged all sorts of things but never followed through. Danny was just one more example of a man who—out of ambivalence, fear, or dissatisfaction—cast aside an opportunity to realize his submissive fantasies.

5

Ongoing D&S Relationships

I n the early phases of establishing an enduring D&S relationship, the partners must work out the same sorts of understandings and agreements that face any new couple. They decide what they like to do, how serious they want to be, how often they want to see each other, what they expect of each other, and so forth. Also, they must discover whether they have enough common interests, shared values, and mutual caring for the relationship to endure. The partners cannot build a strong relationship on D&S alone; they need to develop a mutual love and respect that transcends sexual matters. Just like other adults entering relationships, some D&S couples develop these qualities, while others don't.

AGREEMENTS ON POWER AND ROLE PLAYING

Though D&S and straight relationships are similar in many ways, certain major issues concerning the exercise of power and role playing are particular to D&S partners, and these issues must be resolved successfully for the relationship to work.

In non-D&S relationships, certain expectations about power and roles are generally accepted: men are usually expected to be dominant and women subordinate. To a greater or lesser extent, a man takes the initiative in making a date, suggesting what the couple will do, initiating love making, and continuing the relationship, while the woman generally responds to his lead. Although each couple works out its own agreements, most follow this basic pattern.

However, in a D&S relationship involving female dominance, all such standard roles and divisions of power and responsibility are subject to question. The partners must work out power and role arrangements anew, according to their own preferences as to the extent of the woman's dominance. For example, she may be dominant in the sexual setting only or in nonsexual social situations and in decision making as well. Depending on the individual partners' personalities, abilities, desires, and needs, the power exchange in the bedroom will affect other aspects of the relationship to a greater or lesser extent.

Some women who are sexually dominant seek power in other areas of the relationship, for without such power the sexual dominance appears to them as a kind of play acting in which they act out a male's fantasies. For example, when Angie, a 25-year-old saleswoman, began exploring her dominance with Dick, a businessman in his 30s, she started to make more demands upon him in their everyday activities, and she became more assertive in making decisions. Dick responded by eagerly seeking to please her and agreed with the decisions she suggested. This reinforcement encouraged her to continue to exercise her assertiveness.

In contrast, Anne, a bookkeeper in her 30s, began to feel that her sexual dominance with Paul, a machine-shop owner, wasn't real, because she couldn't assert herself effectively in nonsexual areas. During their early dating, he suggested she assume the dominant role in sex, and she enjoyed the surge of power she felt. But he made the decisions and took the initiative in other areas in their relationship. When Anne sought more power in their everyday activities, Paul resisted. Thus she began to feel that her sexual dominance was merely another expression of his power, and so from time to time she refused to be sexually dominant with him. As their relationship developed, based on the many other common interests they shared, they periodically played with female dominance and then dispensed with it.

Other couples limit their dominance play to the bedroom and otherwise follow traditional male assertive–female subordinate patterns.

Although each couple finds its own way to work out these understandings about when, where, and how the woman will be dominant, there are certain common patterns in the early phases of ongoing D&S relationships. These patterns concern choices in two major areas: traditional male-female social conventions and the division of decision making, responsibilities, and other tasks.

SOCIAL CONVENTIONS

Most D&S couples observe the traditional social conventions governing male-female behavior. The male typically pays for both, takes the initiative in calling, and follows everyday customs of male etiquette, such as opening doors for a woman and lighting her cigarette. Many couples do not see these customs as relevant to the issue of female or male dominance; they are simply following standard social rules. Other couples are cognizant of the power implicit in traditional social and economic roles, and they prefer that the male maintain his leadership even though sexually submissive. As one man put it: "You wouldn't want a man not to be a man, would you?" Quite naturally, he felt, the submissive male should retain his defining male responsibilities.

However, others view etiquette and social roles as a symbolic expression of power. Traditional etiquette, they observe, underscores the female's passive, dependent role. The male pays, calls, or performs tasks for the woman as a way of taking initiative, protecting her, or being assertive. These D&Sers may either assign such tasks to the woman or reinterpret these tasks so that acts of male chivalry are not viewed as signs of his power but rather as signs of his submission and his willingness to serve and please a woman. Thus the male pays for the date or makes the call to reaffirm the woman's role as a superior, desirable sexual being, and to show he is interested in her, wants to be in her company, appreciates her responsiveness to him, and is willing to please. Women in the D&S scene commonly like these displays of chivalry; as one woman commented at a meeting, after a man bent down with a flourish to kiss her hand and ask if she wanted anything, "It shows that they're well behaved."

Some dominant women at times do take over some of these traditional tasks, and most particularly the function of paying. This role reversal involves an exchange of power that is exciting for both the woman and the man. For example, rather than *allow* the man to perform certain tasks he might normally do, the woman may *order* him to perform them. By commanding him to take her out to dinner or by making him pay for an expensive meal, she assumes a dominant position, although he is still outwardly performing his normal social role.

Also, the woman may reverse the roles to dramatically exert her power. For instance, one woman told her submissive partner to give her all his cash as they entered a restaurant. When the waitress handed him the bill, she firmly and loudly announced, so nearby patrons could hear: "Oh, no. I'm paying for this. He doesn't have any money." The man sat sheepishly and humiliated, yet felt a thrill of excitement at this demonstration of her power.

Sometimes the woman may reverse roles because she wants to experience what it's like to be in a different role or wants the male to have that feeling. As an example, one woman took her date out for dinner and dancing and she paid for everything as a gift to him. "I wanted him to have the feeling of what it's like to be taken somewhere himself," she told me. And submissive males generally like women to take the initiative because that helps them feel more submissive. As one male who alternated in playing the submissive and dominant role observed: "When I have to take that first step, it's hard to feel submissive. That's why I like it when a woman I'm dating calls. It helps to put me in a submissive frame of mind." Another man left it up to the woman he was seeing to call when she wanted to see him: "Always feel free to call your slave to serve you."

In short, those in the scene tend to follow the usual conventions about male and female dating, and they don't make this an issue of dominance. But when they do, they play with and modify these conventions to dramatize the power relationships implied by these conventions and use them as another means of playing with female dominance.

HANDLING TASKS AND MAKING DECISIONS

Whereas D&Sers usually follow social conventions, they work out a variety of arrangements for delegating responsibilities and decisions. As the relationship continues, the partners discuss and negotiate such matters and develop unspoken expectations about who will do what. Certainly, all relationships entail some negotiation of roles, but among D&S couples familiar tasks and decisions may become eroticized—a form of dominance that extends beyond the bedroom.

For example, a woman may ask the male she is dating to wash her car, or he may offer to do her gardening. Although these are perfectly ordinary activities, in the context of a D&S relationship they may acquire a sexual or erotic flavor. She may reward him sexually for obeying her wishes or he may perform the task wearing D&S accoutrements that enhance his erotic pleasure in serving her. One woman ordered the man she was dating, who liked occasionally acting as her slave, to weed her garden. Before he went outside, she placed cuffs on his wrists and tied a ring with dangling chains around his penis to stimulate him sexually. She also assured him she would reward him well for his efforts when he finished. When he was done, she calmly walked around the garden like an overseer inspecting his work. Sternly she pointed out this flaw or that, while he followed behind her meekly, excited that he might get his reward and aroused by the anxiety of not being sure. After she nodded her approval, he was ecstatic and bounded upstairs after her into their playroom to receive his reward—a gentle whipping while he was tied up, followed by a chance to orally satisfy his mistress.

Due to this eroticizing of female power, many men in a D&S relationship become quite eager to perform such chores to "serve" the woman. Frequently I heard men in the scene brag about how they did a variety of tasks that they avoided doing in their straight relationships. For example, Brent, a 42-year-old financial planner, had a conventional marriage in which his wife stayed at home and did all the cooking, cleaning, and housework. He "never did a thing," as he put it. But when he dated women in the scene or came to D&S group meetings, he did chores with a flourish. He picked up groceries, helped prepare refreshments, served women food, and helped with clean-up. In this setting he liked playing out his fantasy of serving women, who enjoyed being served. Within the D&S scene, chores were satisfying and erotic; at home they were simply work.

Then, too, many males in the scene enjoy relinquishing their power and having a woman instruct them, because such passivity counterbalances their responsible position in daily life. They can relax as someone else tells them what to do. Likewise, as a counterbalance to their more serious work role, they find pleasure in performing domestic chores.

TYPICAL PROBLEMS

Although partners may enjoy reversing roles and exchanging power, certain problems frequently occur in the early stages of a developing D&S relationship. If the partners are unable to resolve these problems, the relationship usually ends quickly. Though such issues also arise in established relationships, the couple can usually resolve them more easily, because the relationship is on firmer ground.

Four of the most common problems are:

1. The woman has difficulty being dominant enough to satisfy either or both partners. Or she tries to be dominant because she is curious or seeks to please him but doesn't find it erotic. Then, in reacting to her lack of erotic interest, the man finds that his own sexual excitement declines. But often he doesn't understand why and can't express himself. So communication between them breaks down, and they feel dissatisfied.

2. The woman is being dominant, but her partner challenges or tries to test her dominance, either because he is unwilling to be truly submissive or because their notions of D&S clash. Their relationship is a power struggle, rather than a power exchange.

3. The woman is being dominant as she likes, but her partner has very strong and different fantasies of how a dominant woman should act.

4. The male acts so submissively that his partner finds it difficult to communicate with him or maintain interest in the relationship.

Partners usually discuss these problems when they occur and one or both partners may try to change. If they can't, the erotic energy of the relationship soon dissipates, and one or both lose interest. Often, too, the male ends up feeling frustrated—he has failed to find a relationship to satisfy his need to be submissive, while the woman may feel hurt or angry because her partner has challenged or criticized her style of dominance. Let us examine these four problems in turn, looking at several relationships that lasted for about one to three months. In each case, the partners wanted an erotic, intimate, ongoing relationship based on female dominance. But when they could not resolve these problems, the relationship either ended entirely or became a platonic friendship.

INSUFFICIENTLY DOMINANT WOMEN

The story is a common one: a submissive man would like his partner to be dominant, and she tries but doesn't find it erotic, or she has difficulty playing the role because she is used to being submissive or unassertive. Submissive men repeatedly told me about relationships in which they wanted their partners to assume power and encouraged them to take it, but the women tried to do so only to please them. However, once a man realizes that his partner doesn't really enjoy being dominant, the relationship loses its sexual charge for him. In some cases, the women stop trying to play the dominant role. While some men let such a relationship slide along, others end the relationship and look for another partner whose desire for dominance fulfills their needs.

This problem most commonly arises when a woman has not previously been dominant. Her partner not only has to encourage her to be dominant, but also has to train her to assume this role. But generally, the training is not very successful, since most women feel uncomfortable in contradicting the traditional social training that requires them to be passive. Some women are open and willing to challenge social mores, but their partners often complain they aren't dominant enough: they don't go as far as they can; they hold back; they are afraid to administer pain; they resist ordering a man around; and they hesitate to take the initiative and lead. Many newly dominant women agree that as much as they want to be more dominant, they find this new role difficult since it differs so from the way they were taught to express their sexuality.

For example, Dawn, a 30-year-old teacher, reported difficulties in her relationship with Will, also a teacher, because she had trouble being strong enough. She always felt like apologizing whenever she made him uncomfortable or gave him pain, although he wanted her to do so because he found pain sexually arousing. As she observed: "I know I shouldn't apologize, because it ruins the excitement. But I do." Other women worry about being sufficiently creative. "I'm afraid I'll run out of ideas," one said.

The case of Aaron and Eve is typical of relationships in which the woman has difficulty being dominant. Aaron, a lawyer who was 43, met Eve, a secretary in her early 30s, in a bar in San Francisco. They went out a few times—for dinner on the first date, sailing on the second—and on their third date, he slowly began talking about his interest in female dominance by mentioning some activities he liked. He didn't use the words *dominance, D&S*, or *S&M*, so that Eve wouldn't reject his interests out of hand if she had any negative associations with these terms. He liked to be teased with scarves by a woman who treated him firmly, he explained. It was also fun if she held his arms tightly behind his back. And if she put belts or ropes around him, he liked that, as well. Since Eve seemed curious he went on: He found it very stimulating if she whipped him smartly with a crop, too.

Eve offered to try, and when they returned to his apartment, he showed her his equipment, which he usually kept hidden in a bedroom drawer. After he turned down the lights and they undressed, he told her she could do what she wanted with him now. She took a few belts from his drawer, wrapped them around him, and tied his hands with rope, asking several times: "Is this what you mean? Is this what you want?" Uncertainly, she hit him with the crop; but she didn't find the experience very erotic, and neither did he.

On their next few dates, he persevered. Just try it again and it will get better, he assured her. But it didn't; she simply seemed to be going through the motions to please him, and he didn't know how to make her understand what made these activities erotic. In fact, one time, she told him that she thought what she was doing was "quite silly."

Their relationship soon began to fall apart. Eve felt frustrated and confused—she didn't enjoy what he liked and didn't understand why he liked it. Thus she soon began to lose interest in going out with him and doing other things they both liked. And Aaron felt frustrated because he couldn't make her understand. After several unsuccessful sessions, he, too, gradually lost interest in their relationship, for his erotic dissatisfaction colored everything.

POWER STRUGGLES BETWEEN DOMINANT WOMEN AND MALE MANIPULATORS

Sometimes a woman's attempts to be dominant are unsuccessful because her partner is constantly challenging or testing her dominance, although she is firm and experienced as a dominant. If this testing is merely a game, both partners may enjoy it. But if the testing is a sign of a power struggle, rather than a consensual power exchange, the relationship will usually soon end.

A man who occasionally and playfully challenges his partner's dominance is initiating a kind of game in which he dares her to stand up against him and show her power. He usually finds this game erotically stimulating. As one man told me: "I enjoy the spirit of competition or a contest. It's no fun if I just submit. It's too easy if I just give her my power. Anything that's worth having should be worth fighting for." He would regularly devise gamelike tests to measure his partner's interest in their relationship. For instance, when she gave him rules to follow in a session, such as asking her permission to do something, he broke them. Or he begged her to do something he didn't want her to do, such as releasing him soon after she tied him up or stopping a whipping soon after she started. He hoped she would continue doing what she wanted, not what he pretended he liked, to show her power. And sometimes he played the brat, taunting her with pranks, such as tying her boots together, to see how she would react.

Although some dominant women enjoy such an occasional game, most do not want a relationship that is an ongoing power struggle. While they might enjoy a well-timed challenge, they mostly want a submissive male who submits willingly. Few want to devote their energy to persuading or manipulating an unruly male to submit. "If he wants to give me his submission as a gift of himself, fine," one dominant woman told me. "But if I have to spend a lot of time trying to train him to behave, it's not worth it." No wonder the men I met who tried this power game approach reported their relationships usually faded after a few months. The women no longer wanted to play.

If the male's rebelliousness is especially intense, a woman may see it as more than an annoyance. Sensing a potential danger, she may soon end the relationship. A particularly dramatic example is the case of Laura and Chris.

Laura, a sex therapist in her 40s, met Chris, 52, when she answered his ad for a dominant woman in the *Spectator*. At their first meeting, he claimed to be submissive, told her that this was "his true being," and explained that he had wanted to be submissive all his life, though he never had a chance to express this. These claims surprised her, because Chris was a burly six-footer who looked more like an aging football player than a submissive male. Also, he was a retired career officer in the military—an unlikely occupation, she felt, for a naturally submissive male. Yet she believed he was sincere, and as a relative newcomer to dominance herself, she was reassured by his own newness to submission. She felt that they could begin exploring female dominance on the same level.

Chris and Laura began to date about once a week. But soon she noticed that he was trying to lead the relationship, although he had said he wanted her to do so, and she felt that he was challenging her dominance in other ways. For example, he made special cuffs, collars, and chains for her to use on him, rather than letting her decide what equipment she wanted; and when she hit him, he frequently dared her to hit harder, as if he wanted to show her he could endure more pain than she could give. Several times he taunted her: "I want you to make me cry 'Ouch,' and then you can stop." But even when she hit him hard enough to produce bright red welts and draw some blood, he remained silent and stoic. Inevitably, she always gave up and then he baited her: "But I didn't say 'ouch.'"

Laura also noticed that Chris seemed to be testing her limits as a dominant in small ways, too. One night he waxed poetic about female superiority, but later talked about men and women as being equal. Was he challenging her to confront him about his real beliefs, she wondered. Other times, she tied him up, and he led her to think she was in control. But after she was convinced he was helpless, he would dramatically break free, as if to show her she didn't control him at all, but just thought she did.

Her concern increased when he volunteered to train her in women's self-defense tactics. He claimed that if she was going to be dominant with him and other men, she needed to know how to protect herself in case her partner became rebellious. At first, she accepted his offer of training, but as he repeatedly talked about a dominant woman's need for self-defense, she became suspicious, wondering if he was setting her up for a confrontation. When he suggested that she could demonstrate how well she had mastered this training in a simulated rape attack, she got scared. She worried that he might get violent or try to beat her up, using her new knowledge of self-defense as an excuse to turn on her.

When he subsequently urged her to play the submissive role and let him whip her, she refused. Although she had occasionally switched with other men, she was afraid of Chris, of his physical strength and the undercurrent of violence she sensed in him.

Throughout their relatively brief relationship, Laura became more afraid that the situation was building to a dangerous confrontation. She finally stopped seeing him, after concluding that he was probably caught up in what psychologists call an approach-avoidance conflict. "He may want to be submissive; he may say that he does," she explained, "but he seems to have a deep-seated fear of that submissiveness in him, too. Thus, he may turn against his own submission and anyone who makes him submit. I don't want to be there when he does."

Perhaps Laura imagined Chris to be more dangerous or violent than he was. But even if he was not planning a physical confrontation, his actions and Laura's responses do illustrate the failure of a D&S relationship based on a continual power struggle. And whether or not Chris was motivated by an approach-avoidance conflict, submissive men who are so motivated usually cannot sustain a D&S relationship.

POWER STRUGGLES DUE TO CLASHING D&S STYLES

Power struggles also result when partners have vastly differing conceptions of dominance, submission, and erotic activity. Submissive men frequently complain how difficult it is to find an experienced, self-confident, sensitive dominant who firmly and assuredly takes control. These men explain that for them to be happily submissive, their partners must be appropriately dominant, and if they are not, then the submissive should try to direct their activity. In short, they want the women to "make it good" for them, and if she doesn't, they feel they should show her how.

To this argument dominant women, and particularly those relatively new to dominance, complain that although men claim they want to be submissive, some are submissive in a dominant, controlling way. Also, they complain that men often try to manipulate their partners to be dominant in specific ways, rather than leaving it up to the woman to do as she wants. Dominant women sometimes call these men "dominant submissives," because they don't truly surrender their urge to control women.

These opposing interpretations are illustrated by the short-lived relationship of Natasha and Max. They had differing conceptions of dominance, and she viewed his attempts to improve things as manipulative; he saw them as efforts to make things good.

Natasha met Max, an army officer of 35, when she was first discovering dominance. She had encountered it by chance at an evening demonstration held by a social club she belonged to. After a few more demonstrations and workshops, she went to a weekend camp-out sponsored by the SM Church. There she met Max, who had been involved in female dominance for about 10 years, mostly with professional mistresses, and had developed some clear ideas about what he liked.

Max had been attracted to D&S after some self-examination of his sexual experiences. He realized that he preferred cunnilingus to sexual intercourse and that he experienced more pleasure when he focused on pleasing the woman than when he concentrated on only pleasing himself. Also, he recognized that when he assumed the dominant role in relationships, including his marriage, he became very critical and domineering, possibly because these women were not very well educated. Even when he tried to control his judgmental nature, he typically failed, and the relationship usually ended with the woman feeling angry and resentful. Then, too, he found that when he tried to relax and let his partner take the initiative in planning activities or starting sexual activity, nothing would happen. Thus he decided that he needed a more assertive, self-assured, powerful woman who could control him, and he wanted an ongoing relationship—not just an occasional visit with a mistress. He joined the SM Church to find such a woman.

When he met Natasha at the camp-out, he hoped she might be that woman, and he soon became very attentive in a submissive style. He sat down on the ground beside her and massaged her feet; he repeatedly asked if he could get her anything; and when she said yes, he scurried off to bring some food, blow up her air mattress, or do whatever she wanted. "Are you aware of how much power you have?" he reminded her several times.

They started dating, but Natasha had trouble taking the power he wanted to give her, and he had difficulty enjoying the way she used power when she asserted herself. For example, on their first date after the camp-out, Max offered to do anything she wanted, and Natasha asked for some suggestions, since she was relatively new to dominance. But Max refused to suggest anything because he wanted her to take the initiative on her own. "Otherwise you won't be the kind of person I want," he explained. "I want you to be assertive and do what you want and like. Then, I'll like it because you like it." Advancing his theory of what makes submission exciting, he claimed, "The man should forget what he wants. Then, he will get his own pleasure serving the woman."

Although Max wanted to feel he was serving Natasha at her pleasure, he made it clear that he didn't want to appear wimpy, fawning, or obsequious. He still wanted to appear strong and fulfill the traditional male responsibilities, such as being the bread winner and paying for the date. His ego would tolerate submissiveness and role reversal only in some areas. But it soon became clear that Natasha's ideas of how he should please her and his ideas were incompatible. Max continued to tell her that he wanted to do only what she wanted, but he soon began trying to manipulate and direct her. He hoped she would learn to be dominant in ways that he liked; she saw his efforts as his attempt to be dominant, while claiming to be submissive.

A dramatic example of this clash occurred on their second date. Natasha brought over a cluster of black balloons she had gotten from a woman who came to a "Come as a Russian" party the previous night. (The woman had dressed as Russian caviar—in a body stocking covered with a mass of balloons.) Since Natasha enjoyed being dominant in ways that involved fantasy and play, she thought it would be fun to shoot at Max with a water pistol while he was blindfolded and tried to protect himself with the balloons. At first Max said, "If you like it, I like it." But he then criticized her efforts to be dominant in this way as stupid and childish. For him water pistols and balloons were for kids, not erotic or exciting at all: "Pain and humiliation—that's what's real. After all, we're adults. So we don't play childish games. You could simply shoot water at me if it pleased you. So what's the point of the balloons?"

Max then showed her the type of dominance he wanted, using some standard D&S equipment he bought—a crop, a cane, some lacing, and a rope. He bent over, and as he requested, she began to strike him. He moaned, but begged her to go on. After a few more strokes, he asked her: "Do you know you're hurting me?" He wanted her to know he was bearing the pain for her. As long as it pleased her, he liked the stimulation and was erotically aroused. He viewed the pain as an indication of his willingness to serve, and her pleasure in administering pain affirmed his willingness and gave his punishment an erotic meaning. Also, he could proudly display his bruised buttocks to her as a sign of their mutual affection.

As Max later explained to Natasha: "I'm not just a masochist who likes to be beaten up or humiliated by anyone." Rather, he was willing to suffer only for an attractive woman who cared about him and for whom he could show his caring by enduring pain or humiliation. If after the pain she gave him a sexual reward for serving her, the contrast between the mental and physical hurt and the reward was especially exciting. Also, he found the pain and humiliation sexually arousing in themselves becuse he associated them with the sexual gratification he might receive.

However, Natasha didn't find giving pain particularly erotic, and she found it particularly distasteful that Max repeatedly urged her to urinate on him. Further, she felt he was being too assertive in pressuring her to be dominant on his terms.

Yet Max continued to hope Natasha would change, since he had previously experienced some shifts in his own limits, when he encountered activities he didn't think he would like in a sexually stimulating environment. For instance, he once thought urination, or "golden showers," was sick, but when a mistress urinated on him, he found it exciting. Perhaps, at least, Natasha would try some of his ideas: "They're only suggestions," he assured her, "and of course I'm only making them if you want to listen." Then he recommended that she wear tall black boots or high heels, strong colors like blacks and reds, leather garments, and net stockings—all symbols of erotic dominance for him. Yet, even though she appreciated his suggestions and followed some of them, she saw them as another attempt by Max to take power from her and to control her.

Other disagreements arose when Natasha didn't think dominance relevant to an everyday interaction, as Max did. For instance, when they were making plans to go to a party, Natasha asked Max if he would rather pick her up at her house or meet her at a more convenient location. She felt she was only being considerate, but Max snapped at her: "But what do *you* want. You see, you're doing it again. You're trying to throw the responsibility for choice back to me. I'm trying to give you the power and you're throwing it back to me. So what do you want?" "Then you can pick me up," Natasha said curtly. "Good," he agreed.

Yet Max objected when Natasha's decisions contradicted his preferences. After a party, Max asked Natasha if she wanted to come up to his apartment and play. But she was tired and told him she just wanted to go home. Max fell into a silent sulk, which made Natasha wonder again about Max's claims of being submissive. She thought that a "good" submissive should accept her decision gracefully. When she eventually capitulated and agreed to go to his house for a short time, Max immediately perked up: "Wonderful. I'm aroused just thinking about it. You see what power you have to do that." But once again Natasha felt he was the powerful one, for he had manipulated her to do as he wanted.

Natasha's doubts reflected a classic issue in D&S relationships: who is really in control? The submissive, who sets the limits and guidelines for what he likes, or the dominant who is outwardly in charge? Natasha felt the dominant should be in control; but Max felt she should be dominant only as long as he liked what she did. Had they both liked the same things, their relationship might have worked. But since they didn't, the issue kept reemerging—who's really in charge?

At times Natasha did feel her power, when he liked what she did and submissively gave himself to her, and because of such occasions they continued seeing one another. For example, once as they waited in the basement of his apartment building for the elevator at two in the morning, she asked him to bend down and kiss her feet. On the empty elevator, she asked him to take off all his clothes: "So you'll be ready to go when we get inside." He eagerly undressed, exhilarated by the anticipation of a session and the possible threat of public humiliation, however unlikely at that hour, if anyone walked in. Likewise, he enjoyed a session in which she chased after him with a whip, yelling, "Faster...Faster ...I want to see you really crawl," and concluded by caning him. "Don't you see how much power you have now?" he asked her afterward, "You can do anything you want. I'm your complete slave." Yet Natasha continued to doubt. She felt she was merely participating in his fantasy of giving her power, for he still seemed very much in control as he continued to urge her to behave in certain ways.

A few days later, at a workshop for couples led by Mistress Kat and Mouse, their ongoing conflict over control reached a new peak. With the encouragement of other women at the workshop, Natasha dominated Max in a brief, private session in which she whipped him firmly and told him that from now on, "I'm going to be boss." She would do with him as she liked, and he would accept it. He seemed agreeable and even complimented her for being so assertive.

However, on their next two dates, Natasha felt nothing had essentially changed. The first evening began with Natasha ostensibly in charge. She instructed Max to wear jogging clothes, which he did, and she asked him to run in front of her while she chased him with a crop along a path around a lake near his apartment. On their return, she asked him to undress and kneel in his living room. She drew a bullseye on his backside with a crayon and began shooting at his testicles with a dartgun with plastic darts. On the surface, he seemed to like the experience. "It's a ten," he screamed a few times after she scored a direct hit and asked him to rate the sensation.

But when they went out to dinner afterwards at his officer's club, he was once more critical. He hadn't wanted to criticize her during the session, because that would end it, but now he felt he could speak freely. He liked her taking more initiative, and the jogging and shooting were better than the balloons. But still he found these things a little silly. "After all," he asserted, "S&M is for adults, and adult games are more serious." He encouraged her to do something more extreme, like hit him harder, or threaten him with ending the relationship if he did something she didn't like. "You see," he went on, "part of the idea of S&M is for the dominant to make demands on the submissive which become a challenge. They push the submissive to his limits." Natasha thought that her innovative ideas about dominance had tested his limits. But Max wanted more pain, more tests of endurance, more intense experiences of humiliation.

So Natasha suggested an intense humiliation—he could do something outrageous at the restaurant, such as kneeling down so she could hit him. Max became visibly nervous. "No, not here," he quivered. If anyone at the club knew what he was doing, he would be truly embarrassed; these people were not the anonymous public, but fellow army officers who would think he was sick. The thought of doing anything at the club was a total turn-off. To be erotic, the context for D&S had to be appropriate. Thus, again, Natasha found her style of dominance considered wrong by Max.

However, she tried again by following some of Max's suggestions as they waited in line at a movie. She pinched his wrists and bent back his fingers. He was pleased that she did as he asked and was stimulated by the physical sensation and his awareness of the unknowing but potentially disapproving crowd. "I bet everyone thinks we're just another normal couple," he grinned. When they returned to his apartment Natasha said he could give her a massage as a reward for dinner and the movie, and again Max was pleased because she requested something he liked to do—serving a woman in a sensual way. "See how much power you have over me," he reassured her again. But as he walked her to her car, the issue of control resurfaced once more. He admitted he hadn't kept a journal as she requested, and he then again asked her to reconsider urinating on him.

A week later, when the control question continued to be a problem, Natasha finally gave up. Things didn't go well from the first. Natasha arranged to take Max on a hike with a group of friends. When she arrived about six, Max had made the potluck dinner as requested, but he wanted to play before they left. When Natasha explained there was no time, he griped: "You never have any time," and on the way to the hike, he mentioned that he had been thinking of going to a professional mistress because Natasha didn't administer enough pain in their sessions. He griped for several minutes more about his problems at work, and then complained that her clothes weren't very erotic. "Of course not," she snapped, "we're going on a hike."

Later, Natasha suggested that she would play a mistress in their session that night. But he dismissed this suggestion, complaining: "No, I don't want to do that. I don't find mistresses that satisfying. I have to orchestrate everything, and I don't want to do that." Although he *was*, in fact, orchestrating everything, Natasha again decided to smooth things over by deferring to his wishes. "Then, I'll just make sure to give you more pain this time," she said.

During that night's session, he voiced more complaints, perhaps justifiably because of Natasha's relative inexperience with D&S techniques. But Natasha felt each complaint chipped away further at her power. First the ropes she tied around his wrists were too loose, he complained. Then, the tie was too close to his hands, so he could get loose.

But finally the tying was done, with one of Max's hands securely attached to each ankle. Natasha added a large cold chain around his waist and blindfolded him. Then, because Max's constant criticisms and put-downs had angered her, she chased after him with a vengeance. "Now waddle around the floor as fast as you can," she cried, racing after him with the whip and striking him hard all over his body. This time Max didn't criticize her for not hitting hard enough. Now he staggered about, trying to twist away from the rain of blows that kept coming at his buttocks, thighs, shoulders, chest, and back.

She stopped after a few minutes and demanded sternly, "Now lick my feet." For the first time she really meant it, and she felt an intense flush of real power. She ordered him to lie down, ran an ice cube along his back, and struck him several times more with some ropes she twisted together to make a whip. Max endured in silence, though Natasha had given him a safe word to use if the session became too tough. But he didn't use it because he felt that crying out to stop the session would be a sign of weakness.

Finally, Natasha untied him, removed his blindfold, and demanded: "Now wash my entire body." He did this with apparent submissiveness, and Natasha felt she was finally experiencing her power, having pushed him harder than ever before. She savored the excitement of doing exactly what she pleased and not thinking about what would please him. She had heard dominant women describe this erotic rush, and now she felt it.

But the feeling didn't last long, for once again she felt Max's demands compromising her dominance. Could he lick her and orally satisfy her? No, she said, she wasn't in the mood. "But I have this need," he griped. And as she got ready to go, he complained again. The session wasn't at all erotic, he charged, simply full of pain. To make it erotic for him, she should wear the right clothing, use erotic words, touch his penis a little more. Certainly, he wanted the pain, but pain without arousal was unsatisfying. Yet Natasha had gotten really excited by the session.

At this point, their basic incompatibility over the issue of dominance and control was clear. Max liked certain kinds of D&S activities, Natasha others. And while he continued to hope that she would learn to like what he did, Natasha saw their disagreements as evidence of a power struggle. To do what he liked if she didn't want to do it seemed to her to be letting him manipulate her again, and she wanted to be dominant in her own way. Although he suggested they try again, she refused. She wouldn't feel dominant if she gave in to his demands; and he wouldn't be satisfied erotically if she didn't. Theirs was a classic confrontation that occurs when partners' D&S tastes are incompatible. Who's really dominant? Who's really in control?

THE CONFLICT BETWEEN FANTASY AND REALITY

Another common problem in D&S relationships concerns the male who has over the years developed specific fantasies and then seeks a dominant woman to fulfill these fantasies. With his very particular picture of how a woman should be dominant, he has great difficulty finding the "right" woman. The very specificity of his long-held fantasies precludes him from enjoying the reality of an ongoing relationship. This problem is illustrated by the case of Katrina and Alex.

Alex, a pediatrician in his 30s, had long had fantasies, described earlier, that focused on cross-dressing, being forced to play a feminine role, and bondage. As a child and as a teenager, he had dressed up and assuaged his guilt by fantasizing that a woman tied him up and forced him to cross-dress. Over the years, as he continued to fantasize and act out his fantasies by dressing, tying himself up, and occasionally finding a woman to tie him, he developed an increasingly explicit picture of the type of role reversal he wanted and the type of woman with whom he wanted to share these fantasies.

He refined the details of this picture over the years based on those experiences he found especially exciting. For example, after over a decade of privately cross-dressing and tying himself up, he married a woman who accepted his dressing. He persuaded her to put him in bondage for long periods—an experience he found tremendously stimulating, because after long periods of denial, he experienced extreme gratitude and warmth for her when she released him, and he liked the feeling of being totally out of control. Then, after his divorce, due primarily to work pressures, he had his first experience cross-dressing publicly, when a beautiful transvestite he met at a party encouraged him to dress up and go out in public with "her." He then decided there was no point in dressing up only for himself; now he wanted to do it with someone else. But he was not interested in males who dressed up. Rather, he related his experience of dressing publicly to his previous fantasies about being forced to dress by a woman. He wanted to dress up for a woman who shared his interest in bondage and would force him into this feminine role.

Alex had limited success in finding a woman to enact his specific fantasy, though he had no trouble meeting women. But each time he had to persuade his partner to do what he wanted, such as tying him to the bed or locking him in a room, though he disliked having to orchestrate everything, for that meant he was still in control. And some women didn't tie him effectively, so he was able to escape, thus ending any erotic excitement of being vulnerable and out of control. For example, one girlfriend tied him up and left him in the living room while she went to visit friends. But she left a knot in the wrong place, and he was able to undo the ropes. When she returned, he was watching TV and had not experienced the vulnerability and powerlessness he craved.

After a few months, he always lost interest in his girlfriends. After each relationship ended, he hoped he would next meet someone who would find the bondage and forced feminization not just a game but a highly erotic passion. Thus, he eagerly replied to Katrina's ad for men to explore dominance, hoping she might be that woman: "This sounds like the kind of ad I've been waiting to see for a year," he wrote. They met over coffee, and he explained further. He wanted a woman who not only already shared his interests but also could "take the power from me and know what to do with it.... That's what's exciting—reversing roles, so the woman takes this power.... It's making the other person know you have this power, and forcing him to do certain things to get his freedom or desired rewards." At the same time, he wanted this role playing to be part of a complete and ongoing relationship, since this interest was only a part, though a very important part, of himself.

Katrina felt they had much in common, and suggested they try dating. But Alex wavered, unsure. Was that special spark he wanted there? Was his long-term fantasy worth pursuing? Could it be realized, or should he give it up? So far, he had had so much difficulty finding the "right" woman. While he tried to decide, they went out a few times to get to know each other. On one occasion, Alex asked Katrina if she could help him find the kind of woman he wanted, since he didn't know any who enjoyed bondage and cross-dressing. His current relationships with three women weren't working since they didn't share his interests, and he was ready to end them.

At first Katrina was confused by his request, because she thought she might be the kind of woman he wanted; but since she didn't care about having an exclusive relationship, she agreed to help. With these limits for their relationship established, they then shared their erotic fantasies about each other. Katrina described a scene in which one man was tied up in the dining room under the table, while another cleaned her house in the nude. Alex would then appear dressed like a girl, and they would startle the two men by pretending to be lesbian lovers. Alex's fantasy was that he was dressed up and she was disciplining him.

Afterwards, he got his bondage equipment from his car, and they had their first D&S session, based on Alex's long-standing fantasy. Using an assortment of ropes, belts, and ties, Katrina wrapped him up like a mummy, so he would feel the vulnerability he liked. "Now I could do anything," she teased. And he suggested some things she might do. Would she like to make love to someone who could make love like a woman? Would she like him to be her girlfriend? She could then train and discipline him, making him wear high heels, dresses, even a maid's uniform while serving tea. If he didn't behave, she could lock him in the closet overnight.

Or she could order him away, as though he were an absolute nothing. She could force him to go out dressed to various events: to a senior prom, a fancy ball, or a pickup bar. She could even have him act as a hooker. And her commands need not be limited to an evening or a weekend; she could make him come home and dress everyday after work. He would be her ever-devoted girlfriend. Katrina vaguely agreed. When they later made love, both were caught up in the excitment of this joint fantasy and found the experience especially intense.

They dated several more times, but it soon became obvious that Alex's fantasies were so specific that even though Katrina enjoyed having him dress and liked tying him up, she didn't do it exactly as his fantasy prescribed. For example, one night Alex asked her to put him in a new bondage position he had seen illustrated in a bondage magazine. As he suggested, Katrina put him in a collar and ankle cuffs, tied him to a pole, crossed his hands behind his back, and handcuffed them to the pole. She also put on a blindfold and gag. For several moments, Alex felt the intense vulnerability, powerlessness, and constriction he found so pleasurable. But the feeling vanished when Katrina asked him to signal with his feet if he was too uncomfortable. And when she later massaged him, he said she was being too gentle. He wanted a woman to treat him harshly and mean. He didn't want to think she cared. Also, he complained when she released him at his request. "You're not being harsh enough with me," he told her. "You're too solicitous of my comfort."

Katrina assured him she would try harder to give him that powerless feeling of being forced. But his criticism bothered her, since she felt she was being dominant in acting exactly as she pleased. Once again, she was encountering a clash between her concept of dominance and her partner's. Alex's fantasies were so specific that she could not possibly enact them.

Since they weren't fulfilling each other's fantasy needs, the romance gradually disappeared from their relationship, though they continued to see each other. At their last D&S session, Alex asked Katrina if she would try out a training glove on him—a kind of long leather sheath that laces up around the arms to restrain them. He stripped down to his briefs and Katrina laced him in tightly, with his arms behind his back. After a few minutes, he began to beg for her to release him, but she refused, determined not to be accused of being too easy. She would show him her power and he would stay laced until she was good and ready to unlace him. "Look how vulnerable you are now," she teased. He began to plead in earnest, saying his hands were numb, and she released him, feeling a surge of power as she did.

But she felt she was basically an actor in his specific fantasy, that she was really playing his game, not hers. As much as she might enjoy it, she had her own quite different dominant fantasies. Alex, too, was dissatisfied, for he wanted a woman who would be more forceful in asserting her power.

Thus they agreed that she would try to introduce him to other people who might know where he could find his very special woman. But none of the people she asked were very receptive, and some dominant women treated his request scornfully. As one observed: "That's the problem with male submissives. They think they know what they want, instead of realizing that what will really give them pleasure is letting go and letting the woman be really dominant. They always want to keep that control, as much as they say they don't want it. They always want things their way."

Alex's ideal, the product of years of fantasizing, will be hard to find. Alex is still looking, convinced that realizing his fantasy will be worthwhile. But some dominant women would disagree. As one woman commented after hearing Katrina's story: "Sometimes the fantasy turns out to be better than the reality after all. Lots of times when submissives get what they think they want, it turns out they don't want it. Or once they experience their fantasy as reality, they don't want it anymore."

OVERLY SUBMISSIVE MEN

In some relationships, the male's extremely submissive behavior becomes a problem itself, as inadequate communication results from his inability to express or assert himself, or as his partner becomes emotionally drained because she feels she always has to be dominant and take the lead. Dominant women frequently joke about male oversubmissiveness, calling it the "whatever-you-say-mistress" syndrome, for whenever asked for his opinion or preference, the oversubmissive male responds, "whatever you say." Although his partner is seeking information, he responds as someone who has neither opinions nor will. Such men truly have no opinion or are so entrenched in playing the submissive role that they do not offer one.

In a D&S session, complete submissiveness can be appropriate and contribute to the mood of the session. But in an ongoing relationship, it can frustrate and exasperate the woman at those times when she needs the male to voice an opinion or act as a responsible equal. Indeed, although she may feel exhilaration and power when her partner submits totally to her will in a session, she may find it tiring to continually take the initiative in the relationship. "You can't always be on," one woman said.

A representative sample of this problem is the brief relationship between Travis, the biology student in his 20s introduced earlier, and Anne, a market research analyst, age 32. She saw him at a Society of Janus meeting and was immediately attracted by his good looks—tall, dark hair, a little like a young Rock Hudson. She engineered their meeting by sitting in the row directly in front of him during the talk. Afterwards, Travis told her that he would like to become the toy or plaything for an older, more experienced woman, and Anne was intrigued.

When they got together a week later, Travis told her she could do anything with him. At first Anne liked the power and enjoyed being free to try anything she wanted: tying him, slapping him, spanking him, wrestling with him with their arms and legs tied together, and running ice along his back. She had only to ask and he would massage her, wear women's panties under his clothes, put on a collar, or clean her house.

But when she tried to find out what he liked and what he didn't, he repeatedly said, "Oh, I liked that....I like anything. I like whatever you do." Similarly, when they did everyday things together, she found it almost impossible to get Travis to voice an opinion or make a decision, even when she truly wanted him to respond. They went shopping for clothes, and several times she asked for his advice about which garments looked best on her. But inevitably, he demurred. "Oh, no....I don't know....It's so hard.... I can't tell....I like everything....I can't decide." No matter what the topic, she felt as if she were carrying on a monologue. Travis would meekly agree and mostly listen, almost never initiating a conversation on his own. As physically attractive as she found him, she began to feel he had all the personality of a wall.

She prodded him to express opinions and be assertive, but he held back, afraid he would say or do something that might displease her. He only wanted to be liked and gain approval, and he lacked the confidence to take a stand. Travis wasn't merely playing the role of being submissive; he thought that by doing whatever she wanted, he would surely please her. Unfortunately, Anne wanted more than this, though she initially found his eager submissiveness delightful and charming and she enjoyed showing off how he willingly obeyed her commands. For example, at one Janus meeting, Phil, a dominant heterosexual male, demonstrated the obedience of Judy, the submissive woman he lived with, by snapping his fingers. She got down on her knees and waddled toward him, still on her knees, until he snapped his fingers for her to get up. Anne boasted that Travis was equally well behaved, and she snapped her fingers. Although they had never done such a routine, after a moment Travis knelt down and did not get up until she motioned him to do so.

But after a while, Anne found their one-sided relationship exhausting and boring. There was no challenge, no interpersonal interplay, no intellectual stimulation. Her initial enthusiasm for dominating and playing with him waned, and her erotic interest cooled. Travis sensed this and he lost interest, too. After a dance party at which they barely talked, they returned to Anne's apartment for drinks. Travis massaged her feet as she requested, and she started drifting off to sleep. Suddenly, Travis stopped. "I've got to get up and study early tomorrow," he said and left.

They continued to run into each other occasionally at D&S meetings and were friendly. But neither phoned the other for a date; they both knew the relationship was over.

Thus, just as a relationship in which a submissive man engages a dominant woman in a battle for power can flounder, so can one in which the woman perceives the man as overly submissive. In one case, the woman finds the male seeking to be too powerful and so a threat to her own dominance; in the other, she considers him not powerful enough, and so she loses interest. Certainly, overdependence or passivity by one partner can ruin any sexual relationship; but personal inequality between D&S partners is particularly problematic because the use of power is central to the relationship. As Anne's responses show, if the polarization of power roles is complete and ever present, the dominant partner will soon lose interest. Although a dominant woman enjoys being with a submissive man, rarely will she be satisfied by a man who seeks to be only her toy, not her adult partner.

6

Loving Couples

P artners in a long-term relationship involving female dominance have resolved the kinds of problems discussed in Chapter 5. Past the early stages of establishing an ongoing D&S relationship, they have come to accept and enjoy each other's styles of D&S, and they have developed a close understanding of each other's personalities, needs, and preferences. As they claim, D&S partners are often especially close. Their experimentation with power, roles, and fantasy contributes to an intimacy that produces closeness in both sexual and nonsexual areas. D&S is only one aspect of their ongoing relationship, and they share in many other ways as well.

Some D&S couples remain monogamous, but many explore other types of sexual play with other individuals and couples. Although these partners have a primary commitment to each other, they may decide to play or have sexual intercourse with others. Each couple develops its own ground rules, which may often change as the partners' desires and needs evolve. Even within the primary relationship, patterns of dominance and submission shift as personal preferences and everyday experiences influence each partner's desire to be dominant or submissive. After a difficult day at work, a man may feel like being more submissive at home, because he wants someone to nurture and protect him. Or he may feel like becoming more dominant to release his aggression, anxiety, or tension. Each couple handles these issues differently, and generally the woman is not always dominant either sexually or socially. Almost always some shifting of roles takes place.

Similarly, a couple's sexual behavior and amount of time devoted to D&S sex vary. For some couples every orgasm, whether it involves penetration or not, must be preceded by a session of D&S play, and they may play extensively with D&S without penetration or orgasm, since they enjoy the sensual, stimulating quality of such activity. Other couples occasionally try D&S, but participate in a great deal of straight sex, too.

Such variety occurs in the social sphere, as well. In some couples, the male has primary responsibility for such domestic chores as cooking and cleaning. Other couples share these roles, while still others follow tradition

77

in assigning these tasks. The same holds for decision making and for balancing out the degree of dominance or assertiveness each partner expresses in sexual and nonsexual areas. The most common overall pattern is for the man to be socially dominant in most traditionally male-dominant areas, while his partner is sexually dominant. But many relationships are egalitarian or hard to classify. In a minority of relationships, the woman is both socially and sexually dominant.

In general, the couples I met can be grouped into four major categories:

- Couples who were married and exclusively monogamous; some socialized with other D&S couples or went to meetings of D&S groups, but their D&S play was exclusively with each other.
- Couples who were married, monogamous, yet involved in playful, though not sexual, sessions with other couples or individuals.
- Couples who had an open marriage that permitted both play and sexual activity with other individuals and couples.
- Couples who were unmarried and involved in playful or sexual activities with others.

Although logic would dictate a fifth category of unmarried couples who were monogamous and living together or seeing each other steadily, I did not meet any couples in that category. All the unmarried couples I met were nonmonogamous.

MARRIED AND EXCLUSIVELY MONOGAMOUS COUPLES

Most married and exclusively monogamous D&S couples seem like everyday middle-class "folks" with typical middle-class values. They work at professional or white-collar jobs and live a stable, respectable, comfortable lifestyle. Those who have a traditional male-dominant or a more egalitarian marriage experiment with female dominance only at times, and mostly in sexual matters. In a few marriages the woman is largely in command at all times.

However, whatever their style of dominance, these couples face two key issues because they choose to remain monogamous. First, they need to prevent their D&S play from becoming monotonous or routine by keeping it constantly new and exciting. At times, couples encounter difficulties in doing so, and then they often temporarily cease D&S activities. Second, these monogamous couples are highly aware of the fluctuations of power in all aspects of their relationship since they confine their D&S activity to their own relationship, and sometimes they make special efforts to highlight the gain or loss of power.

Tipi and Tom, both in their 30s, have a traditional male-dominant marriage and play with female dominance occasionally. He owns a machine shop, while she attends school and handles the financial details of his business. When I met them, they had been experimenting privately with D&S off and on for about two years.

For most of their five-year marriage, Tom had been the traditional male, much like the men he knew socially or through work. Tom shared the values of his fellow blue collar workers and emulated the image of a strong, aggressive, "masculine" male. But in the third year of marriage, Tom read some D&S magazines that recalled some of his childhood fantasies. At first, he was strictly interested in being dominant, and he persuaded Tipi to participate as the submissive in some of his fantasies, most of which involved tying her up. One time he suspended her for several minutes from two cranes in his machine shop. She found these experiences erotic, and he encouraged her to become dominant and carry out his submissive fantasies of being bound, whipped, and ordered around. Initially, he orchestrated most of their activities; as she learned to play and enjoy the dominant role, she sought to take more initiative and proposed new ideas—such as sketches for new equipment Tom could make in his shop.

Sometimes Tom resisted—he wanted to be submissive when he wanted to be. So Tipi wasn't sure if she was truly dominant or just playing the role when Tom wanted her to; and at times she worried about running out of creative ideas. As a result, their play with dominance went through a series of ups and downs. She would periodically dismiss play with dominance for awhile, but then Tom would urge her to try again, and eventually she would give in. This recurring play with dominance also made them more aware of how they shared power in their relationship as a whole, and Tom became more open to performing domestic tasks at times, although he continued to play the traditional male role most of the time. For example, when Tipi invited friends over, he now helped her serve them; and he was more cooperative when she asked him to do things around the house. Tipi viewed his cooperativeness as a sign of her power. She hadn't earlier thought much about who did what activities, but now she saw how many of their interactions represented a power exchange, and she occasionally asked him to perform a task, such as getting something from the store or wearing a particular shirt, so she could feel her power.

At other times they didn't play with D&S at all for extended periods, because they were very busy with other things. When Tipi first returned to school, she had little energy to be dominant. At about the same time, the workload at Tom's machine shop increased, and he became less interested in D&S, too. But inevitably they returned to it, and when they did, they once more worked to keep it creative and exciting. And they continue to examine the role of power in all aspects of their relationship.

Nancy and Tony, both in their 30s and working in management and sales, have a more egalitarian relationship but encountered similar issues. Like many couples, he was the one first interested in dominance; after they began dating, he interested her in it. But unlike Tom, Tony eagerly urged his partner to be mostly dominant in their sexual activities, and she readily assumed this role. After a year of dating and then living together, they married.

Nancy continually seeks new ways to make her dominance exciting, usually by keeping Tony guessing about what she will do next. She surprises him each week with an erotic postcard as a gift. She tries out new techniques she learned at a D&S organization they belong to; one was spider bondage—an aesthetic way to tie up a person in a web of ropes. One time, she ordered Tony to go to work wearing women's panties under his clothes. Another time, she denied him sex for eleven days to make him especially frustrated and sexually eager. And she frequently reads D&S magazines for ideas.

In nonsexual matters, though, theirs is basically an egalitarian relationship in which they are quite aware of one another's use of power. They usually make large decisions jointly, such as deciding where to live, what kind of place to rent, and how to decorate it. And they share or exchange many household tasks, depending on the pressures each is experiencing at work. But still they view aspects of this apparently egalitarian relationship in terms of dominance and power. For example, in describing an evening together, Nancy will say: "When I came home, I asked Tony to cook, because I was feeling dominant. But then, Tony suggested a movie, and I went along with him, so he was more dominant then." Thus their consciousness, some would say *over*consciousness, of the power exchange informs their everyday decisions and actions, although, like Tipi and Tom, they usually put active D&S practice aside when they are too busy with everyday activities.

Katherine and Carl have a marriage in which Katherine is dominant most of the time, sexually and otherwise. Both in their 40s, she is an administrator and he is a building contractor; they have been married for about four years. They met when Carl, recently divorced, was sharing an upstairs room in the house with Katherine and her first husband. From the first, Katherine took the initiative. Bored with her husband, she began dropping enticing sexual hints to let Carl know she was interested. He responded, and they began a torrid affair while her husband was still in the house. Once Katherine's divorce was final, she and Carl got married.

Katherine most often takes the lead, and, like Nancy, she is always searching for new sources of sexual stimulation. Often she and Carl shop for new gimmicks and toys, and frequently she brings home surprise gifts—a new leather whip, nylon cord, or Q-tips for poking and prodding.

Sometimes she threatens Carl with devices he fears, such as a cattle prod, though she never uses them. Katherine is always planning something new: once she dressed him in baby clothes; another day, she had him perform cunnilingus while she was eating dinner; and once she treated him to a day of D&S on a deserted island.

In nonsexual matters, Katherine makes a point of being dominant, while Carl agreeably submits, finding it a relief from the responsibilities of work. For instance, she has him do most of the domestic chores, such as cooking, taking out the garbage, doing the dishes, going to the grocery, and serving dinner when company comes. In turn, he asks her permission to do things, and when he fails to do so, as happened once when he went shopping for D&S toys alone, she shows her annoyance by either symbolically punishing him, though with something she knows he likes, such as a light whipping, or more firmly punishing him by withholding sex play.

Though she is dominant most of the time, still there are times, as with the other married couples, when she doesn't feel like playing with D&S. Most typically, this occurs when she has had a hard day at work and comes home exhausted, wanting to be pampered herself and not wanting to give any orders. On one such evening, she wanted Carl to take over. He sulked and whined disappointedly for a while, expecting her to play her more usual dominant role, but eventually he acquiesced. Once refreshed, Katherine resumed her typical role.

MARRIED, MONOGAMOUS, AND PLAYFUL COUPLES

Like the married and exclusively monogamous couples, these married, but playfully monogamous couples seem quite ordinary and middle class. But they differ in their style of dominance play. Whereas the former strive to keep their strictly monogamous D&S activities stimulating, the latter look to other couples and individuals for much of the variety and excitement they find in D&S. Thus they are somewhat less concerned with generating variety in their relationship, for they gain much of this by playing with others. However, they establish clear limits on how intimate they will be with them. They engage in D&S play with others but reserve sexual intercourse for their spouses. By combining the variety of outside play with marital faithfulness and loyalty, they seek to maintain and strengthen their marriage.

Like other D&S couples, these couples sometimes confine play with female dominance to the sexual sphere; in a few marriages, the woman is dominant socially as well.

One such couple, who mainly view D&S in terms of sexual play, are Herman and June, who have a mostly egalitarian marriage. In their mid-40s, a former teacher and a financial planner, they have been married for almost 25 years, and they have two children, both now in college, from whom they hide their D&S activities. Occasionally, however, they have had to lie about traces of their activities left about the house, such as a whip left in the living room. "I got it for riding," Herman told the children.

When they first married, they lived in a small Midwestern town and had a conventional monogamous marriage. But, after a few years, Herman, who had cross-dressed as a teenager because he liked the feel of women's clothing and enjoyed becoming the woman of his dreams, admitted his interest to June and began dressing for her. After awhile, he asked her to dress up in corsets, garters, and fancy clothing; then he gradually stopped dressing himself, preferring to dress her as his female ideal. To get more ideas about dressing, they began reading about D&S in general, and, after a while, June would dress up and begin to play the dominant role using some D&S accouterments, most notably a crop and some bondage equipment, to emphasize her dominance. Through their explorations, Herman discovered that he liked enemas—the pressure of several quarts of water in his rectum was erotically arousing—and soon many of their sessions consisted of June dressing up in attractive corsets and heels, using light bondage and physical teasing, and giving Herman an enema.

In search of variety they became interested in meeting other couples and individuals through D&S organizations and ads. In these play sessions, they explore new activities that they don't generally use when alone. But, by prior agreement, these scenes never involve actual sexual contact. Herman sometimes desires this, but he honors their decision to confine sexual intimacy to their marriage and maintain their commitment to the ideal of monogamy. They also agreed not to incorporate D&S dynamics into other aspects of their lives. They make most decisions jointly and apportion household tasks according to traditional roles. For example, June does most of the cooking and makes most everyday purchases, while Herman does the gardening and fix-it chores around the house. In sum, their basically egalitarian outlook includes adherence to conventional social roles.

In contrast, Bella and Benji, who also like to play with others while remaining sexually monogamous, have a highly unconventional marriage in which Bella is the socially and sexually dominant partner. Now in her mid-40s, Bella once worked as a nurse, and Benji, in his late 30s, formerly worked as a photographer. They have been married about a year and a half and consider themselves a perfect match. This is Benji's first marriage; he never married before because he had not met a woman who would accept his interest in dressing up. Bella has had two unsatisfactory marriages—her first husband tried to control her completely, and her second was uncomfortable with her sensuality. But with Benji she feels she can be both dominant and sensual.

Within a few months of their marriage, they decided to leave the conservative Northwest, where they had both grown up, and move to more liberal California. Bella finally felt free to express her long-repressed dominant sexuality. She began to work as a part-time professional mistress, while continuing to do nursing on the side. Benji decided to give up photography, which now bored him, to be her manager. For them, the change has been ideal. Bella explores a wide variety of erotic experiences in sessions with some dozen clients a week. Her clients understand that these sessions are not to become sexual, and with Benji nearby she has had no problems. Working together this way, she and Benji feel a special closeness. Importantly, too, Benji can now freely dress up, and Bella encourages him in this because she likes having him as her "girlfriend" with whom she can share many feminine interests. Benji also enjoys being even more submissive than he formerly was. And they both value their commitment to traditional monogamy, even though their relation is unconventional in other ways.

COUPLES IN OPEN MARRIAGES

Couples who have open marriages are quite different from the monoga- mously married. They are not only sexually involved with others but also highly adventurous in exploring female dominance and other forms of D&S inside and outside of marriage. Also, they are very nontraditional in their role relationships, in their occupations, and in their general lifestyles. These couples seek variety in many areas, with D&S as only one aspect of their experimentation.

Nonmonogamous couples strive for a nonpossessive relationship in which spouses offer one another their primary emotional and sexual satisfaction. Occasionally, one partner may become jealous of the other's extramarital activity, but most couples choose open marriages only if they are sure that jealousy will not be an ongoing problem. Further, most nonmonogamous couples develop special ways of showing their primary commitment to their marriage, such as staging a special ceremony to reaffirm their love.

One example of an unconventional open marriage is that of Diana and Drew. Both in their late 20s, they lived together for about a year before deciding to get married. Drew is an entrepreneur and small businessman, always involved in new projects—doing credit investigations, running a print shop, and publishing several lifestyle journals. Diana is an art student and sometimes works as a mistress. They belong to the Pagan community, a group seriously involved in Witchcraft, and they regularly participate in and sometimes lead ceremonies.

Their religious beliefs inform their practice of dominance. The Witchcraft tradition holds that the goddess is preeminent during the spring and summer—from the spring equinox to the fall equinox—whereas the god reigns during the dark time of the year, in the fall and winter. Thus, during spring and summer, Diana is dominant sexually and socially most of the time; in fall and winter, Drew assumes the dominant role. Similarly, their marriage ceremony incorporated pagan rituals. Diana and Drew wore white silk costumes and capes, and a Wiccan priestess married them, while four couples, dressed in red, yellow, green, and blue robes to represent the colors of the four directions, looked on and recited poetry to bless the union.

Diana and Drew likewise explore D&S with a creative flair, and they often share some of their techniques with the D&S community. At one SM Church meeting, Diana demonstrated aesthetic forms of bondage using an intricate interlacing of ropes. At other times, they organize D&S poetry readings and write D&S poetry. Recently they moved from a house in a small Bay Area city to live in a tent on some country land they purchased.

An equally unusual open marriage is that of Devora and Ken, both in their 30s and married for ten years. She is a former secretary now working as a mistress, and he is an audio engineer. Theirs was originally a conventional marriage, but, when Ken became interested in swinging, Devora agreed to try it. They met a couple who were active in D&S and owned a club where they threw D&S parties and where several mistresses worked. Ken visited some of these mistresses a few times, and Devora, with Ken's encouragement, decided to work for this couple. She was bored with her secretarial work, felt it didn't pay well, and realized she could earn much more as a mistress doing what she felt was very easy work.

Thus, in the fifth year of their marriage, Devora began working as a full-time professional dominant. Concurrently, she and Ken, both as a couple and separately, started to play with other couples and individuals and to participate actively in D&S organizations and experimentation of almost any sort. Devora's work as a mistress gives her a certain expertise, and she teaches courses on S&M techniques. Sometimes they take part in elaborate D&S scenarios, some of which they organize or inspire. For one birthday, Devora was the star of a kidnap fantasy, in which four members of the SM Church "kidnapped" her from her home, blindfolded her, tied her up in the back of a car, and led her to a D&S party, where they "served" her up to the guests as the cake, complete with icy white frosting sprayed all over her body for the guests to lick off.

In spite of all their playing, Devora and Ken maintain their primary commitment to each other and generally are not prone to jealousy, since they believe each should be free and independent. Also, they trust that their primary commitment will continue, even though they each occasionally have more-than-casual extramarital relationships. Thus, while Devora was having an intense three-month affair with another man, Ken regarded it as simply "another fling" and trusted that she would get over "her grand passion." He did not view this other man as a real threat to his marriage, and one night Ken agreeably shared his bed with Devora and the other man. After the affair ended, the three of them remained close friends.

As a symbol of this mutual commitment, Devora and Ken staged an elaborate recommitment ceremony at the end of their tenth year of marriage. They rented a wooded park site, invited three dozen guests—about half of them involved in D&S, the rest close friends—and at dusk emerged from a large medieval-style tent dressed like a wedding-cake couple—she in a frilly white dress and white hat, and he in a light gray suit with tails. They followed a small procession of friends, dressed in colored robes, and two English Morris dancers into a circle of about 20 well-wishers gathered around a fire. There, before a Wiccan priestess, they repledged their marriage vows. For everyone present the ceremony reaffirmed the success and vitality of an open experimental relationship. Devora and Ken's active participation in nonmonogamous D&S had not diminished their strong, primary commitment to one another.

UNMARRIED COUPLES

All the unmarried couples I met, whether their relationship was relatively casual or close, were actively involved in sexual play with others. Most couples have an understanding that each is free to do whatever he or she wants with others, although a few couples reserve their female dominance activity for each other, to keep that part of their sexuality special. All these relationships are generally free spirited, nonmonogamous, and nonpossessive. Most couples would agree with a woman who explained that: "The D&S lifestyle doesn't fit well with monogamy, since people like to play with other people. Being totally committed to one person would cramp a person's style."

Some couples combine this free-spirited approach with an otherwise conventional lifestyle. They have typical middle- or upper-middle-class occupations—as doctors, architects, teachers, secretaries, computer programmers, and the like—and present a fairly ordinary outward appearance to their straight friends, relatives, business associates, and neighbors. Others have somewhat more offbeat jobs and lifestyles: one woman runs lingerie parties; another works as an occasional mistress; and a few men float from job to job.

Some members of these couples both engage in D&S sexuality with others and have relationships that do not involve D&S. Others frequently play with various D&Sers in multiple combinations—in triads, foursomes, and in open party scenes. To an extent, open marriage couples experiment in these ways, too, but the unmarried couples experiment even more and seem open to try almost anything. Like the open marriage couples, they combine this intensive play with a strong closeness and intimacy with their primary partner. Some of these unmarried couples have occasional problems with jealousy, as do couples with open marriages, but generally jealousy yields to nonpossessiveness and playfulness for them, too. For example, Jesse, a 32-year-old credit investigator, for a year seriously dated Dorothy, who worked as a mistress and saw several men. At times he envied the other men in her life, because he cared for her so much, but he dissipated these feelings by reminding himself that he had no right to have them. Even after Dorothy began a committed relationship with someone else, Jesse put aside his jealousy to organize a birthday party for her.

The following four couples, each of whom has been together at least a year, are representative of long-term unmarried relationships. All partake of the openness and experimental playfulness that characterizes the scene, but each has particular preferences in D&S activities and in the dynamics of their relationship.

A couple combining the conventional and the offbeat is Marvin and Melody, introduced earlier. He is a highly respected internist of 40, she a former housewife in her 30s who now sells lingerie through home parties. When they met, both were married to others, and Marvin was a friend of Melody's husband Frank, also a doctor. At first, the two couples socialized as an ordinary foursome, although Frank and Melody had a straight monogamous marriage, and Marvin was not yet willing to share his D&S interests with anyone. But then Frank decided that he wanted an open relationship; soon after, Marvin's marriage began to break up, and he started to see Melody. After they had dated for about a year, Marvin slowly shared with Melody his interest in D&S. At first he told her his male-dominant fantasies and then gradually encouraged her to take the dominant role since he preferred to be submissive. Though new to dominance, Melody was soon eagerly participating in his fantasies, using whips, piercing, chains, ropes, and other paraphernalia and techniques.

Marvin and Melody see each other about once a week and spend some weekends and an occasional week together, although Melody remains happily married to Frank. Marvin's divorce, his second, is final and he is enjoying his freedom. In addition to his ongoing relationship with Melody, he is casually dating a few other women and occasionally participates in encounters with males and couples. Sometimes he and Melody go to D&S gatherings attended by the other women he is dating. But, while Marvin sees other people and Melody has her marriage, they agreed that neither would engage in another sexual relationship involving female dominance before discussing it with the other. Each can freely engage in nonsexual erotic female dominance play with others, but they reserve the combination of female dominance and sex for each other, since they see it as somehow very special and intense.

Similarly, Sharon and Lance—the office administrator and real estate contractor introduced earlier—date and play extensively with others, both as individuals and as a couple. Sharon met Lance at a Society of Janus meeting soon after she had broken away from a triad relationship in which she was feeling oppressed by being submissive. Lance had already been involved in female dominance for about five years, mostly with some professional mistresses who later became friends, and for years he had had strong fantasies about bondage with chains. Through their experiments, Sharon found she liked both the dominant role and the chains, though she continued to be socially submissive. Within a few months, they came to think of themselves as a couple. Sharon became active in helping Lance organize the SM Church, and they saw each other frequently, several times a week. After a year, they decided to live together, while each continued openly to have relationships with others.

At times, each meets the people the other is seeing, and occasionally they assist each other in arranging to meet new people. Frequently they invite individuals and couples to participate in their scenes. For instance, when they ask another woman to join them, Sharon binds Lance in chains and orders him to crawl for her, while she lashes him gently with a whip; then she invites the other woman to participate in chaining and lashing him. Typically, these play sessions with other couples are brief, perhaps an hour or two, but they sometimes have long extended private sessions in which Sharon keeps Lance in chains for one or two days. For one of the most dramatic of these sessions, she staged a kidnap and took him bound in chains to an S&M retreat in northern California for a weekend.

Their relationship works very well, enabling them to live out their long-standing fantasies through a D&S lifestyle. Even when they participate in ordinary activities, such as going to movies or attending the opera, they typically view their experiences from a D&S perspective. For example, as Lance once observed after seeing a movie: "There was lots of D&S in it. The kidnappers tied up the hero, and then one of the women threatened him. Nobody admits it, but that's female dominance." Also, they often talk about their shared dream of creating new communities based on the women having total power over the men, who would serve as their worshipful "slaves."

Another unmarried and playful couple is Danielle and Harvey, who live next door to each other. Danielle, a real estate salesperson in her late

20s, had discovered she liked dominance after working as a mistress at the suggestion of her dominant ex-husband. She met Harvey, a chef in a restaurant in his early 30s, when her ex-husband took her to an organizational meeting of the SM Church shortly after their break-up. She had seen Harvey before at the club where she worked as a mistress, although they had never had a session and had never struck up a friendship. Harvey mentioned that he was looking for someplace to live, and since Danielle was in the process of moving into a new apartment and knew the apartment next door was empty, she suggested that Harvey might live there, too. He moved in and they soon became very close. Not only do they participate in frequent sessions, most of them focused on Danielle whipping, spanking, tickling, and teasing Harvey, but they share many interests: listening to music, smoking marijuana, going to films, and visiting. They see one another almost every day, although both have other relationships. Danielle sees several single and married men for occasional sessions, and she plays with a number of men at SM Church gatherings. Occasionally, too, she has play sessions with some women she met through Samois, an organization of gay and bisexual women involved in D&S. Meanwhile, Harvey casually dates a mixture of straight, dominant, and submissive women, and from time to time plays with a few men, some of them transvestites.

At times, Danielle and Harvey participate with others separately, at times together, and they play in both private and public sessions. When Danielle teaches courses and heads workshops on D&S, Harvey is one of her most willing subjects. And often she uses his apartment for D&S parties and programs. Also, like other playful D&S couples, they frequently help each other meet prospective new partners. For instance, when Natasha attended an SM Church campout for the first time, Danielle asked Harvey to look after her and make her feel at home. In short, Danielle and Harvey have chosen an ongoing D&S lifestyle. Yet, despite all this activity, like most D&S couples, they keep up the appearance of being quite ordinary people.

In contrast, Kat and Mouse, a former social service director and social welfare professor, both in their 30s, not only live this playful lifestyle but also openly organize D&S activities. Mouse had had fantasies of being both dominant and submissive since he was about 15, and he began to explore them tentatively with a few mistresses and women he dated while living in Washington. Through a mutual friend he met Kat, who was then unacquainted with D&S and had been brought up as a properly demure and well-behaved Southern girl. They were strictly friends for about three years, since they were dating other people and Kat had moved to the Bay Area.

On a visit to California, Mouse called Kat and suggested getting together. Soon after they became lovers, and Mouse introduced Kat to

D&S. Initially, as they were making love, he put his hand on her throat, as if to strangle her. She wondered why he was doing that, and she felt a strange mixture of fear and excitement that was very arousing. After examining these new feelings, she decided to explore D&S with Mouse.

At first, she was submissive to him. Then, at his request, she began to work at the Chateau, a B&D establishment, to learn about dominance and submission. Three months later, Mouse moved to the Bay Area, and they started living together. Mouse had strong submissive fantasies, and now that Kat had learned dominance, she quickly assumed the dominant role. She took to it readily, feeling it tapped her deep urges to be assertive and strong, and it allowed her to release her devilish, wicked, and selfish side, long repressed by her conservative upbringing.

Soon D&S became integral to their lives. For several months they gave an erotic S&M sex show at a local club; she began working as a mistress giving private sessions and started writing a column on dominance for the *Spectator*, a sexually oriented paper; and together they offered workshops on D&S and worked to organize a high-quality S&M stage production. Within their relationships, they are especially interested in exploring the psychological dynamics of the power exchange and in examining their responses to various types of role reversals and D&S activity. For a time, Kat was strictly dominant, and Mouse tried being a house husband, providing much of the care for Kat's child by a former marriage.

They also play extensively with other people in their sessions together and separately, because their goal is to explore the full range of D&S experiences. They meet most of these people through the D&S scene: men Kat has met when working as a professional mistress; respondents to her column; and members of various D&S groups. From the beginning, both have kept journals to record their experiences and feelings. These journals help them to become more aware of their feelings, understand their D&S experiences better, and provide ideas for their sessions together.

After a few months of D&S activity, they noticed that Kat was becoming generally more aggressive, both sexually and socially, while submission led Mouse to become more passive and, for a short time, less articulate and verbal, as he turned more inward. But then their relationship shifted again, for, as it continued, Kat occasionally felt like being submissive in their sessions, though she continued to think of herself as mostly dominant. Concurrently, Mouse wanted to explore dominance outside their relationship and began casually seeing several submissive women. Also, they participated as a couple in triads in which they both dominated another woman, and sometimes in foursomes as well.

Throughout their relationship, Kat and Mouse have experimented extensively with all sorts of D&S activities: pain, bondage, urination, and suspension, among others. They participate in a variety of D&S parties,

weekends, and week-long scenarios. Although their public advocacy of
D&S through workshops they organize makes them an atypical couple,
their attitudes reflect the same interest in experimentation that characterizes
other unmarried couples in the scene. Some unmarried couples occasionally
play with D&S, others make it part of a total lifestyle, but all share the
desire to experiment, explore, and play.

PART III

JOINING THE SCENE

7

Workshops for Dominant Women and Submissive Men

en and women new to female dominance often feel uncertain or
confused about assuming unconventional sexual and social roles.
Although interested in experimenting with dominance, some men are
uncomfortable about having and expressing submissive feelings, while
some women find it difficult to take and use their new power. Both men
and women may want emotional support from others who have similar
feelings or are in similar relationships. And both may seek more information
about D&S techniques and the dynamics of the D&S relationship.

To help relative newcomers understand the emotional, psychological,
and physical facts of D&S, Mistress Kat and Mouse (the former social
agency director and social work professor introduced earlier) conduct
workshops, classes, and support groups. Their approach to female
dominance, shared by many but not all members of the D&S community,
holds that the submissive male should surrender control and allow the
dominant woman to satisfy herself; though she should consider her
partner's limits and preferences, she should focus on pleasing herself;
dominance will then be erotic for her, and her pleasure will bring about her
partner's. A woman should not merely play out her partner's fantasies—to
experience her power and to give her partner the physical and psychological release that comes from abandoning control, she must assume her
partner's consent and enact her own fantasies and desires.

A WORKSHOP FOR WOMEN

A representative workshop Kat and Mouse conducted occurred one
Saturday in February 1981. Fifteen women met with them in a building that
had once been a small coffee house. At the fringe of the Haight-Ashbury,
once famous for its hippies, and now a multiethnic neighborhood
struggling back to middle-class respectability, they gathered for an

93

introductory workshop on dominance. The long narrow room had large cushions along the walls, and toward the rear was a cushion-lined adult "playroom" about 8-feet square, separated from the main room by a line of wooden bars, which made the playroom resemble an adult crib.

Most of the women had recently been introduced to dominance by a man they were seeing, and they were uncertain about playing the dominant role. Among those present—some of whom we have met earlier—were Laura, a former sex therapist who wanted to become more assertive in daily life; Katherine, the administrative assistant who was dominant in her marriage and eager to discover new techniques; and Vicki and Fern, friends of Kat who worked as occasional mistresses and wanted to learn more.

Kat and Mouse began by telling how they had discovered D&S (see Chapter 6). In this workshop, they would share what they had learned from their year and a half of experimenting. But first they wanted the women to explain why they had come to the workshop. Each woman took her turn speaking; most said they wanted to become more comfortable with the dominant role, to hear new ideas, and to gain support from other women. Brenda, a 25-year-old secretary, remarked: "I've always been socially dominant in organizing things, running a house and a business. But sexually, I've been taught to be passive. So it's awkward in relationships. I'd like to be more comfortable with my own feelings." And Nancy, a saleswoman, observed: "In my relationship we switch, and we both push each other to our limits. But it takes a lot of creative energy to be dominant. I want to be able to keep growing and exploring."

Mouse then described his approach to D&S as a consensual and balancing or compensatory activity. Seeking to allay the unease caused by societal taboos, Mouse explained that a consensual exchange of power serves balancing functions for men and women: "Both have a need to experience the other side of their personality. It's a need for balance. Exploring female dominance helps to readjust the present imbalance." By exchanging roles, "men can have the experience of being overwhelmed, of letting something happen, of having no goals, and of releasing their emotions through worshipful love; and women can learn to unlock their emotions from their sexuality so they can have heartless, selfish, whimsical, expressive sex, and experience creatively orchestrating it. Then, for both, this role reversal releases lots of new energy."

As Kat described it, this new energy was a rush of mutual, telepathic excitement, much more intense than the arousal of ordinary sex. "It feels like a release of blocked energy, which is heavy, physical, and frequently genital or pelvic." She found it hard to describe this energy, though she felt it addictive and sometimes a bit frightening in its intensity. Mouse added,

"We aren't exactly sure why this energy works. But it's something real and fun that taps something very deep."

They explained the many ways that people can spark this energy:

1. Pain: "A person can enjoy much more intense stimulation when sexually aroused, and one gets a spaced-out feeling when submissive that magically turns pain into pleasure."

2. Humiliation and bondage: "They're pleasurable because they're a more intense way of experiencing exercising power or being out of control. Humiliation makes the power more 'feelable,' and in bondage, the person feels vulnerability and a loss of security. There's an excitement in feeling out of control."

3. Unusual imagery, toys, and paraphernalia: "They help free people to feel 'into' it and experience more extreme feelings, just as uniforms and paraphernalia help us to get into other roles."

4. Cross-dressing: "It helps men feel more submissive and feminine."

5. Urination: "The extreme insult. It plays up the other's power."

6. Enemas and dildos: "The rectum is normally a forbidden part of the body. So invading it is another form of expressing power...and the stimulation itself can be erotic."

Not everyone likes all these ways of being dominant and submissive. But Kat and Mouse urged tolerance of others' likes and dislikes. In addition, ideas that now seemed unpleasant might later, as Kat and Mouse discovered, be appealing.

Kat devoted the rest of the morning to tips to the women on how to be effectively dominant, whatever techniques they used. "Find that edge where your partner feels he can't take it anymore. Then get him to cross just beyond that edge—that's exciting.... The key is using reality to create an illusion....Be aware of your partner. Though I may appear uncaring or mean as part of my role, part of me is always asking: 'How is my partner? Can he take it?'....Have the appropriate attitude. Be playful, adventuresome. Feel free to explore your own sexuality and your capacity to be cruel....Let the suppressed parts of you go. There's an excitement, a release in doing something forbidden."

Kat's emphasis was on releasing one's deep feeling to experience sensuality and pleasure: "Do what you feel like....Do what you want, but make it consensual. Trust the energy. When you're both really open, the communication is almost telepathic....S&M sex is very intimate. You'll share parts of yourself you don't ordinarily show....Get in touch with your dark, hidden side." To find that side, Kat suggested: "Do what makes you feel sexy....Fantasize....Become an actress. Create a character. Give your dominant part a name.... Ask questions and find out about his fantasies. It's a source of your power, knowing that secret part of him. But *don't act out his fantasies unless you like them. Just do what you feel like doing....*

"And make it real. Do more than he expects, such as hit him harder to feel your power and take him out of control.... Try using threats, though you don't have to follow through. Create stories, use words to turn him on. Use clothes, costuming, equipment, body language, and facial expression to emphasize your message and intensify the experience. For example, bite, bare your teeth, hiss at him.... Learn to say no and tease. He can't always have what he wants. Only when you're willing. That adds to your feeling of power and his feeling of being out of control.... Use humiliation or pain. Make him value the pleasure he gets.... And watch for that rush; it's like riding a wave. If you feel it, your partner will, too.... Focus on your own pleasure. Do what you feel like doing. Yet remember him and what turns him on, too, since there has to be a mutual exchange."

Afterwards, some women felt relieved, now that they had a better idea of what to do, and they felt more confident in taking command. Reassured that they were not doing anything their partner didn't like, they felt freer to explore their desires. But other women had lingering doubts and concerns. In being dominant they experienced a powerful, sometimes oppressive, feeling of responsibility for their partners as well as feelings of power, and they worried about going too far or trying something that their partners would reject. Kat acknowledged the oppressive, responsible aspect of power and the women's fears of doing the wrong thing, falling back into the passive female role, and feeling pressured to be creative. Being dominant would not always be easy, and women might find it easier to alternate periods of dominance with periods of "straight time" when they put playing with power aside to relate on an equal basis with their partners. She concluded by restating the erotic and psychological rewards of being dominant—a more creative, vital, exciting sex life; a more intimate and deeper relationship; and a sense of personal balance—rewards that one's partner will also experience.

After lunch Kat demonstrated how people's deep-seated energies are released by D&S to create mutual pleasure. She wanted the women to observe graphically how she and her partners enjoyed a session, even though these activities might seem painful or disagreeable to some. Franklin and Daniel, two submissive men Kat worked with, had volunteered to assist her.

For the first demonstration, she stood holding a crop behind Franklin, a tall, burly, light-skinned black man in his 40s who worked in electronics. Once a professional client, he had become Kat's friend. Now, at her command, he bent down on his hands and knees with his backside in the air. Kat pulled down his pants, and rubbed her palm across his backside a few times. She explained, "I feel a rush with each stroke of the crop, and I associate this with the knowledge I'm creating pain. It's like his pain is a gift to me. Then, each time I hit him, he feels the same kind of rush. It should be telepathic, and, if we're on the same wavelength, he'll experience about the same level of rush as I do."

She used a ten-finger code to illustrate. With each stroke, they each raised one to ten fingers to indicate how intense their rush was—the more fingers, the greater the rush. At first, as Kat cropped Franklin, each held up only two or three fingers. But as she continued to hit him harder, the number of fingers each held up increased almost in tandem. "You see," Kat observed, "that's telepathy." She concluded by rubbing Franklin's backside gently and offering him her hand to kiss. "You want to give him some pleasure as well as pain to give him something to look forward to—a reason to endure the pain."

Next she introduced Daniel, a short, thin, frail-looking man who considered himself a poet. He had written her in response to her column, offering to submit completely to her as her "slave" who "wished to serve" by doing whatever she wanted. Kat played with him occasionally, and he was the man described in Chapter 4 whom Kat "loaned" to Natasha. But the ten-finger demonstration was less successful than the first. Kat explained that the "telepathy" wasn't there because "Daniel has trouble trusting me completely and relaxing. So he's resisting."

The next demonstration was designed to help the women relax, focus on experiencing their own pleasure, and forget about their partners' feelings. Kat instructed Daniel to lick a small framed pane of glass. "Just focus on how nice it might feel and how willing the man is to do this," she urged. At her command, his licking became faster or slower, in imitation of a man performing cunnilingus. "Just imagine you're satisfying a woman" Kat told him. The women watched thoughtfully. Many had never experienced such openness about sexuality of any type, and they watched with avid curiosity. The demonstration also enabled them to feel more comfortable later talking about their own sexual experiences and difficulties.

Kat next sought to dispel the image of giving pain as an act of cruelty, using Franklin as her subject again. "As this demonstration shows," Kat said, "pain given correctly and in the right context is erotically stimulating." She put a clothespin on Franklin's nipple as he knelt before her with his shirt off. She again used the ten-finger code as she squeezed the clothespin. Though Franklin breathed heavily and gulped occasionally, he held up nine or ten fingers most of the time. "You see," Kat interpreted, "it's exciting to him. You need to trust that, when you're excited, your partner is. You need to trust that mutuality and that rush, for you're tapping a deeper source of D&S or S&M energies when you release your dominant side and he releases his submissiveness. The energy bubbles out like a gusher and you feel that rush."

But one cannot analyze or intellectualize the energy, Kat warned, for that would destroy it. One can only feel and through these feelings experience a kind of catharsis or cleansing in which one can release feelings of love, self-interest, whimsy, caprice, even anger at men. But the dominant woman must also stay in control, retaining a fine balance between assuming power, surrendering to the rush, feeling loved, being responsible, and making sure the activity is mutually arousing.

Kat's message highlighted some of the paradoxes and sometimes hard-to-reconcile aspects of D&S. Yet the women found it reassuring, for they had experienced these paradoxical elements. In the discussion session that followed, they examined these paradoxes and their insecurities in taking the dominant role. As relative newcomers to dominance, these women needed reassurance that their behavior and feelings were natural, that assuming power was acceptable and erotic, and that men like it, even when the women themselves weren't sure.

To conclude the workshop, Kat talked about types of equipment and how to use them creatively and safely. She flourished whips, crops, ropes, cuffs, and other equipment as she spoke. "You must be responsible. If you're careless, you can hurt or turn people off.... Try it on yourself first. Know what you're doing to someone else.... Build up to it; as you do, the person can take more.... Hit where the flesh can take it and know where you want to hit. Other cautions included: "Tie your knots carefully. Don't leave someone tied up alone or too long"; "If you use cuffs or manacles, be sure you know where you have the key." With care and awareness, Kat and Mouse emphasized, the dominant woman could transform ordinary sex into an unusual, extraordinary, exciting, creative realm of pleasurable experience.

A WORKSHOP FOR MEN

The focus in the men's workshop, held a few weeks later, was quite different. The women's workshop had been designed to help the women overcome the difficulties of using power and to show them D&S techniques. But with the men, Kat and Mouse emphasized learning to submit by letting go and allowing things to happen. They encouraged the men to share their fantasies and discuss their submissive feelings, thereby providing peer support for one another. Some of the men present had for years bottled up their fantasies, but in this safe, supportive environment, they felt free to share.

Early in the workshop, Kat and Mouse discussed a major difficulty some men have with female dominance—the men want to be submissive in a specific way that will fulfill long-standing fantasies. "You have to drop that image," Kat and Mouse argued, because it "destroys the woman's ability to be truly dominant. Then the 'heat' or eroticism disappears from the exchange of power." Rather, the men needed to learn "to give in, release control, and trust the dominance of the woman." As Mouse expressed it in a handout he distributed during the workshop: "The submissive becomes a leaf in the rapids, mindlessly flowing with the power of the river.... You've got to let go of your fantasized wants and follow her dominant will.... Don't try to make it happen. Let it happen to you."

But although the men affirmed their strong need for erotic submission, even when able to satisfy their sexual drive through straight sex, they still had qualms about both surrendering control and putting aside their long-standing fantasies. When Kat and Mouse urged them to yield their decision-making power and cultivate the qualities of humility, shyness, and uncertainty, they resisted. As American men, they had been trained since infancy to be strong and aggressive. How could they accept their own submission? How could a man reconcile powerlessness and his masculine identity?

Thus most of the workshop concerned the psychology of submission and how to surrender control. Kat and Mouse sought to help the men feel comfortable learning to submit, so they could then satisfy their desires. They emphasized that submission is not a form of spinelessness or self-obliteration. Kat advised, "Be loving, respectful, admiring; but don't be a wimp. Be willing to serve, but don't be too eager. Share your fantasies, but don't demand that she enact them." Moreover, the men were counseled to make their partners comfortable with their dominance. A man should show patience and tact in asking his partner to take the lead, and he should not be overly critical: "Remember it may not be easy for her to be dominant. Respect her erotic tastes and styles. Don't leave her with egg on her face." If a man wants his partner to be dominant, Kat explained, he has to support her dominance in various ways: reassuring her that he wants to please, reminding her she has the power, and truly giving up his control and power.

Various exercises were used to teach the men about submission. In one, the men gathered in pairs or small groups to talk about submitting without focusing on their wants. In another, they role played talking to a woman about wanting to submit. To help them relax while awaiting their partner's actions, Kat had them close their eyes and sit back, while she circled around lightly cropping them, pinching them, stroking them, or teasing them about all the things she could do to them. Since they didn't know if her next action would bring pleasure or pain, they had to abandon all expectations and let go.

After the exercises, they talked about their feelings and repeatedly revealed their ambivalence: "I want to submit. But can I trust my partner?" "If I give up my power, what then?" "Suppose she doesn't do what I want her to do?" Despite the ambivalence, these men did want to be submissive, and Kat and Mouse encouraged them by reminding them that submission is "a way of satisfying inner needs, discovering a deep and fulfilling intimacy with another person, balancing the feminine and masculine energies, and experiencing an intense erotic pleasure....But to make it happen," Kat stressed again, "You have to relax, let go, and let it happen."

A WORKSHOP FOR COUPLES

About a month later, Kat and Mouse held follow-up workshops for couples who attended the women's or men's workshops. Six couples were present, most of whom had been together at least six months. The married couples, introduced in Chapter 6, were Katherine and Carl, the office administrator and real estate contractor, married two years; Nancy and Tony, both in sales management, who married shortly after the workshop; Tipi and Tom, the graduate student and machine shop owner, married a year. These six people had been exploring female dominance for at least a year; they had signed up for the workshop to learn new approaches and to examine specific issues concerning dominance. Among the unmarried couples were Misty, a researcher, and Andrew, an accountant; Will and Dawn, both teachers; and Wilma and Gary, a nurse and dentist respectively.

Everyone sat on pillows in the same long room where the individual workshops had been held. At Kat's request, people described their experiences since the previous workshop. In general, the relationships seemed to have improved: the men were more comfortable in letting go, and the women found it easier to assume power. "I'm more relaxed about letting things take their natural course," Will observed. "I know I pushed too much in previous relationships." "I'm letting things flow more," Carl said. "I feel more in control," Wilma remarked.

Yet there were some problems—most notably, some men continued to try to control how their partners expressed their dominance, and some women had difficulty being dominant. For example, Tipi complained that Tom wouldn't let her be dominant: "I told him to do something, but he didn't do it." "I didn't feel like it," Tom shot back. "If I'm in the mood, I like her to be dominant. But I wasn't in the mood just then." Kat tried to explain why Tom's attitude hindered their pleasure: "You have to leave it up to her for the real submissive experience. She has to feel dominant, too. She can't just turn it on when you want it."

The men then met separately with Mouse for a general discussion, while the women divided into two groups of three. Each woman was to gather enough information about the other two in her group so she could later intelligently interview their partners. After those interviews, the women would reconvene to discuss ways to improve each relationship.

Katherine, Tipi, and Misty retreated to the playroom. Tipi began by describing her difficulty in assuming power. "Tom says he wants to be submissive, but then says 'I want you to do this.' I can't feel real power in the relationship.... I'm still curious about dominance, but I could drop it. So far, power's not erotic to me, but maybe I could learn to like it. If I'm going to continue being dominant, I want to learn to like it for myself. Not just for him."

Katherine explained how completely dominance influenced her life with Carl: "I make him call me mistress. I torment him with verbal threats to keep him in the mood. He's never sure if I will do something or not. And knowing he likes it gets me stimulated, too." Then Misty outlined her partner's main complaint that she wasn't dominant enough and described her difficulties being dominant: "He says I don't hit him hard enough. And he tells me he has certain fantasies I don't want to do."

Then the women each met with one of the men to conduct an interview. Kat's guidelines for the interviews instructed the women to ask the men the following kinds of questions: Is he satisfied with his role in the relationship? With his partner's role? What is his ideal relationship? What are his fantasies? What excites him the most sexually? In what ways is he fulfilled or unfulfilled? What problems does he see?

During his interview, Tom complained that Tipi wasn't dominant enough when he wanted her to be. "She's wishy-washy. I'd like her to be stronger." Why? Because, he explained, "It's a change. It's exciting to think about. It gives mystery." Yet he wanted her to dominate him in a certain way: "It's fine as a play. It's okay to say for now we're changing roles. But she needs too much mental preparation to get ready. I'd like her to be more spontaneous." Because of this conflict, they had dropped D&S activity for awhile, and they were busy with other things. But Tom still desired to be submissive if only Tipi would take the power. "Maybe she could come up with a plan," he suggested. "I'd like her to take more initiative, but announce it in advance."

In contrast, Carl reported no problems other than an occasional difficulty in "letting things happen and flow." He was especially interested in expanding their female dominance lifestyle even further. He described what he and Katherine did to make their relationship work and viewed their successes as the result of their mutual trust and their enjoyment of variety and the mental stimulation of dominance power games.

"I feel I can totally trust my partner now.... I'm more interested in the mental stimulation, not so much in the pain. But the pain makes the domination more real. I enjoy humiliation in the head. So we play dress-up games. It's erotic to feel funny and ridiculous. For example, I'm dressed up, but it seems I'm not. Outside I look manly. But underneath, I'm wearing women's underwear or a corset.... I think the main problem we've been working on is my letting things flow. I've tried to put aside my preconceptions and let things happen. I try not to be so helpful anymore. I've decided that, whatever happens, she does it, and it's okay with me."

After these interviews ended, the two women's groups reconvened to help one another design a brief encounter for their respective partners. These encounters were to enable each couple to confront barriers to the expression of dominance in their relationship. In these encounters, the woman could work alone with her partner, or she could involve other women, even the whole group.

First the group discussed Tipi and Tom's relationship. Katherine made many suggestions about how Tipi could get Tom to submit: "Tom needs submission. He wants it. You've got to get him in a submissive position, and tell him: 'We'll be dominant my way, or not at all.' Maybe some of the techniques I use with Carl might work. I intimidate him with verbal comments. He doesn't know if I will or I won't. And I buy things I never use, like a bull whip, just to torment him."

Tipi responded by describing a struggle she and Tom had had over her attempt to shave off his mustache after she tied him to the bed. He liked being tied up, but when she tried to shave him, because she preferred him without a mustache, he got furious, struggled, and yelled at her. She desisted and didn't try again. But she continued to think about the experience as a symbol of the basic problem of their relationship—his unwillingness to let her be truly dominant.

Again, Katherine had some advice. "That's just it," she pointed out, "he says you can do whatever you want. But then, when you try, he won't let you. He has to experience that loss of control. You have to experience that power. So tell him, 'This is my afternoon. I can do what I want.'" Bolstered by Katherine's encourgement, Tipi agreed to do just that.

Then Katherine and Tipi talked about how Misty might be more dominant with Andrew. They recalled her comments that Andrew kept suggesting she do something she didn't want to do, and they proposed that she forcefully tell him in the planned encounter that she never wanted him to mention it again. "And tell him you're going to do exactly what you like," Katherine added. "You don't care if he likes it or not. It's going to be your way from now on. Let him know who's the boss."

The group didn't have time to discuss Katherine's situation at length. But she already knew what she wanted to do: "He's been having trouble letting go. So I'm just going to put him in a hood and tie him up. That way he's especially vulnerable and out of control."

The whole group then met in the main room to begin the encounters. Several could go on simultaneously, and they could be done privately or before the whole group. Each was to highlight a key issue in the couple's relationship.

Nancy started off by asking Tony to stand up and strip down to his black T-shirt and pantyhose. She placed a pig's mask on his head and, as everyone watched, led him to a post in the main room. She tied him up using a technique called "spider bondage," which she had recently learned at a Society of Janus meeting. As she draped the ropes around him, she created a dramatic spiderweb effect by interlacing the white ropes against his black shirt and tights. She explained that Tony had been overly pushy and "piggy" in pressuring her to be dominant in the past week, when she felt tired from her new job. So now she wanted him to stay there quietly for the rest of the afternoon and think about how he had been a "pig."

Then, Dawn, who found it difficult to hit Will as hard as he liked, took Will into the front room to get a demonstration of whipping from Kat. She felt she needed peer support so that she would feel it was permissible to whip him; thus she invited the other women to watch. Kat directed Will to bend over. She pulled down his pants and snapped her whip against his backside again and again, gradually building up with harder and harder strokes, until reddish marks began to appear. After briefly stroking them with her hand and brandishing the whip a few more times, she passed the whip to Nancy and Wilma, who had been in Dawn's group, so they could whip Will, too. If these other women could hit Will and he enjoyed it, then Dawn would feel free to hit him, as well. When Wilma handed the crop to Dawn, Dawn shooed everyone out, so she could have her private session with Will.

While everyone waited in the main room for Dawn to finish, Nancy added a few final rope ties to Tony and left him alone again. When Dawn returned to the main room with Will, both were smiling broadly, apparently satisfied by their private session. Will sat down gingerly on one of the cushions. "It's sore," he grinned, expressing a kind of pride. Dawn had finally hit him hard enough, his look implied.

Then, Wilma took Gary into the front room, and Kat demonstrated more hitting techniques, since Wilma, like Dawn, had difficulty being dominant. However, Gary wasn't overly cooperative; he moaned dramatically from time to time and kept wriggling about. Kat decided he needed to learn to behave and keep quiet. She instructed him to keep still and to moan only when she ordered him to do so. One time she told him to moan; another time she told him not to. "The idea," she explained to Wilma later, "is to control everything that starts getting in your way. Then, you show you have control over that, too."

Meanwhile, Katherine took Carl into the back room for a private session. She ordered him to strip to his shorts and put on a big black leather face mask that had holes only for his mouth and nose. She encased his hands in a long black snug-fitting glove and attached a chain. And she threatened to shock him with an electric cattle prod, which she buzzed menacingly around his head.

Just as Wilma brought Gary back into the main room, Katherine led Carl out by his chain. She wanted him to feel totally under her power. Her procedure seemed to have this effect. He walked behind her quietly, his shoulders drooping, his head down, and he looked perfectly subdued. Then, to further highlight her power, Katherine demanded: "Now stick out your tongue to show us all." Everyone laughed when he did. In turn, his willingness to appear foolish at her command emphasized her control.

For her session with Andrew, Misty took him into the back room. Then, as the women suggested, she informed him that she was in charge. She ordered him to strip to his briefs and snapped a blindfold around his head. "I can do whatever I want. And I'll do what I like because it pleases me." To demonstrate, she demanded that he crawl around the playpen, chased after him with a whip, and ordered him to kiss her feet. He could make suggestions, but, if she said no, he was not to raise the issue again.

Then Misty invited Kat, Katherine, and Tipi in to demonstrate how well Andrew was following orders. At her request, he crawled about some more and kissed their feet. Then Kat hit him sharply again and again, commenting on how red his backside was getting and that he would have something to remember this workshop by.

A bit later, Misty and Andrew returned to the group. He wore a blindfold, had a dog collar around his neck, and his hands were tied with rope. Misty led him out on a leash, and he sat down quietly at her command until she removed the blindfold, indicating the session was over.

Next, Tipi took Tom into the back room and bound him with heavy handcuffs, chains, and ropes. As he sat motionlessly against the wall, she slipped out quietly and picked up a bowl of water, a razor, and some shaving cream, which one of the men had secretly obtained for her at lunch. She had a strange, wicked, self-satisfied grin on her lips as she walked in, and everyone expected to soon hear Tom yelling and thrashing. But the back room was very quiet, and a few minutes later Tipi came out followed by Tom, his mustache replaced by a content look.

In the discussions that followed, the women and men gathered into separate groups with Kat and Mouse. Generally, the women claimed to be more comfortable now with the dominant role. Wilma felt supported by the group; Dawn thought she had greater control; Tipi felt reassured that she could be in charge after all. "I didn't think I could do it," she remarked. "But I did." To which Nancy added, "As strong as his will is, your must be stronger to take control."

Meanwhile, the men shared their feelings about surrendering control. In general, they had liked the experience; they found it freeing to have someone else in command. Tony observed that this was the first time he had gone public with his submission, but he felt safe doing so and would do it again. Will said he discovered he was an exhibitionist; he loved the public exposure. Gary and Carl agreed that the workshop left them feeling sexually stimulated. Andrew rated the encounter "a 9½ on a scale of 10"; enduring the pain was his way of showing Misty he cared.

The workshop ended with everyone in the same room sharing a few additional fantasies and suggestions on techniques to try: "You can take a teaball, put spikes on it, and put it around a penis or a nipple"; "I have this fantasy of making a hydraulic bondage/torture device that could be used to slowly stretch a man's genitals." People also discussed what they told outsiders: "We try to keep it quiet. We use other words than S&M to describe what we do"; "We only tell people selectively, if we think they'll understand"; "Our friends are aware we're into something unusual, but they're not sure what. If they ask, we just say it's 'creative sex.'"

The workshop had served to support and motivate the participants. For the couples relatively new to D&S, it was an initiation into the larger D&S community, and some subsequently participated in other D&S activities. But even those who did not felt more comfortable at having met others with similar likes from whom they gained social support and approval. Those couples who had been involved in D&S for some time gained from the workshop renewed energy and impetus; they, too, forged new links with the D&S community.

All the couples seemed very much to need this encouragement and support, since they mostly practiced their activities in a half-hidden fantasy world. They could tell few people, and, when they did, they chose their confidants carefully from among relatives, family, and friends who would understand. The workshop was another step into the open by making what had been private a bit more public; it was a way of "coming out" into the larger local D&S community.

A SUPPORT GROUP FOR DOMINANT WOMEN

To offer the women continuing affirmation, ideas, and support, Kat launched a group for dominant women, which gradually became a consciousness-raising group on general issues concerning D&S, role reversal, and women's assertiveness. Like the workshop, the support group provided a source of contacts and invitations to events in the scene as well as the social support the women needed to keep them active. Over the six months that the group met, a nucleus of eight women and a half-dozen occasional members shared their experiences, discussed their problems, exchanged ideas for D&S techniques, and learned new ways to relate to men.

The group met for the first time three weeks after the couples workshop. Katherine, Tipi, Misty, and Nancy, who all had been at that workshop, attended, along with Frances, a legal secretary in her 20s, and Andrea, a social worker of about 35 who had attended the workshop for women. The meeting began with each person describing what had happened since the workshop. What had she gained? Did she feel more comfortable being dominant? Were there any changes in her life?

The women involved in strong ongoing relationships generally praised the workshop as a source of new inspirations and ideas that had led them to make firmer commitments to D&S and to their partners. Tony had asked Nancy to marry him, and she was trying out new techniques. One day she painted his toenails while he slept to surprise him when he woke up. She tied some jewelry around his penis, so it jangled loudly as he walked. And when they shopped for the wedding ring, she ordered Tony to stand in front of a lingerie shop, while she made the selection. "He felt both embarrassed and excited by having to stand there," she said.

Andrea reported that she had become more forceful, which so thrilled her boyfriend of about a year that he proposed. And Katherine said the workshop stimulated her to try some new ideas: "I tied up Carl in the livingroom and read aloud to him from an old etiquette book about a male's proper behavior with ladies. He loved it."

However, the same problems resurfaced in other relationships. For example, Tipi complained that Tom was still not letting her be truly dominant; he still wanted her to be dominant his way. Immediately after they returned home from the workshop, she had disappeared into her office to be alone and think. When she came out, she wanted to be soft and gentle, but Tom expected her to be firm and tough. "Why aren't you different after the workshop?" he asked as she tried to snuggle up to him. "But I am," she protested. For her, being dominant meant she could be soft and gentle when she wanted to be. Tipi said that, despite their successful encounter at the workshop, she felt no closer to "being boss."

The women tried to support each other in confronting these problems. For instance, Kat urged Tipi to be soft and gentle if she wanted to be. "Being dominant isn't always being tough and mean. A dominant woman can be tender, too. It's all in your attitude. It's doing things your way." After praising Tipi for asserting herself in saying she wanted to be gentle and soft, Kat urged her to persevere. Of course, she assured Tipi, breaking old patterns was hard. But ultimately it would be worthwhile.

Next, as they would continue to do over the next few months, the group shared ideas and fantasies of dominant activities. Katherine, especially, had dozens of ideas, just as she had in the workshop. She described a rubber blindfold: "Sometimes I make Carl get into the shower with it on. Then, I shampoo his hair, and he has the feeling he'll drown."

One afternoon she took Carl into the woods, pulled down his pants, and hit him with stinging nettles. She often teased and threatened him and left him wondering whether she would do something or not. "He never knows. For instance, once I put some sticky Q-tips by the side of the bed, but said nothing. So he wondered. Maybe I would poke him, prod him, stick them up his ass. I didn't do anything. But the anticipation, the not knowing, can be very exciting."

As the sharing continued, Frances offered to get everyone nipple clamps: "They're great. You can make them more intense by attaching weights." She passed around some key chains, one with small pliers at the end, the other with a small wrench: "You put this on someone and press." Nancy described how Tony had once been her pleasure slave for the day. "I dressed him up in a garter belt and stockings, and hung tools from his cock. Then, I ordered him around and made him please me sexually. He'd like to do it all the time, but I pace it, so his anticipation builds up. And I don't have the energy to do this everyday."

The women also shared fantasies—some plausible, others impossible to realize; but, then, one of the attractions of D&S is the chance to imagine the bizarre or fantastic. Tipi said she would love to have Tom be a coffee table in her living room for an afternoon; she would invite some women friends over to have their coffee on his back. Katherine fantasized about having Carl crawl around under the table while she entertained a group of women friends; as they appeared to be having a perfectly normal conversation, he would crawl over to each woman and orally satisfy her.

The discussion then shifted to practical concerns, such as preparing for a session and safety. Frances wondered how to signal her partner when she wanted to be dominant. "Try a collar," Kat suggested, describing a technique some of her acquaintances used. "If a man wants to be submissive, he puts out a collar, and if his partner agrees to be dominant, she takes it. Or if she wants to be dominant, she puts it out, and if he puts it on, that means go ahead." Or even better, Kat recommended, "Try surprise, since signaling leaves the power in the man's hands, because he can choose whether to pick up the collar. But a dominant woman should be dominant whenever she wants, and he should be ready to submit."

Then Andrea asked questions about safety: How tight can you tie the ropes? What about gags? How long can you keep someone suspended? Frances observed that some of her friends in Gemini, the organization of dominant men and submissive women, had developed a safe gag made from a piece of foam rubber stuck on a stick. "It'll absorb the saliva and it can't drop back into the mouth." And Kat reassured the women that with the proper safety precautions, dominance was perfectly safe. "You can pretend you're doing something dangerous, like leaving him alone with a gag on to create excitement. But then, you stick around."

The first meeting concluded with the most experienced women—
Katherine and Nancy—reassuring the others. They, too, had felt unsure at
first, but had overcome it. As Katherine explained: "When I started out
being dominant, I felt inferior at first. How could I compete with Carl's
vivid imagination and elaborate fantasies? But we don't have to compete, I
realized. We're not fantasies. We're real." To build up confidence, she
suggested, "Start off with small things like putting an apron around him and
telling him: 'It's your turn to do the dishes.' Then, gradually, you build up to
making him submissive in other ways. That's what I did."

The second meeting, a month later, was attended by Nancy, Katherine,
Tipi, and Laura. Kat opened the meeting by announcing she had a "boy"
who would like to meet a dominant woman—"He's about 28, a travel agent,
who lives with his folks, maybe a little cocky, but otherwise submissive,"
and Laura scribbled down his number.

Nancy talked of looking forward to her pending marriage to Tony, but
she still reported problems in getting him to be submissive. "He still tries to
manipulate me. He tells me his fantasies and hopes I'll act them out." But
she was working on showing him that she was still boss. "I made him put on
a panty girdle and I said I would do nothing until *I* wanted to."

Katherine described Carl's recent resistance. "He still slips out of it.
For instance, I forbid him to go into dirty book shops without me. But it's
hard to enforce." And one day he bought a slapper, although they had
agreed that Katherine should buy all the equipment. She had tried various
ploys to discourage his "naughty boy" behavior. She teased him with mock
sexual threats—one night running her nails lightly between his testicles and
whispering sinisterly: "You know, I'd like to slit you." She refused to do
what he asked for days or weeks until she was ready and threatened to do
uncomfortable things like removing the hair on his legs with bandage tape
or making him wear hair rollers, stockings, and a girdle.

While these strategies worked for Nancy and Katherine, Tipi was still
having difficulties, so she was thinking of ending their play with dominance.
"In some ways, Tom's like a pussy cat," she explained. "I usually get my
own way at home, handle the finances, and tell him what to do. Yet I still
have to let him believe he's in charge, and he wants his friends to think so,
too. So when his friends are around, I wait on him. But he still has fantasies
of being forced to do things—he imagines being deflowered and raped.
He'd like someone to jump out of the closet and fuck him. Yet, he still won't
do certain things I say. So it's hard to feel dominant. And until I do, we
won't play."

Kat agreed that this problem was a common one. "Men keep falling
back into trying to direct the action, though they still have this driving need
to submit. It's so hard for them to let go of their wanting and relax." Daniel,
the would-be poet who had performed for her class, now seemed to regret
having given her some original poems and telling her his deep secrets. He

also seemed reluctant to do the little chores he once had eagerly performed, such as weeding her garden. "He's still having trouble learning to accept his submission," Kat remarked. "He wants it. He needs it. Yet he can't seem to relax and trust." She concluded, "Many men want to be submissive, yet are scared or ambivalent, so if the dominant female relationship is ever going to work, the female must be strong." Being strong meant women needed to "deal with specific behaviors" that challenged them: "You have to stop him to keep the power. That dominant power has got to be real."

After a discussion of each woman's situation, the meeting concluded, like the first, with new ideas. Katherine passed around a *Tit Torture Catalog* that illustrated dozens of nipple clamps and bondage devices with chains that connected one part of the body to another. Frances recommended a few places to get equipment, a leather shop, a swing house, and a romantic hideaway with mirrored rooms. At the end, Laura suggested a shopping trip to buy erotic clothing and explore pornographic bookstores.

The following weekend, Laura, Katherine, and Misty began their afternoon at a riding shop, a popular place for S&M equipment. Laura was particularly interested in the crops. She had never owned one before, but wanted one now to get tough with Rod, her military man. After looking through several crops, she decided on a long, thin one, because "It has a certain flair." When a salesperson came over to help, Laura said: "No, just looking." Then, like many D&Sers, who like being involved in something forbidden which outsiders don't know about, she enjoyed thinking about the encounter. She giggled to the others, "He thinks we're interested in horses. If only he knew what we're really doing with the equipment."

The next stop was the Salvation Army, Goodwill, and other thrift shops—a common source of offbeat and cheap clothes and equipment for many D&Sers. On the way, the women fantasized about what they might do with their purchases. Katherine suggested a B&D party to show off their fashions and equipment and exhibit their slaves. Laura mused about bringing two submissive men at the same time to show her power. Also, Laura found that the chance to get new clothes was especially important, for the new outfits she acquired—which included a sleek black silk jumpsuit, slinky black dinner dress, and a tight red jacket—differed dramatically from the soft pastels and gentle earth tones she wore before becoming interested in dominance. Now she wanted strong and flashy clothing to look the part.

At the adult bookstore, looking through a few female dominance magazines, Laura commented on the different styles of dominance the women in the group were developing. "Some like the fantasy. Katherine likes teasing and making it a total lifestyle. And I still feel very much a novice. But I like the physical part and switching around."

By the third meeting, the group—which included Nancy, Laura, Katherine, and a new woman from Kat's workshop, Bridget, 28, who juggled several odd jobs, including answering obscene phone calls and working as a mistress—was feeling more confident and assertive. The women had overcome most of their difficulties, and the discussion now focused on reporting successes. Kat set the tone by describing her plans for a stage show to introduce female dominance to the wider public. She had located a potential director and was looking for potential investors, while Mouse was writing the script. She had overcome her problems with Mouse's occasional resistance by exploring other types of role reversal. Now she was sometimes submissive to him, and he was exploring dominance with other women.

Her relationship with Daniel seemed to be ending, and Kat was ready to let it go. He had become confused about their relationship, since he had seen both her "mean dominant bitch persona" and her more gentle, warm, and loving side. He wasn't sure which one his relationship was with, though Kat had told him, "It's only with the dominant me." And although his wife had originally been supportive, she had become upset because Daniel's activities had been intruding on their private time and space at home. Daniel hadn't asked Kat to release him. "But I think he's building up to this," Kat said, "though he doesn't have the nerve yet. And I think it's time to let him go."

Next Nancy described her wedding, held on a boat that sailed around the bay at dusk. Most of the 30 guests were friends not involved in D&S, but she and Tony turned the event into a pageant by asking everyone to come dressed as a favorite romantic fantasy. They presided as Anthony and Cleopatra and even received a few S&M gifts.

Bridget talked about her own growing confidence. Her initial involvement in D&S was as a submissive, when her female love, Nadia, who was running a B&D house near San Francisco, suggested she work for her as a submissive. Bridget willingly quit her studies for a teaching credential and began working. Because many men wanted a dominant, Bridget uncertainly began to work as a dominant, too: "I used to blindfold them right away, so they couldn't tell if I did anything wrong." Gradually, she gained confidence and enjoyed being paid to order men about. Her various relationships—heterosexual, gay, dominant, and submissive—seemed to increase her self-assurance and strengthen her self-image.

Laura, too, exuded new confidence, for she found that her experience with sexual dominance enhanced her assertiveness in nonsexual matters. She was now more forceful in expressing herself and standing up to people. She was about to leave the man she lived with, whom she had been upset with for a while, and she had finally told him about the men she was dating and her D&S activities. "Before, I wanted to keep my new world to myself, because I was afraid Ralph might impinge. Now I don't care what Ralph knows." She was also more assertive with the two submissive men she was dating and at work. She summarized her overall sense of release and change, saying "Once I used to keep my spoiled child or bitch part down. But now I'm allowing that out, and it feels great."

The women's growing assertiveness was also reflected in their talk about their partners' limits. Kat noted that some cultures, such as some Hindu and American Indian groups, ascribe a spiritual quality to experiencing great hardship or pain. Laura said she once worried about tying her partner too tightly or putting clamps on his nipples. But a few nights earlier she just did what she wanted and noticed that her partner's arousal matched her own. And Bridget commented that she now did whatever she liked as long as she could see that the man was excited.

To close the meeting, Kat played an erotic fantasy tape, made by a woman in the group, that matched the women's growing self-assurance and assertiveness. On the tape, a mistress played an army officer disciplining a soldier who had gone AWOL: "You stupid grunt, how could you run away? You worm, you're nothing but a lowly soldier....Now, I want you to crawl, I want you to grovel in the dust....Can't you do anything right? I'll have to punish you for that...(Slap, Whack)."

With each new insult, each thrashing, each demand to make the hapless soldier obey, the women chortled and roared. The tape, with its good-natured humiliation of the soldier, helped them feel their power and reinforced their sense of being dominant. The soldier enjoyed being humiliated, and they responded to both his humiliation and his enjoyment. Also, listening and laughing together, the women felt validated, encouraged, and supported.

By the fourth meeting, the women, now even more secure in their dominance, talked about choosing the times when they wanted to be dominant and how to use their power creatively. For example, Katherine commented: "In my new job, I have to do a lot of boring administrative work, and when I come home, I don't feel like being dominant. I just want to be pampered. I want Carl to do things for me. But quietly. I don't want him to tell me about it. He wants to be rewarded, punished, and teased. But I'm simply not into it. So I don't do it." However, since she felt she was in charge, she could decide how and when she wanted to be dominant.

The nonmonogamous women said they were enjoying expressing their dominance in new relationships. Those that had a primary relationship still wanted variety. "I like a real smorgasbord," said Bridget, now seeing several men and women. And Kat and Sharon, who had primary relationships, agreed. "My relationship with Lance is still very hot," Sharon said, referring to the man she later rented a house with. "But I want to play with other people, too."

But at the next monthly meeting, the talk shifted back to the difficulties of dominance, reflecting the up-and-down pattern dominant women commonly experience. For a time, they feel satisfied with their level of dominance or want to increase their involvement, and their partner or partners are generally cooperative. But then, their interest in being dominant declines for a while, or their partners resist. Then, they pull back for a time until their energy and interest revive. Now, it seemed, the women were in this dormant phase. The confidence that characterized the two previous sessions was lacking.

Some of the women made suggestions for dealing with a partner's resistance. "Use your mind to control," Kat recommended. "When a person starts to resist, I nip it in the bud. Your power is in his wanting to be with you. Make your will bigger than his." Sharon suggested: "Get restraints that don't need tying. Or the next time he tries to resist, say: 'Shut up.'" And Inge, 30, a full-time mistress and friend of Kat's, advised: "Tell him what you want from the first. For example, when I start a session, I say I want to find you on your hands and knees when I come back. You see there's a ritual to all this. When you move from everyday life to the erotic, ritual helps you go from one to the other. So try combining ritual with a show of force."

Tammy, 34, an occupational therapist and newcomer to the group, expressed her doubts most pointedly: "I know intellectually what to do when I take over the dominant role. But when it comes to actually doing it, I feel stymied. It's as if I'm putting on another personality, and I'm not comfortable with it. I feel safer in my head. So right now, it's all fantasy pictures—I feel like Scheherazade." Her boyfriend recognized her inse-curity: "Instead of calling me Mistress Tiger, he calls me Mistress Pussy."

Inge described her feelings of burnout after seeing several customers a day for over a year. "Mostly I get sick of hearing some of my customer's outrageous requests," she said. "Like this surgeon who's into scat asked me to give him some shit he could hold in his mouth, because his turn-on is feeling intensely degraded. Then, when I actually gave him some, he had the nerve to ask: 'Is it yours?'"

Yet, in spite of the doubts, the meeting ended on a more optimistic note with another discussion of new ideas to inspire sexual creativity, capped by Inge's suggestions: "How about Saran Wrap? I wrap them up in it sometimes. And I keep a can of shellac around and say sometimes: 'You need a shellacking.' Or try putting on leathers. Pretend you're a prison guard."

The last meeting reflected this spirit of optimism, too, as the women focused on what worked in their relationships. For example, Katherine described her latest exploits with Carl, which included: reading a "sexy book" to him for several nights while he licked her to stimulate her sexually; encasing him in Saran Wrap and cropping him while he lay on his back like a mummy; and putting him into bed in diapers to enact a baby fantasy.

Thus the meetings reflected the members' shifting rhythms of dominance and submission. And the meetings provided the women with an important source of support, validation, and reassurance. They openly discussed their problems, fears, and failures; they shared their successes, discoveries, and fantasies. As their self-assurance and confidence increased, their need for the group declined. Thus, since they had come to feel comfortable with their own dominance, after some six months, the group disbanded.

8

Foursomes

Though D&S activity is very private for most couples, getting together as a foursome is a common occurrence for some in the scene. Unlike swingers, D&S foursomes generally don't engage in sexual intercourse with one another's partners. More typically, a foursome experiments with a wide variety of D&S erotic foreplay in a "scene." This play may lead to orgasm, especially for the male who receives stimulation, but usually orgasm occurs without penetration and is produced by paddling, manual manipulation, licking, teasing, and related activities. And, unlike swingers, D&S couples usually do not exactly swap partners. Rather, the dominants typically control their submissive partners, and when any member of the foursome wants to do something to the submissive, he or she joins the activity the dominant has already started, asks permission, or waits until the dominant relinquishes control over the submissive.

Many couples make foursome arrangements at D&S groups, like the Society of Janus and SM Church, or at private D&S parties. Some also answer the ads in sexually oriented newspapers and magazines. Couples living far away from urban centers are especially likely to use advertising, since they have difficulty meeting others in their area and are usually willing to travel up to a few hundred miles to make contact. But couples in major cities and their suburbs do advertise and respond to ads, too.

The first meeting, however initiated, usually leads to a session, though couples sometimes get together just to talk about D&S. Couples usually spend some time getting acquainted and then propose ideas for the scene, much as individuals do before their first session together. Couples discuss their likes and limits, and the foursome usually arranges a signal, perhaps a safe word that any member can use to stop an undesired activity. Most view structure and control as essential, particularly in the first session.

SENSUAL AND EROTIC PLAY

One couple that was especially active in seeking out foursomes was June and Herman, the former teacher and financial planner introduced in

Chapter 6. An example of a representative evening of sensual and erotic play occurred after they placed an ad in the B&D magazine *Kinky Contacts*. Misty and Victor, a 45-year-old surgeon new to the public D&S scene responded with photographs and a brief descriptive letter, as do most respondents to these ads. About a week later, Herman wrote back and gave his phone number; as the dominant in the relationship, Misty called to set up a date.

At first, they briefly discussed their interests in D&S and assured one another of their sincerity—a major concern of couples meeting other couples. Then they arranged to meet at June and Herman's spacious suburban home near San Francisco one evening in late May when their two children, who didn't know about their activities, would be away. Herman then proposed a program for the evening that would gradually and comfortably lead to erotic play. The four would start by chatting over wine and hors d'ouevres in the livingroom and looking at B&D magazines. June would be dressed in regular clothes, but with an exotic corset underneath. When everyone was ready, Herman would take Misty upstairs and dress her in an exotic corset and heels. Then the scene would begin and would include both men's favorite activities: a spanking for Victor and an enema for Herman. The evening would conclude with a buffet dinner.

The four exchanged several more phone calls, and in a letter Herman provided new details: "Since June's a former teacher, she has some special 'tests' prepared for Victor, which may produce some equally special punishment in case of failure! We'll have the black corset and accessories ready for Misty, and June will wear a white outfit, in keeping with her 'nurse' activities. I'll pick up some extra goodies on my day off Friday— wrist cuffs, mainly."

Misty and Victor arrived the following Saturday at about 7:30 p.m. As Herman had requested, Misty brought a suitcase with fashionably erotic clothing—black heels, bright red shorts, an orange jumpsuit—and a camera. Victor brought his favorite paddles and crops. For him, the evening was to be his first public D&S experience. Until then he had been very secretive about his D&S activities, going to mistresses occasionally. But now he was searching for organized groups, since his wife was interested only in being submissive privately, though she knew about and accepted his outside activities.

The evening began like an ordinary social occasion. The couples sat down on a sleek white sofa in the living room and began eating taco chips and cheese dip and talking casually about their work. But slowly the conversation moved to their interest in D&S. Victor described having attended an English boarding school, where he first discovered spanking to be erotic when he was disciplined or saw other boys being hit. June and Herman mentioned their interest in costuming, enemas, and verbal teasing. They briefly discussed the outsiders' image of S&M—"People seem to think it's all whips and chains, but there are all kinds of people with all kinds of tastes," Herman observed.

Then Herman led Misty upstairs to help her dress. When they returned, she wore a stiff black whalebone corset with garters under her short orange jumpsuit, thin black mesh stockings, and heels. After a few moments of conversation, June announced that it was time to begin. "I think you should go upstairs now and get ready," she told Herman firmly, yet playfully. "Is everything prepared, Mr. H?"

He assured her it was and the three followed him upstairs to the bedroom. A large orange enema bag hung from a stand next to the bed. Herman undressed and lay down, fully nude, alongside it. Victor, who knew nothing of enema play, stood watching curiously. June moved the stand closer to the bed, turned to Victor, and instructed him: "Get undressed. Then lie over the towel I've laid across the trunk." She gestured towards it at the foot of the bed. As he undressed, she removed her outer clothing, and stood in her white corset, bra, and stockings, and black heels. Misty took off her jumpsuit.

June snapped leather cuffs onto Victor and suggested that Misty paddle him to keep him entertained, while she went over to "play nurse" to Herman. She assumed the solicitous but stern tone of the nurse, asking, "Did you eat anything today?"

He replied as her meek, submissive patient. "Oh, no. No, mistress."

"But you did," she accused him. "I saw you eat two crackers."

He admitted he had, and she picked up a crop and teasingly brandished it over his head. "Now I told you not to do that. That's going to be punished." He admitted also to having eaten something in the morning—"But just a little." She waved the crop in the air even more menacingly, advising him: "You'll have to take the full four quarts for that," meaning that she would put four quarts of water in the enema bag and siphon these into his colon. Although she called this his "punishment," Herman loved receiving enemas, finding the heavy fullness in his lower abdomen uncomfortable, yet so sexually stimulating that after two to three quarts he usually experienced a strong orgasm. Sometimes, for variety, June gave him wine enemas to make him high or other exotic combinations of materials, but this time she used only soapy water.

She began by putting a small leather "cock-cage"—a harness-like device designed for stimulation—around his penis, tapped it gently with the tip of her crop, and told him firmly: "Now I want your cock to stay erect for all this." She then asked Misty to come over and help—a practice common in foursomes, whereby the dominant women work together with one male at a time.

As June inserted the enema tube, Victor squeezed out of his cuffs and came over to watch. When he asked a question, June shushed him gently. Questions or discussion would detract from the experience; afterwards, they could talk. Soon Herman began to protest he couldn't take any more. "Of course you can," she teased, and continued. But once he started to protest seriously, she stopped, aware he had reached his limit.

Herman later explained that usually he could take more, but he needed to be stimulated beforehand. This time June teased less than usual because others were present. And since this was the first time the foursome had met, he felt more constrained than usual.

The women now turned their attention to Victor. Just as June had planned the enema to suit Herman's likes, she had designed a spanking scenario for Victor. "Lie down on the trunk again," she told him. He lay down on his stomach, and she hit him lightly with the rattan cane he had brought. Misty picked up the paddle and joined in. From time to time, Victor would indicate: "harder," "more to the right," "try the other side now." Although submissives often like to relax and enjoy, at times, particularly if the dominant is a novice or a new partner, they offer suggestions to let her know what they like.

Next, June proposed a spelling bee for Victor. "You will be punished, of course, if you don't spell a word properly," she advised. "But I'm a lousy speller," Victor said good-naturedly, anticipating an erotic spanking as his punishment. On the first round, he misspelled *valence*, and she hit him once for each letter in the word. He protested kiddingly, "But you didn't pronounce it properly." She hit him again: "That's for insubordination."

Next Victor suggested they switch roles—a frequent occurrence in D&S scenes—since he wanted to spank June, who had said she enjoyed being submissive on occasion. At first, June declined, for she was the teacher. But then she agreed and lay down across the bed. Victor began paddling her, while Herman moved in front of her and began pulling on her breasts. Everyone intuitively understood that Herman could do this, since he was her husband, but that Victor and Misty, as relative strangers, were limited to less intimate forms of erotic stimulation. Though no one said anything, everyone had a clear sense of what was permissible—a common characteristic of these scenes where limits are known, or sensed and respected.

Again respecting these implicit rules, Misty waited for a lead from Herman, who would play dominant to June's submissive. He suggested she massage June's feet. June found their combined efforts wonderfully stimulating and proposed that Victor have the experience as well. They switched again; June paddled Victor while Misty massaged his feet, and Herman began massaging Misty's arms and legs with a rabbit skin. The unspoken understanding was that the massage would be enjoyable and sensual, yet not sexual, because they were relative strangers.

After a brief photo-taking session, everyone put on their regular clothes, went downstairs, served themselves at the buffet, and sat down to dinner. Their D&S session was over, and they ate and chatted like any two couples having a social dinner on a Saturday night, although their conversation focused on the session. Everyone agreed it had been a good beginning, though not that intense erotically, since they didn't know each other that well. But in future get-togethers, they could explore more and develop more elaborate role-playing scenes, as June and Herman had done with other couples. The conversation then moved to other D&S topics— some erotic films Herman had seen, a television program on S&M, a weekend retreat June and Herman were planning, and their desire for a local party place for D&S couples. When Misty and Victor left at about 1 a.m., shortly before the children would return, Herman proclaimed it a wonderful evening: "Let's do it again," he said.

TALKING INTIMATELY

Not all first meetings include a role-playing encounter, even when the participants are active in the D&S scene and hit it off socially. Instead, the evening may focus on the couples sharing their D&S interests, as occurred when Suzanna, 36, who hoped to be an actress, brought Alex, a pediatrician who liked cross-dressing and bondage, to meet Bella and Benji, introduced earlier. Suzanna had met Bella and Benji at the Society of Janus and suggested that the four get together, since the two men liked to dress up. When Suzanna mentioned the invitation to Alex, he was immediately enthusiastic and had wild visions of how the evening might turn out. He fantasized that the two women might attack him and tie him up at the end of the evening.

But the evening turned out to be a time for talking. Bella explained that her early interest in sensuality had been repressed until she met Benji, who had not found a woman who accepted his interest in dressing until he met Bella. Alex passed around photographs showing him dressed up as different types of women: a hooker in a miniskirt, a career girl in a suit, and the girl next door wearing slacks and a blouse. Bella praised him, "You really make a terrific woman. I'm sure you could pass." Alex glowed with pride and gave her one of his photos. Then Benji showed photos of himself wearing a wig, corset, and heels.

As Alex and Benji talked about liking to have a woman force them to dress up, because such coercion allowed them to cross-dress without guilt, Bella commented on the intimacy of the conversation: "It's wonderful to be able to talk like this—so openly and honestly." And later she described the ins and outs of being a mistress, which she characterized as "another form of nursing." But when Alex asked which of her clients' fantasies she found most exciting and said he would like to see her playroom, Bella demurred.

These fantasies were private and her playroom was just another room; the toys were all put away. As much as Alex and Suzanna tried to prod the evening toward a role-playing encounter, Bella and Benji only wanted to talk. "It's wonderful to talk so freely," Bella remarked repeatedly.

Yet, while Alex enjoyed this, he had hoped for something more. "I kept hoping you both would grab me and take me inside," he told Suzanna as they left. "I kept hoping something would happen, but nothing did."

MISFIRES

At times, these role-playing encounters misfire. Sometimes couples who have recently met or who have different ideas about what is erotic are uncomfortable with the sudden intimacy of a foursome. Other times the energy or chemistry of the encounter goes wrong, just as in a one-on-one encounter, when an activity turns from excitement and pleasure into unerotic discomfort or pain. As in any social encounter, foursomes can fail for a variety of reasons.

One evening Natasha, the graphics designer, brought Alex to see June and Herman. Alex was extremely interested in meeting them when he learned they had a small business making corsets, for he hoped to try some on. Also, Herman's former interest in cross-dressing was an area of commonality. And professionally and socially, the four knew many of the same people.

After an hour of conversation over a sumptuous buffet dinner and wine, everyone was eager to begin the session June and Natasha had planned. The scenario was based on an African ritual fantasy, using African music and incense to set the mood. June and Natasha now prepared the upstairs den, placing candles and incense around the room, a furry mat by the door, and African records on the stereo. They undressed to reveal their costumes—June wore a black corset, stockings, and heels; Natasha a simulated leopard-skin bra and bikini. As the men entered the room, Natasha beat on an American Indian drum, swaying sensuously, to accompany the African ritual music pounding in the background. "Come in," she told them, "and kneel on the mat before your priestess." As they did, uncertainly, she instructed them: "Keep your eyes down, and take off your clothes."

At first, Herman and Alex were startled by the unusual and unexpected ritual, and they laughed nervously. But they good-naturedly stripped down to their briefs and knelt quietly before Natasha. June brought her two large scarves, which Natasha used to blindfold the men. The women led their partners to a ladder, and asked them to lean against it, and tied them up, slowly draping the ropes and seductively brushing against them in time to the thump of the drums.

Within minutes, the carefully crafted scenario began to unravel. Alex felt dizzy and faint from the smell of incense and from the disorienting experience of standing blindfolded against the ladder. Natasha untied him and laid him down, still blindfolded, on the bed. He urged them to continue without him. So Natasha joined June in decorating Herman's face and chest with lipstick, powder, and eyeshadow. June attached clothespins to his nipples, and Natasha rubbed ice across his chest—practices Herman usually liked. Then June began blowing hot air at him from a hair dryer, while intoning in the spirit of the ritual: "Now feel the hot dry wind of the Sahara. The winds are whipping across the desert as you walk." At this point Herman crumpled, too, complaining of dizziness. June untied him; he washed off his warpaint, returned, and sprawled in a chair. Meanwhile, Alex sat up, feeling better and relieved that Herman had felt faint, too.

The fizzling of a scene sometimes ends a new relationship when it is based on enacting a scene. But these four had enough other common interests to keep the evening going. They had a brief, though somewhat tense and embarrassed, discussion about what had gone wrong to learn from the experience. Everyone agreed that it must have been the combination of the heavy dinner, wine, incense, darkness, heat, and the men having stood up blindfolded. The discussion then turned to corsets, when Alex asked if he could put one on. Suddenly everyone relaxed. At once, June hopped up, scurried into another room, and returned with a bright red corset with black fringe. Excitedly, Alex stood in the center of the room as June laced him up. He savored the feeling of being restrained, while seeking some reassurance at publicly enacting a long-held fantasy: "Do many other men get corsets? Do you know any women who like their men in corsets? I'd like to get one."

Thus, even though the scenario misfired, the corset demonstration saved the evening, and the two couples talked about getting together again to try another scene. The next time, though, they would plan more carefully.

NO-SHOWS

Since planning a D&S scenario can be erotically stimulating in itself, some couples go no further than this planning, although they act as though they want to participate. Such planning may be extremely elaborate, as the couples repeatedly confer about the scenario they are arranging. But, in the end, one couple may back down because they are afraid of the actual encounter or are interested only in planning it, or both.

This happened to June and Herman, when they met Edward, a sales manager of 35, at a Society of Janus event. He told them he and his wife, Ann, were very active in the scene and would like to get together with them. Enthusiastically, June and Herman agreed, and over the next two months, Herman and Edward had about a dozen conversations during which they carefully crafted the scene. Each time they spoke, the planned session became more elaborate and exciting.

When the appointed night finally came, June and Herman drove over to Ann and Ed's, about an hour away. They arrived at about 8:45 p.m., some 15 minute late, and found the house dark, though as they rang the bell, they heard paper rustling. Ed had said he would be returning from a business trip that night. So, thinking he could be late getting back, they drove off to have coffee, and phoned at 9. At first, they heard the answering machine's recorded message, but in the middle of the message, it sounded like someone was yanking out the phone, and the message abruptly clicked off. Puzzled, they drove back. As they pulled up, Ed walked out of the garage in his bathrobe. "Sorry, it's all off," he snapped, heading for the front door. "You were 30 minutes late." He slammed the door behind him.

June and Herman drove home completely baffled. Thinking about it later, Herman toyed with two explanations. Perhaps Ed and Ann were excited by the fantasy of a foursome, but did not really want or intend to act. Or possibly Ed had talked Ann into participating although she was hesitant to do so. Then, when he and June were a few minutes late, Ann had had second thoughts. "The experience isn't so unusual," Herman observed. "We know other couples who encountered similar situations with people who got cold feet. But at least they could have invited us in for coffee and told us they weren't up for a session that night. After all, we had a long drive to get there. They could have given us that courtesy, and we would have understood."

9

The Organized Scene & the SM Church

A small but growing number of people—perhaps 10,000 to 20,000 across the country—actively participate in various organizations and informal social networks that are part of the organized D&S scene or community. The total membership of such groups and networks is difficult to estimate, because groups overlap and thousands of people drop in and out. But the community includes social and educational clubs, commercial establishments that sponsor occasional parties, and at least one church whose founding principle is female dominance. Most of these organized groups are located in major cities, notably New York, Chicago, Los Angeles, and San Francisco. This chapter focuses on one group—the SM Church—in the San Francisco Bay Area, which hosts five major nonprofit D&S social organizations.

In the Bay Area, about 1,000 people a year are more or less active in D&S groups; perhaps 500 or so of these are involved to some degree in heterosexual female dominance, though most experiment with other types of D&S, too. For about 40 or 50 of these people, D&S has become an everyday lifestyle, and they not only live it in their relationships, but they play an active leadership role in D&S groups. Perhaps another 100 or so are more or less regulars in these groups; and about 150 or so attend group activities occasionally. Others drift in and out of the organized D&S scene.

This organized scene consists of activities sponsored by the following groups: the Society of Janus, a broad-based umbrella organization that primarily sponsors educational activities concerning all aspects of D&S; the SM Church, the one organization devoted exclusively to female dominance, with about 150 members; Samois, an educational and social organization of about 200 gay or bisexual women interested in D&S; the Gemini Society, a group of about 50 dominant males and submissive females; and the Club 15, a group of about 100 gay males who enjoy heavy D&S.

These five groups are organizationally distinct, each with its own rules—for example, in Gemini the women must behave strictly submissively and the males dominantly at group functions. But the groups have overlapping membership and at times sponsor activities together, since so many members enjoy switching roles.

SOCIETY OF JANUS

The Society of Janus was founded in 1975, modeled after the first D&S group in the country, the Tyl Eulenspiegel Society in New York. Almost all its original members were gay men, but with growing public interest in D&S, the group has had an influx of single males, couples, and a few single women with various D&S interests, including female dominance. To remedy the imbalance of males to females (a problem common to sexually oriented groups, since women are much less likely than men to join) the Society began a female recruitment project, which brought in a few women, though the problem remains.

Because of the diversity of its membership, Janus primarily emphasizes the educational aspects of D&S, rather than the social, preferring to leave social activities to the more specialized groups defined by D&S orientation. Thus, through mid-1982, the group's major activity was holding a monthly meeting on a topic that would appeal to all segments of the D&S community: pain, piercing, bondage, safety, toys, or styles of dominance and submissiveness. As the character of the group has been shifting and a more heterosexual group has emerged, recent activities have included parties and special events such as a bondage contest and a slave auction, as well as more frequent meetings.

THE SM CHURCH

The SM Church is the major Bay Area organization devoted to female dominance. Uniquely, it combines an interest in erotic female dominance with ideas about female worship, spiritual development, and ritual. While most of its 150 members and several hundred visitors and subscribers appear only occasionally at Church activities, the Church has an active nucleus of about 25 people who regularly plan and participate in group events. Church events include a weekly class on sexual fantasies, monthly parties, and a bimonthly Church service. The service resembles the traditional Christian rite, except that it incorporates ideas about the power of the Goddess and includes some D&S symbolism in the communion ceremony. Communicants must kneel and are tapped on the shoulders and head with a whip, a symbol of purification.

The Church's beginnings were relatively informal. In 1977 several men who frequented Backdrop, a commercial B&D house, and several women who worked there decided to organize activities apart from Backdrop. This group included most of the officers now active in the SM Church: Lance, Harvey, Ken, Devora, and Danielle. The women planned to work privately as mistresses and the group wanted to throw D&S parties. They felt that by forming a church they might gain legal protection for their activities, and they hoped the SM Church would enable people active in D&S to meet others.

For its first few years, the Church remained small and informal. Then Diana and Drew, who were interested in Witchcraft as well as D&S, joined the group and taught the others about Goddess worship and the female principle in nature. Members began to realize there was more to female dominance than throwing D&S parties, and they sought to explore the philosophical, theological, psychological, and social aspects of female domination. They developed a philosophy that incorporates Goddess worship, D&S, and a concern for issues related to the feminine principle, such as ecology and nature. Diana, who had been initiated as a Wiccan priestess, taught classes on Witchcraft rituals, and the Church officers read widely about the Craft and ancient matriarchal societies.

The Church continued to sponsor parties and other D&S events, and many of its members, most notably males, remained primarily or solely interested in such activities. But the Church organizers worked to develop the Church as a respectable, serious, and public organization. They initiated Church services and educational programs that addressed not only the sexual, but the spiritual, social, and political implications of female dominance. Thus the Church eventually coalesced into a major force within the D&S scene and a central focus of female dominance activity. Concurrently, those who participated actively within the Church began to think of themselves as a small community or family, with close links to others in the scene.

SM Church Beliefs

The Church's beliefs invest female dominance, usually a purely erotic and sexual activity, with spiritual meaning. The essential premise is that the female should be an object not only of erotic interest, but also of spiritual worship, for her spiritual nature is superior to man's. These views derive in part from the Wiccan and Pagan beliefs about the Goddess. According to Witches and Pagans, the Goddess is a manifestation or symbolic representation of the feminine principle in life, embodied in the forces of nature associated with fertility, growth, and reproduction, and related to such qualities as receptivity and intuition. Throughout history, this principle has been represented by the particular Goddesses worshipped by different cultures; but fundamentally the Goddess represents a primary force in nature.

Also, the Wiccans, Pagans, and Church organizers believe that the Goddess was once worshipped in ancient pre-Christian societies, many of which were matriarchies. They claim that matriarchal organizations and beliefs were more harmonious and peaceful than the later patriarchal Christian societies. As Lance, one of the Church officers, once suggested in a Church service: "People then were more in tune with themselves, with others, and with nature. They were more willing to cooperate and work together. They were more intuitive—more in touch with the magical and psychic aspects of life. And they were more in harmony with the natural rhythms of the universe, because they practiced seasonal rituals, in which they recognized the changes in nature."

The SM Church attempts to revive the old traditions of Goddess worship through ceremonies, rituals, and literature, and the organizers frequently talk about organizing a small-scale matriarchal religious community, though this is more of a collective fantasy than something likely to become real. Thus, despite its nonreligious origins, the Church has become quite serious about its beliefs, though its approach is more of a search or quest than adherence to codified dogma. As the group's monthly newsletter explains: "Our primary purpose is the historical review of the ancient Goddess-oriented religions in the search for an alternative sociotheological model to offer a better harmony between humankind and nature. Simply stated, our purpose is the 'search for the ancient Goddess.' Thus, our purpose is more of *quest* than of *belief*."

The Church organizers are tentative in their approach, since they are still learning about Witchcraft and Goddess worship. They are tentative, too, because D&Sers come from many religious traditions, and most are no longer practicing believers and some actively oppose organized religion. The SM Church thus offers its beliefs but does not require participants in Church services or group rituals to affirm those beliefs. Indeed, most members and guests don't believe, yet they attend even overtly religious activities because they view these events as ritual dramas or as opportunities to socialize with other D&Sers. Yet, while the ceremonies may be strictly pageantry and drama for most, the organizers and a few other active members have begun to feel a true spiritual power in the Goddess, much as anyone new to a religion slowly discovers personal meaning in its symbolism.

In fact, some have used this symbolism in personal rituals. For example, to help raise money for the Church, Lance and Sharon performed a ritual. They lit candles, wrote what they wanted on a piece of paper, chanted and burned the paper in a small dish of incense to the Goddess. Yet, not totally convinced the ritual would be effective, they talk of it as a scientific experiment. "We're not sure if the power is real or not. But we did the ritual anyway, since we're doing anything we can to make the Church work."

The Organization of the Church

The SM Church is still quite small, since only about 30 of its 150 members attend activities regularly. Yet it has a rather elaborate organizational structure, which is intended to facilitate the group's expansion and also reflects a common tendency within the D&S community to develop grand scenarios with numerous roles, rituals, and dramatic performances. Thus, although most Church business could be handled informally, particularly since all the leaders are close personal friends, the Church leaders prefer a more grandiose and theatrical structure.

At the top of the Church is the five-member board of directors: Lance, the president, who sometimes calls himself Cardinal Lance when he plays his role; Drew, the vice-president; Sharon, the secretary; Devora, the treasurer; and Danielle, the officer of external affairs, who is in charge of most programming and miscellaneous functions. Under the board is the advisory council, made up of other Church officers and assistants to officers. The council's three members are all in close relationships with members of the board. Ken, Devora's husband, is the officer for grounds and maintenance; that is, he makes sure the Church office is in order. Harvey, who lives next door to Danielle, is the assistant to the officer of external affairs, and Diana, married to Drew, is the dean of the Athenian Institute, which sponsors the classes offered by the Church.

While this structure may seem quite ordinary for an organization, it seems unusual in that the two highest positions in a group devoted to female dominance are held by men. From time to time members raise this question, too: Why aren't the women in charge? This issue, as we have seen, is a central one in the D&S community. Does the real power reside with the dominant, who is ostensibly in control, or with the submissive, who sets the limits? Thus, in some ways, the Church may represent a submissive male's vision of being submissive to the Goddess, a vision that empowers men to have a significant role in designing and guiding the structure. But Church organizers also claim practical reasons for having male leaders. They hold that male leadership confers respectability in the larger community, since most established churches are headed by men. Since the Church is so unconventional in other ways, a traditional structure is a useful community relations strategy.

Further, in practice, the women do have much control, since the women officers—Diana, Devora, Danielle, and Sharon—lead most of the church services and classes. Also, the board recently created The Sisters of Morgana, a spiritual advisory council of three women, to increase the women's influence and role in providing spiritual leadership. The board consults the Sisters on all religious questions, such as the content of the Church service. Again, this structure may now seem unnecessary, since the three Sisters, Diana, Devora, and Sharon are already on the board or advisory council. But everyone enjoys structure, and they hope for a membership large enough to preclude the doubling up of roles.

Church leaders frequently discuss various ideas for expanding the Church. For example, they organized a 12-week novitiate training program for males who wanted to join the community and sought to prepare them for membership by teaching them Church doctrine and philosophy, techniques of submission, and proper conduct in rituals. But only half a dozen men enrolled in that program. So expansion seems to be one more wonderful fantasy, exciting to envision, but largely unattainable now.

Church Activities and Services

Female domination, whether through erotic D&S, religious worship, fantasy, or ritual and performance, is central to virtually all Church activities and informal get-togethers among Church members, though outside the Church, members may interact as equals or the males may dominate. Church services honor the Goddess, and seasonal and other rituals emphasize female power, both spiritual and erotic. Other Church activities include fantasy classes, which help members better understand female domination; technique classes, which offer information on equipment and D&S techniques; and occasional parties and gatherings. All these partake of three key mainstays of female dominance: erotic D&S, Goddess worship, and fantasy.

The group started holding Church services in mid-March 1981 as part of an effort to appear more respectable to the community as a whole. Members wanted an open, public ceremony to which they could even bring straight friends and relatives. Accordingly, the Church leaders incorporated some traditional elements of Christian worship in their service: reading a litany, singing songs, and having a sermon, offertory, and communion. But the service also focuses on female dominance, for it is led by a priestess, and the litany, songs, and sermons praise female power. The service also includes a subtle hint of D&S activity: those who wish to receive communion bend down at the feet of the priestess, who taps them lightly on the head and shoulders with a small flail, asking: "Are you willing to suffer to learn?" Only after this D&S version of penance can the communicant, now purified, receive the bread and wine of communion.

Services are held two Sunday afternoons a month. Typically, the priestesses first place on the altar a candle, incense burner, cup with wine, ritual knife, and small basket with bits of bread. The participants, mostly Church regulars, and a few guests file in, and the head priestess—either Diana, Danielle, Devora, or Sharon—turns to the altar, holds the knife aloft, and blesses the room, dedicating the service to the Goddess.

Then the priestess leads the group in a song adopted from the pagan tradition, which expresses love for the Goddess and extols the benefits associated with the feminine in nature: having a rich harvest, healing, working magic, and understanding the rhythms of nature.

....Around and around and around turns the good earth,
All things must change as the seasons go by.
We are the children of the Lord and the Lady.
Whose mystery we know, but will never know why...
....We live in the love of the Lord and the Lady;
The greater the circle, the more the love grows.

The litany (or responsive reading) that follows praises the Goddess, her love, and the honor and respect due her and the natural world, which is her body:

...We are now joined here together (priestess reading)
TO WORSHIP THE GODDESS (congregation reading)
...For she is the Great Mother
AND HER LOVE IS POURED OUT INTO THE UNIVERSE...
....And we must love all nature and care for the planet in which we live
FOR THE EARTH IS INDEED AS THE BODY OF THE GODDESS...
....She has been with us from the beginning
AND SHE IS THAT WHICH IS ATTAINED AT THE END OF DESIRE. SO MOTE IT BE!

After the priestess announces upcoming programs, a priestess or a guest speaker gives the sermon—or, more accurately, a brief sharing. For example, in one sermon, Danielle explained that the Church was dedicated to help women develop socially, personally, politically, and spiritually, and gain a stronger tie to the natural environment. Another time Lance discussed the advantages of matriarchal societies ruled by such powerful women as Cleopatra, Elizabeth, and Nefertiti.

After the offering comes a reading from an ancient legend that praises the power of the female as Goddess. According to this legend, women "would solve all mysteries, even the mystery of death." This is why, when the Goddess journeyed to the underworld, Death knelt at her feet, much like a submissive man might kneel before a dominant woman, "because she was so beautiful," and shared with her all his secrets. Also, the reader describes a woman's incredible powers over men and all life, for, as the priestess read:

....Mine is the secret door which opens upon the door of youth, and mine is the cup of the way of life....I am the gracious Goddess, who gives the gift of joy unto the heart of man....I am the Mother of all living, and my love is poured out upon the earth....
...So call unto thy soul; arise, and come unto me; for I am the soul of nature, who gives life to the universe. From me all things proceed, and

unto me all things must return....Let my worship be within the heart that
rejoiceth; for behold, all acts of love and pleasure are my rituals.

The communion service, described earlier, follows, and the service
then concludes with a song adopted from a traditional Witches' ceremony,
also acknowledging the Goddess's power: "O She will bring the buds in
spring, and laugh among the flowers...." The priestess then walks past the
congregation, gently kissing or hugging the person at the end of each row.
This person then embraces the person sitting to his or her side, symbolically
passing along the group's love and warmth. The group considers this
gesture an appropriate closing for a Church oriented to erotic activity and
love.

After the formal service is over, the regulars usually head off to a
restaurant for lunch, though at times, after services the Church sponsors a
special activity, such as a demonstration of bondage.

Rituals, Religion, and D&S

The worship of the dominant woman as Goddess is also enacted somewhat
less conventionally through seasonal rituals borrowed from the Witchcraft-
Pagan tradition and through elaborate ceremonies that are a cross between
religious services and D&S parties. These activities provide an occasion for
members to express their creativity and love of pageantry and drama.

A Spring Equinox ritual, held at dawn after an overnight campout to
celebrate the birth of the year, was typical. Those who wanted to
participate in the rituals took a class led by Diana; other Church members
and guests attended to observe. Diana served as high priestess, and the
other Church officials assisting—Devora, Danielle, Lance, and Sharon—
appeared in long, colorful robes. Diana prepared the ritual table with the
usual tools of the Craft—the knife, wine cup, incense, candles, and platter
of cakes, and placed four small tables around the perimeter of a large
circular area to mark each of the four directions. The four officers and four
participants gathered in a circle, two beside each of the small tables.

Diana opened the ceremony by standing in front of each couple,
holding her knife aloft, and asking the Goddess of that direction to be
present at the ritual. Each participant read a short litany honoring the
seasonal changes and the coming of spring. Diana swept the center of the
circle with a broom to symbolically sweep out the old year and sweep in the
new. After more chanting and reciting, she instructed everyone to search
for Easter eggs, which symbolized the birth of the year. When they
returned with their eggs, placing them in the center of the circle, Diana
handed everyone a seed, faced the sun, chanted some more, and asked

everyone to plant his or her seed in the ground to honor the Goddess and send forth wishes for a successful new year. The ritual closed with the traditional Pagan spiral dance, in which participants join hands and race about in a circle, followed by the sharing of cookies and ritual wine, and the hug of peace, in which each participant in turn hugs the person to his left.

The Church also conducts special "high" rituals that incorporate some D&S activity as part of a unique dramatic pageant; only Church regulars may attend. Each of these is designed around a special theme; for example, a special ritual was held to celebrate the roughly concurrent birthdays of five church regulars—Lance, Harvey, Marvin, Luke, and Dick. Six women and eleven men attended the event, choreographed by Danielle. The women dressed as priestesses in long dark robes, while the men wore only chains around their waists. As Danielle explained the symbolic rite of purification and dedication to the Goddess, the mood changed from one of light kidding and joking to one of mock seriousness, reflecting the intermixing of Goddess worship, the eroticism of D&S, and the celebrativeness of a party. Some found the atmosphere especially erotic, others felt a sense of spiritual uplift, and others were mostly amused. Some experienced all three feelings.

Danielle turned off the lights, and by candlelight the women led the men upstairs to the livingroom, now the Sacred Triple Goddess Temple, where the ceremony would take place. The men knelt in a semicircle, as the women gathered around the altar and consecrated themselves as priestesses of the Goddess. "Gracious Goddess," each woman recited as she dabbed oil on her forehead, "Bless and purify me that I may never search for evil, never listen to gossip, never give voice to evil."

Then the women took turns putting on a ring symbolizing the authority of the Goddess. Sharon announced that the men would now be purified and strengthened by looking within to help them in honoring the Goddess, "for that is the pathway to Wisdom." The women would instruct them how. Accordingly, as the men quietly complied, the women placed each man on his stomach, facing the altar, and bound his feet to his hands. Their intention was that this bondage should make the men truly experience their humility before women and feel the power of the Goddess, represented by the women as priestesses. At the same time, the bondage inspired erotic feelings and made the men feel foolish as the object of good-natured fun. As Sharon read solemnly about how this bondage would help the men meditate more intensely to better reach an altered state of consciousness, Melody whispered to Katrina: "Don't they look cute, like you just want to hit them."

After the men meditated several minutes "on the vision of the Goddess," the women told them to wriggle out of their bonds and took

turns selecting one of the men to experience the high point of the
ceremony—a ritual scourging—which mingled a bit of spirituality with
some good-natured teasing and D&S.

As the women called each man to come forward for his scourging,
Danielle read with authority: "The last stage of your purification has
arrived....You must call upon your strength to help you gain the
Center...the union with the Goddess....So kneel. It is now your time to
receive the ancient purification of scourging."

However, some of the men jumped up in a joking and half-serious
way, showing this wasn't a totally spiritual endeavor. When Danielle called
on Lance, he responded with a broad grin: "But suppose we're not ready to
have the Goddess purify us?" She tried to bring the ritual back to its
ostensibly serious purpose. "Then you're not ready," she told him, "and you
will need to be purified twicefold later." Her implied message that he
would be punished more severely when he was scourged did not displease
him, however, since he found whippings sexually stimulating.

The purification ceremony itself was pure D&S, though the litany
provided a spiritual veneer. As each man stepped forward, the woman who
selected him led him to a hook by the fireplace, retied his hands in front of
him, attached them above his head to the hook, and whipped him several
times with a long black cat-o'-nine-tails. The five men celebrating their
birthdays were whipped by the other women, too. After each ceremonial
whipping, Danielle intoned solemnly: "Now the weight of your impurities
have been removed from you. You are in union with the Goddess. Now
return to your place and meditate upon your joy."

To remind the men that this was more than an erotic experience,
Devora concluded with a brief communion ceremony. "The Goddess has
purified you, and you are blessed," she said as she passed around a basket
of bread and goblet of wine. "We have traveled from afar to this Sacred
Triple Goddess Temple and have found what we were seeking—
purification. We can now return...and continue to grow spiritually with
our Lady's guidance. So mote it be."

Thus the ritual had involved a mixture of spiritual expression, fantasy,
drama, and erotic stimulation conducted in the form of a religious
ceremony. But while the women kept reminding the men that the ritual was
a spiritual experience, the men were especially interested in its erotic and
D&S content. Thus one man who wasn't among the birthday celebrants
complained, "No one hit me hard or long enough."

"But it wasn't your birthday," Danielle explained.

Fantasy Classes

Danielle also offered sexual fantasy classes, which met weekly in an ideal
setting—Harvey's next-door apartment, which had postcards and portraits

of attractive women all over the walls, a small altar with a statue of a man kneeling before a dominant woman in the livingroom, and a bedroom designed for D&S play, with wall and ceiling mirrors, suspension hooks, chains attached to the bed, and D&S gadgets hanging from the walls.

Initially, the class was intended for the sharing of erotic fantasies, many of which members had kept hidden for years. And often they acted out these fantasies. For instance, Bertrand, a retired teacher in his 70s, described his long-held fantasy of being hit by the female teacher who punished him as a child. A woman in the group demanded that he crawl over to her, and she disciplined him on the spot. Harvey said that after seeing a fraternity hazing in *Animal House*, he fantasized about being teased in a sorority initiation. The three women in the class asked Harvey, Bertrand, and another man to crawl into the bedroom, bend over the bed, and say "Thank you, mistress; may I have another," each time they hit them, as in the movie.

But gradually the class evolved into an educational support group, too, as a core of regulars began to come every week. Some classes dealt with D&S techniques, such as giving pain and tying ropes, and others were devoted to recurring issues, such as the difference between fantasy and reality and D&S etiquette. Class members occasionally attended D&S movies, and about once a month played a Truth, Dare, and Fantasy game, which enabled them to ask probing questions, share fantasies, and dare each other to perform assorted D&S activities in a gamelike setting. And most members participated in various D&S and everyday activities together, too.

D&S, FANTASY, AND ORGANIZATIONAL STRUCTURE

Although the mixture of fantasy and D&S can transform otherwise ordinary events into special occasions, the participants' intense interest in fantasy and drama also contributes to some organizational problems for the SM Church and the D&S community as a whole. One organizational problem is that a fantasy can become so attractive that planners only fantasize and do not develop realistic or feasible ideas. Church leaders frequently fantasize about community structures that never materialize, such as the community Lance calls Walden II, which would be fully devoted to dominance and male submissiveness. Similarly, the leaders often share elaborate visions of the Church becoming a national group with thousands, even hundreds of thousands of members. But for the most part such fantasies outstrip probable reality, and as a result Church leaders sometimes act on unrealistic fantasies and dismiss more feasible ideas.

The second major problem shared by the Church and other D&S groups is the relative scarcity of women members, which causes many men to drop out in frustration. The Church officers tried to resolve this problem by creating a special structure that reflected the usual attendance at meetings—about three or four males to every woman. As they conceived it, the new groups, called *curias*, would function as matriarchal communities, with a few women in charge of about nine to twelve men. But few men signed up for these groups. One reason? They didn't want to join a group with so few women.

10

The Party Scene

For those persons actively involved in the public D&S community, parties are a central part of the scene. D&Sers find them not only erotic and enjoyable times to socialize, but also occasions for individuals to receive self-validation and social support from others with similar interests.

D&S parties range from privately arranged informal gatherings with seven or eight people to vast, sometimes elaborately staged, productions sponsored by D&S organizations for 50 or more people. But almost all feature some fantasy play, which may be as simple as private or public paddlings or as elaborate a fantasy drama as the organizers can devise: a "slave auction," ritual, or pageant organized around a specific theme. Many come to participate; others just watch.

Theme events are particularly popular for large parties sponsored by organized groups, with the theme providing roles for guests to play. For example, at an SM Church "Ladies of the SS Night," the dominant women dressed up as Nazi commandants who treated the submissive, mostly naked males, like prisoners and slaves. At a fancy Roman toga party to celebrate the reign of Empress Theodora, the women played queens and princesses who ruled lowly male subjects. At some parties participation in the fantasy theme is optional; at other events, participation is required and observers are prohibited.

At many parties, although all sorts of playful or erotic D&S activities occur, there is no actual sexual contact; but at others, sexual encounters do take place. It depends on the ambience of the party, the desires of the guests, and the attitude of the host. Most typically, sexual activity occurs at the smaller more intimate parties or at the end of a larger party, when most guests have left and an intimate core group remains. But sometimes a small group breaks off from a larger party to explore sexual or D&S activity in another room. The host may designate special playrooms or bedrooms for such play, while reserving the livingroom for social mixing. But if the host permits and guests are uninhibited, scenes may occur virtually anywhere.

Often, some or all participants come in costume or wear appropriate D&S appurtenances, such as studded belts, collars, cuffs, boots, and leather. Some bring favorite toys, such as whips and ropes, or the host may

135

provide these. Costumes and such are encouraged, because they help everyone get in the mood and feel appropriately dominant or submissive. Also, some partygoers enjoy these garments or toys for their fetish value— just seeing them is exciting and arousing.

As Danielle, who threw frequent parties for the SM Church, explained: "It's harder to get things started when people come to a party wearing their street clothes. But say a woman brings a costume with her. When she goes into the bathroom to change, she is thinking about the new role she will play. When she comes out, she's transformed and ready to be dominant." And when the males undress or put on their collars, it helps them feel submissive. Also, when many or all participants are in costume or bring toys, the spirit of role playing becomes contagious and it becomes easier for everyone to feel free to act out their fantasies. Danielle added that the mood of a party also depends on how long the guests have been active in the D&S community. The more novices or outsiders, the less likely D&S activity is to occur.

PARTY ETIQUETTE

The type of D&S activity and its participants are, in turn, governed by a code of etiquette widely accepted by regular partygoers. The principal rule is consensus, which means that everyone participating in a scene must agree about what is to happen. Thus, if a person wants to start a scene or join an ongoing one, he or she must ask permission. To join, typically, he or she must first ask the dominant person who appears to be in charge and then ask the submissives and any other participants, too. Obtaining permission is crucial, and to intrude on a private scene is an extreme breach of etiquette, for an intrusion not only makes the participants uncomfortable but also may douse their erotic energy, thereby ending the scene.

Thus partygoers do not enter a closed room, though, if the door is open or the scene is public, anyone is free to watch. Indeed, some D&Sers are exhibitionists. But if the participants become nervous, an observer should move on. If the observer wants to become at all involved, including making remarks as well as physical touching, he or she must first ask permission. Partygoers who do not ask face varying consequences, depending whether they are regulars, who should know better, or newcomers, and depending on how angry the intrusion makes the others. They may verbally admonish the intruder, eject him or her from the scene or the party, or even, though rarely, fight back.

For instance, at one party, Luke, a 55-year-old retired gardener who liked to disrupt people to provoke a punishment, first hopped into a hot tub without asking permission of those already present and later interrupted various conversations. The people he disturbed tried to be polite; they said nothing but just glared at him silently. Luke ignored their dirty looks and continued to misbehave until Danielle, one of the party's organizers, took him aside and told him he would have to honor D&S etiquette or he would never be invited to another party.

At another party, the reaction to an offender, a naive outsider, was more immediate and dramatic. Angie, a dominant transvestite, brought her three slaves, dressed in bathing suits and collars, to a huge public Halloween costume ball. She led them behind her on a leash, and as she stood showing them off while they knelt beside her, a male stranger suddenly bent down and slapped one of them playfully. Bertrand, the slave he hit, was furious— not only had an outsider hit him, but the outsider was a man, and Bertrand was submissive only to women and male transvestites. He reared up, grabbed Angie's crop, hit the man squarely across the face, and snapped at him: "If you do that again, I'll kill you." The man cowered away. "It serves him right," Bertrand said later. "He had no business to intervene. So that taught him a lesson. I even left marks."

Permission is also required for taking photographs. For obvious reasons, partygoers allow only persons whom they know and trust to take photos. Some partygoers refuse all photo taking, but others like being photographed.

Party etiquette extends to the use of alcohol and drugs. At most parties, guests drink a moderate amount of wine or punch. But they typically avoid heavy drinking because alcohol, they explain, interferes with sensual arousal and safety. For the same reason, they tend to avoid the use of the more powerful drugs like LSD and mescaline. As one woman put it: "You're playing with human bodies. You need to be in control."

However, partygoers generally consider acceptable the limited use of certain relatively mild drugs, such as marijuana and cocaine, as long as the user retains control and acts responsibly. At most parties, guests freely pass around marijuana; cocaine is less in evidence, since it is mostly reserved for smaller groups of intimates, because of its high cost. Not everyone uses drugs, and no one is pressured to indulge or abstain.

Party etiquette also requires guests to remain nonjudgmental regarding others' interests and sexual preferences. At many parties guests may include men and women with various predilections for being dominant, submissive, or switching, and for being heterosexual, homosexual, or bisexual. And even at parties designed for people with certain orientations, such as the SM Church parties for dominant women and submissive men, other types of activities may take place, since as noted, D&Sers often switch roles. At times, this variety can make for a very "hot" party, with all sorts of activities happening simultaneously. But if the party is large, such variety can sometimes prove inhibiting, since guests have a difficulty finding others who want to stage a scene they will like. As one woman commented: "Suppose you're into bondage. You don't want to do a scene with someone who's into heavy pain." Also, while a large party can sometimes loosen people's inhibitions, its size can create an impersonal mood that constrains participants.

Thus many D&Sers prefer smaller, more intimate parties, or parties where the guests have similar or complementary orientations. The SM Church, for example, takes this approach and tries to limit its parties to dominant women and submissive men. As Danielle summarized: "We've found that D&S parties work best when all or almost all of the people have the same interests. People know their place, and it's easier to get them into playing fantasy roles. They get into the party mood more quickly, and the scenes become hotter, too." Such limits also prevent conflicts between dominant and submissive men or between dominant men and women, she claimed. For example, the presence of dominant men could make submissive men feel guilty or unmanly about their submission, thereby reviving the conflicts many experienced in coming to terms with their need for submission. Or the dominant men could begin "coming on strong" with the dominant women, which would disturb some women. Thus the Church invited only trusted dominant males, if any.

At parties whose guests have various D&S orientations, both the males and females may take the lead in starting a scene. But at a party for dominant women and submissive men, the men usually wait for the women to begin. "It's hard to feel submissive," one man said, "if I have to take the initiative to get things going." If the women don't act forcefully enough, the party may be slow in getting started. For example, at one party, Devora was dancing sensuously in front of a half-dozen men seated on a couch. She repeatedly asked for a volunteer to join her, but no one responded. Frustrated and annoyed, she marched out of the room. But, in fact, the men wanted to join her, as they later explained. They were simply waiting to be chosen or commanded; they didn't feel volunteering was something a submissive should do.

The host or hostess also plays an important role at parties, because the host establishes the rules, and these guidelines are especially important to guests in a situation where there may be some play acting and a change of roles. The host signals where and when D&S activities can start, explains any house limits on the type or intensity of play, and indicates whether sexual activity may occur. At small parties among people who already know each other, the host may not need to do much. But at larger parties, many hosts plan special activities to get the party started. A host may ask a few participants to come in costume and act out a brief scenario to get others in the mood, or he or she may invite several people known for being able to break the ice.

At one large party, the host asked Baby Robin, a professional sports announcer and former wrestler from New York, to make a special entrance. So Baby Robin wore a cape and a gold women's bikini as he ran into the living room, where people were casually talking. He waved his arms with a flourish, as his cape flapped behind him, and Katrina chased him with a whip. After she strung him up in the suspension cuffs dangling from the livingroom ceiling and cropped him briefly, a few other guests joined in. Such a dramatic approach usually livens up a party, Baby Robin observed. "People often sit around waiting for someone else to do something before they feel free to get involved themself. That's why the host usually invites me and a few other people to come in costume. Then, we are, as it were, the first act, and the others naturally follow."

Some hosts use games or, more rarely, introductory rituals to help guests feel free to play. Especially popular is Truth, Dare, or Fantasy—a game in which one player challenges another to choose to answer truthfully any question he or she poses, to perform a dare, or to make up a fantasy on a topic he or she selects. The dares usually involve D&S activity (tie someone up, take a whipping, take off your clothes), with the darer respecting the other player's likes and preferences. The first players tend to choose truth or fantasy, particularly if they don't know each other very well. As the game continues, dares become common, and the party becomes more active and uninhibited.

Like any host, the organizer of a D&S party keeps an eye on how things are going and makes sure that no one is getting drunk or unruly. At a D&S party, this control is particularly important because unruly guests are not merely embarrassing but potentially dangerous. Thus the host must make sure that the dominants are behaving responsibly, so that no one will be hurt. Disruptive guests are quietly taken aside and advised to behave, or more rarely, to leave.

A host must also informally monitor inexperienced dominants. At an SM Church party, Devora, one of the hostesses, had to rescue Harvey, who was tied to a table in the basement, from serious harm. Rita, a relatively inexperienced professional mistress from Nevada, was hitting him with a chain and causing painful bruises. He protested, pleading in the usual submissive style: "Please, stop, have mercy, mistress." But Rita continued to hit him, thinking he was only protesting in jest, as a good submissive. When Devora came downstairs, she stopped Rita at once, led her away, and released Harvey. "Don't ever hit someone like that," she later admonished Rita. "Not with a chain."

TYPES OF PARTIES

Just like relationships between individuals and couples, D&S parties vary widely in what happens. But, overall, these parties can be categorized into four main types.

1. The primarily social party, which includes some D&S activity.
2. The mixed party with participants of varying sexual orientations.
3. Theme or fantasy parties.
4. Smaller, often impromptu, parties, which include intense D&S scenes and sometimes sexual activity.

Though there is no hard and fast line between categories, this is a convenient way to think about parties.

The Social Party with Some Female Dominance Play

Some parties are much like ordinary social or cocktail parties, except that many guests come dressed in role—dominant women in sleek, sensual clothing and high heels or boots, submissive men wearing a collar—and others bring their toys. During the evening, some guests play in public or break away from the party to play, while others continue conventional socializing.

At one such party, most of the dozen women guests sported the dominant look—for example, Bella wore tight black silk pants, a skin-tight black top, silver chain belt, and black high heels; and Devora wore a bright red gypsy blouse, black toreador pants slit up the side, and high black boots. A few of the dozen men wore symbols of submissiveness—Laura's current lover, Barry, wore a thin studded collar, and a small pair of handcuffs dangled from Harvey's collar—though otherwise the men dressed casually.

The party began with the guests milling about and chatting about general topics, current events, and new films. Gradually, conversation shifted to the D&S scene. Bella had recently started working as a mistress and was glad to have left her straight job as a nurse; Susie, a male transvestite, who came to the party dressed, talked about some male strip clubs "she" had visited; Kat mentioned her plans to raise money for a high-quality S&M stage show. Other guests shared D&S fantasies about scenarios and future plans. Herman and June described an expensive home they had visited. In one magnificent room with tall windows, they could envision wall-to-wall and ceiling mirrors, hooks for suspension, and other designs perfect for D&S scenes.

As the guests became more comfortable, Angela, the hostess, a photographer of 30, played a fantasy tape in which a dominant mistress ordered one of her slaves about and disciplined him with a whip when he didn't behave. As the tape played and most of the guests watched, she and Harvey enacted the two roles, with Harvey stripped down to his gold G-string and crawling about on the floor. Since Angela was the hostess, this D&S performance signaled that the guests could play now, and while most remained in the living room talking, some disappeared to the playroom and bedroom downstairs.

Victor, who liked spanking, invited Laura downstairs to paddle him with one of his paddles and afterwards he paddled her. Soon after, Laura paddled Barry. Meanwhile, Angela turned on soft red lights and a strobe in the playroom and put on a New Wave record. Devora, waving her crop about, stripped sensuously down to her one-piece black bathing suit, threw her clothes seductively at one of the men, and sashayed out. Then, Angela, wearing a black and red corset, net stockings, and heels, began dancing with Alvin, poked him a few times with the crop, and finally pushed him down on his knees, and stood above him, with one foot on his back, as if he were her conquest.

In the livingroom, meanwhile, as some guests talked, Herman and June began their scene. Herman stripped to his briefs, June to her corset, and Herman lay across her lap, his face in her crotch. From time to time, she brandished a whip over his head, as he licked her thighs and under her corset. Soon Sharon began whacking him lightly with a crop. Then, June, as the dominant in the scene, invited Misty over, and Sharon handed her the crop, while she began to massage Herman's feet.

When this scene ended, Sid, a doctor in his 50s who was watching quietly, asked Sharon to paddle him on the buttocks. He had never done anything publicly before, but now wanted to try. Sharon agreed, and he took off his clothes and knelt in the middle of the room. As some watched and others talked, she slapped him with the paddle.

Overall, this party was relatively low key, with some intermittent D&S activity and much typical party conversation. But shortly after midnight, when most of the guests left, those who stayed on to help Angela clean up—Danielle, Harvey, Brent, Laura, Barry, and a newcomer to the scene, Thomas—had their own D&S party. Danielle suggested playing Truth, Dare, or Fantasy to get things going, and explained the rules. As the six became less inhibited, the women mostly played dominant and the men submissive. For example, Danielle ordered Harvey to come over and kiss her feet; Brent dared Danielle to crop his backside six times; Laura told Thomas to undress and she walked around to inspect him; and Barry asked Angela to help Brent get dressed, which she did, but in a suitably dominant way. She ordered him to lie on his stomach and squirm into his pants, socks, and shoes while she held them, and she concluded by snapping a pair of handcuffs around his ankles. Some players used the game to allow others who liked to switch roles to do so. For instance, Thomas, who considered himself a dominant male, though willing to be submissive, dared Brent to tie up Laura's hands with ropes and lead her around the room, and later he dared Laura to reveal her bare backside to Danielle, while Danielle gave her ten whacks.

MIXED PARTIES

Some parties are for guests who have a wide range of D&S interests and orientations. One such party sponsored by the Society of Janus began as two separate parties—one for the dominants, the other for submissives. The two parties were planned for the same evening at the same time to give the dominants and submissives a chance to get to meet and talk with others of their own D&S orientation. But it soon became apparent that the participants wanted to play, not talk. The dominants decided to crash the submissives' party after the submissives rejected their order to join them.

When the dominants arrived, a few submissives were experimenting with suspension on hooks the hostess had recently installed. The ensuing party included all sorts of public D&S activity. Baby Robin, a heterosexual male who fancied himself an exhibitionist, dressed as a French maid and darted about emptying ashtrays. Warren, a bisexual who liked to switch roles, cropped Sammy, a usually heterosexual, submissive male, who twisted about with his cuffed wrists attached above him to the suspension hooks; then Marvin, who was usually submissive and heterosexual but who switched, took over. Later, Warren took a turn in the harness, and a half-dozen D&Sers with varying sexual orientations cropped him, too, a few of them pulling off his pants. In the end Warren teetered off to a chair, smiling radiantly, as several men sitting nearby complimented him: "You really took a lot; you took that well."

Meanwhile, Paul, a submissive heterosexual male of about 50, looked for women to participate in his infantilism fantasy. In one hand, he held several dozen 3x5 and 4x6 cards he had previously stamped with a list of punishments he should receive for wetting his pants and statements about his need for diaper training, and he wandered about asking women to sign his cards, later inspect his diapers, and mete out the appropriate punishments. And Luke, who liked to have women hit him and enjoyed being the center of attention, suddenly pulled down his pants. Several women with different orientations—one mostly dominant, one mostly submissive, and a bisexual switch—hit him, too.

In short, the mixed atmosphere of the party encouraged a variety of scenes and permitted people to try new roles. Usually submissive males and females tried being dominant, while typically dominant people became submissive, too. Also, gays and heterosexuals interacted with each other, and switches and bisexuals had plenty of opportunities. But since many people didn't know each other well and the range of interests was so broad, the intensity of the erotic activity was relatively low. Most was public, lighthearted, and erotic but nonsexual (that is, no intimate sexual touching, intercourse, or orgasm).

In contrast, at mixed parties where guests know each other well, people break up into smaller scenes catering to particular interests, and the play can become more erotic and even explicitly sexual. At another Society of Janus party, for example, while most guests engaged in casual erotic play in the livingroom, a half-dozen friends gradually drifted into the bedroom and closed the door. At first, they sat around talking. But then Mouse, normally submissive in his primary relationship, noticed his good friend Phil lounging on the bed while Tammy, a submissive woman Mouse dated occasionally when he played dominant, joked with the group. Mouse sat down beside Phil, motioned for Tammy to come over, and while the others continued talking, he ordered Tammy to take off Phil's pants and orally satisfy him. As she did, he lifted up her skirt and caned her backside from time to time. The conversation ground to a halt as everyone watched. Tammy continued, oblivious to them until she had finished; she looked up, suddenly aware of the group, and everyone clapped. For a moment, she blushed, then acknowledged their appreciation with a quick little bow.

FANTASY AND THEME PARTIES

Parties can become quite elaborate, designed around one person's fantasy or a theme selected by a group. Frequently, birthdays are a time to satisfy somebody's fantasy. For instance, for her thirtieth birthday, Devora, who worked as a professional mistress and was usually dominant in her marriage with Ken, wanted to be mostly submissive. Danielle organized the party accordingly.

The night of the party, Dorothy, who worked as a mistress with Devora, and two male friends, Serge and Dick, started the evening with a "kidnap." After Devora saw her last client for the day, the two men suddenly appeared and informed her: "You're coming with us." Since Devora knew one of them, she played along. The men blindfolded her, hustled her into the trunk of a car, tied her up, and drove her to the site of the party, about an hour away, at Marvin's house in San Francisco. They led Devora directly to the bathroom, where Danielle, Sharon, Lance, Marvin, Melody, and Jesse were waiting. They stripped off her clothes, sprayed her with whipped cream, and sprinkled her with nuts, like a big birthday cake. Then, they placed her on a double bed in the basement, where the five men eagerly licked her clean, as Danielle, standing nearby in a long white ceremonial robe, orated grandly: "This is your preparation. You are being made ready for your rebirth."

Next Serge and Dick led her, still blindfolded, to the hot tub on the deck, as Danielle followed, announcing, "You are now to be purified."

When they pushed her in and pulled off her blindfold, Danielle proclaimed, "You are now reborn."

Devora gloried in playing out the submissive role for the rest of the party. She fetched drinks and helped serve refreshments. When the group played a round of Truth, Dare, or Fantasy, the other players dared her to be submissive in various ways—such as letting the men hit her or kissing everyone's feet—instead of giving her the usual dares to be dominant. Knowing she was normally dominant, her friends didn't ask her to be too submissive. When Marvin hit her, he did so lightly, so the strokes were symbolic rather than painful. Also, he feared later repercussions if he broke an unspoken rule about acknowledging her primary dominance. "I didn't want to hit you too hard," he told her later, "because I was afraid of what might happen afterwards. I was afraid you might really try to get me then."

Some fantasy parties are extremely elaborate, and sometimes the celebrant asks a few close friends to enact part of a special fantasy before the other guests arrive. Jesse, for example, wanted for his twenty-ninth birthday party to enact a fantasy of being captured by women, who would rape him, baby him, and afterwards proclaim him king—a concluding gesture that was especially important to him, since he had grown up hearing tales about his aristocratic ancestors in Europe. He wrote his close friend Dorothy a letter describing exactly what he wanted: "We'll go walking on a beach.... Five women will abduct me. They'll force me to suck and kiss their tits and pussy, and then they'll force me to be a baby to them.... They'll put me in a bubble bath, and after I am purified, they will take me to a priestess, who will crown me king.... Then, the party will begin." He also told Dorothy whom to invite—Sharon, Devora, Dick (a male he had a relationship with as a bisexual), and Angela, whom he dated occasionally.

While pretending not to be planning a surprise, Dorothy organized an elaborate event with Sharon's help. They arranged to enact his fantasy and afterwards have a party with about two dozen guests.

When those participating in the fantasy arrived, Dorothy led them into an upstairs bedroom and showed them Jesse's letter, while he waited downstairs, unaware of what was happening. When everyone was ready, she blindfolded him and guided him in. As he neared the foot of the bed, Dorothy signaled and everyone pounced. They flung him to the bed, stripped off his clothes, snapped on leather wrist and ankle cuffs, and tied the cuffs to the ends of the bed as Jesse chortled with pleasure.

They massaged and tickled him, and since he had said he wanted to be babied, Devora sat beside him and let him suck on her breast. Meanwhile, Sharon, Dick, and Dorothy shaved off his pubic hair so he would be smooth as a real baby. They sprinkled baby powder over him, rubbed him with oil, snapped on a large linen diaper, and fed him from a bottle and jar of baby food, as he cooed and laughed like a baby. Then, saying he "didn't like his vegetables," they turned him over and spanked him.

Next they plopped him in a bubble bath, washed him down with a sponge, dried him off, and guided him, still blindfolded, into another larger bedroom where Dorothy stood behind an altar with a single glowing candle. She had removed her street clothes and now wore a black bra and panties. Sharon and Devora stood beside her like ladies of her court.

Dorothy ordered Jesse to kneel down on the cushion before her, removed his blindfold, and began solemnly reciting the coronation ceremony outlined in his letter:

By the fire that gives you strength,
By the water that quenches the fire and carries away your anger,
By the earth that shares the secrets of being,
By the wind that purifies,
And by the air that shares its magic,
I ask you to drink of the blood of life,
And I crown you king...

She handed him the chalice, and he took several sips. She placed a crown on his head and told him to rise. As she read on, "I give you the scepter to rule over your people," Devora placed a black cloak around his shoulders and Sharon brought him the scepter. Finally, Angela and Dick brought over his birthday gifts, and after he opened them Dorothy suggested he put on some briefs and join the party.

Jesse soon involved the other guests in his fantasy. He wore his cape and crown throughout the party, and he began "initiating" some of the arriving guests into his court. One after another, he called them forth, asked them to kneel before him, and knighted them by tapping them on the shoulder three times and giving them an appropriately aristocratic name—Countess Wilhelmina the Second, First Squire Charles, Baroness Alicia. "I dub you once, I dub you twice, I dub you three times.... Rise, you are now a member of my court."

When Jesse finished this ceremony, Dorothy, now wearing a tight black slitted dress, led him to a pair of cuffs hanging from the ceiling, strapped him in, put on a collar symbolizing submission, and invited the guests to give him his birthday whacks—29 and 1 to grow on. In keeping with unspoken D&S etiquette, only those who participated in the earlier fantasy and Serge, who knew Jesse well, gave the whacks. The other guests watched, sensing that the hits were ceremonial in nature, an extension of the private fantasy enacted before they arrived. Afterwards, as Jesse continued standing with his arms aloft and his wrists firmly in the cuffs, Dorothy kissed him long and sensuously as his birthday reward.

The party then became a more typical D&S party, with conversations about D&S, small public and private scenes involving light bondage and hitting, and for the four couples who stayed to the end, some sexual activity, including oral sex and intercourse. As at other parties, many people switched roles. In the early part of the evening, most of the women were dominant in the scenes, but by the end of the party they were being submissive too.

The most elaborate parties resemble staged productions and require extensive planning. Participants usually come in costume, either exotic D&S clothing or a costume based on the theme of the event. The SM Church stages about a dozen such events a year. In one of the most elaborate of these pageants, a Theodora party, one woman played the role of the Roman Empress Theodora, and the others were officials of her court who helped her enforce discipline: a sergeant of the guards, a jailer, and an executioner. To start the ritual, the men undressed and were chained together in a downstairs room. The sergeant of the guards blindfolded them and led them, one at a time, upstairs. There the jailer and executioner hit them, draped them in chains, forced them to lick their feet, and gave them other orders, before dismissing them abruptly: "Okay, you can go now," and sending them to wait in the dark in another room. Then they selected a few favored slaves to play with in twosomes and small groups.

At other parties, the women were commanders of the SS and guards of the Spanish Inquisition who disciplined the men as their hapless prisoners, exotic women of the jungle who captured male slaves, goddesses the men had to worship and serve, and kidnappers who held the men hostage. Also, the Church sponsored a few slave auctions, where the women used play money to bid for the males, then took them off for erotic play.

SMALLER AND IMPROMPTU PARTIES

Small, intimate, sometimes impromptu, parties are a common part of the scene. A small group—perhaps a half-dozen to a dozen or so—decide to get together; a few people drop in to visit; or a group decides to head for someone's house after a formal program—and in moments a party has started.

Though socializing may be central to small parties, often the setting is conducive to a D&S scene or series of scenes involving some or all participants. At times these scenes become very intense and far more sexually explicit than the light and public erotic activity at the larger parties. Small parties may include a great deal of sexual touching, orgasm, and intercourse. Some parties are much like swingers' parties, as guests experiment with a variety of private, semiprivate, and public sexual activities, though combined with some D&S activity too.

As an example, Jesse, an SM Church member, organized an "insiders' party" at Marvin's for Church regulars and a few other active participants in the D&S community. Sixteen guests attended, including Lance, Sharon, Danielle, Harvey, Brent, Angela, Devora, Ken, and Kat and Mouse, and their two playmates for the night.

At first, the party proceeded like a typical D&S party, with people talking about their D&S experiences and participating in casual and public D&S activities. For instance, as several people munched hors d'oeuvres in the kitchen, Danielle playfully pulled down Harvey's pants and cropped him on the buttocks. Brent and Haskell squatted on the floor in the living room massaging Sharon's feet. Kat ordered Alan, her evening's playmate, to hold a strawberry in his mouth without swallowing it until she told him to do so.

Gradually, the atmosphere changed, and the D&S activity began to shift from erotic to explicitly sexual. First, Kat, Mouse, and their playmates disappeared upstairs, where they frolicked about on Marvin's king-sized waterbed. One at a time, others in the party began to join them. Angela appeared after Mouse, who was submissive to Kat but looking for other women to dominate, sent Janice downstairs to hand Angela a scrawled note that said: "Take off your clothes and crawl into the master bedroom on your hands and knees." Angela knocked on the door, but refused to crawl, and Mouse invited her in. A few minutes later, Marvin knocked, and he joined the group on the bed. Mouse told Janice to crawl over to Marvin and embrace him sensuously, then pull him down to the bed and strip off his clothes. As she began licking his body, Haskell came in and joined the group, too.

Yet this was not an ordinary group sex scene, for there was no sexual intercourse. Instead, the two dominants choreographing the scene, Kat and secondarily Mouse, used D&S techniques to heighten the sexual arousal. After Mouse directed Marvin to lick Janice between her legs, he told Janice, "But don't come. We just want to tease him." As Marvin approached the point of ecstatic release, Kat stood up and announced: "Okay, it's time to go. I think Janice has been well worked up. Now you," she turned to Mouse, "can take her home and fuck her." Mouse lurched up, pulled Janice away from Marvin, and got dressed. Meanwhile, Marvin lay on his back, clutching the bedsheet, breathing heavily, and moaning: "How could you do this?" Yet, as he later commented, he found his frustration oddly enjoyable, for it prolonged his arousal.

Soon afterwards, Marvin went downstairs and found that Devora was receptive to continuing the session. He led her upstairs to what soon became a semipublic session, for in a few minutes, Danielle and Harvey joined them and watched from the sidelines and Jesse briefly stopped in to observe, too. While Marvin and Devora noisily achieved several orgasms,

Danielle and Harvey cheered them on, announced the "latest score," and clapped when they stood up and took quick bows like two performers. Meanwhile, in the basement, another couple had a private D&S scene that ended in very ordinary and very private sex.

In short, this small, intimate party became intensely sexual. But no one was pressured to participate, and several people did not. While Marvin and Devora were staging their performance, her husband, Ken, was conversing happily downstairs, and several couples only socialized throughout the evening.

An example of an impromptu party created by people with very different D&S interests occurred after a Society of Janus meeting. Several people were sitting in a bar discussing the meeting: Chris, a dominant gay male; Bridget, a bisexual woman who liked to switch; Phil, a dominant straight male; Judy, Phil's submissive lover; Warren, a mostly submissive bisexual; and André, a switch-hitting gay. Chris suggested a party, remarking that his submissive gay roommate, Al, might enjoy being dominated by Bridget for a change, and Phil and Judy said they would enjoy seeing his playroom. So at about 11 p.m., the group drove to Chris's, raided the icebox, woke up his two sleeping roommates, and made for the basement playroom.

At first, Bridget teased Al—wouldn't he like to be dominated by a woman? But when he demurred, claiming to be too sleepy, Phil volunteered to do a scene with Judy. This was not a scene most of the participants would do themselves—a dominant male in charge of a submissive female—but they were eager to watch, perhaps to learn and expand their own D&S repertoire by observing others.

With everyone seated at the sides of the room, Phil began the scene by clicking his fingers, his usual signal with Judy. At once she crawled over and knelt at his feet awaiting his orders, no longer Judy, but his slave. She looked up and said softly, "Your slave is willing to serve her master." He strung her up in a pair of cuffs dangling from the ceiling, removed her red jumpsuit, leaving her wearing only a garter belt and stockings, and began to whip her lightly across her buttocks, thighs, breasts, and back. Occasionally, he moved a vibrator between her legs. Soon she began to moan, begging him as she usually did in their scenarios: "Oh, please, please, Master. May your slave come? Your slave begs to come." He let her beg several times, for he liked to hear her, and finally held the vibrator firmly between her thighs, "Yes. Come. Come. Your Master gives you permission to come."

He repeated this sequence several times, explaining how much he enjoyed having her beg and then letting her come. He then released her and asked her to go to everyone in the room, kiss their feet, and thank them for "watching your humiliation." She did so, referring to herself always in the third person—"Thank you for watching this slave's humiliation." Phil then snapped his fingers and counted to three to end the session: "Now you're Judy again."

The scene had been an unusual one for most of the observers, since they didn't practice heterosexual male domination. Yet, in keeping with the D&S community's spirit of tolerance and experimentation, they enjoyed the experience, while Phil and Judy found having observers to be a new source of stimulation for their usual session.

PART IV

PSYCHOLOGICAL DYNAMICS OF D&S

11

Power: Its Use and Meaning

The power exchange is central to every D&S encounter, and those who regularly engage in D&S are highly attuned to the exercise of power in all aspects of their lives. Thus this chapter is devoted to a discussion of the dynamics of power; Chapters 12 and 13 discuss three other hallmarks of D&S activities: pain, eroticism, and fantasy.

THE DYNAMICS OF THE POWER EXCHANGE

For the power exchange to work, the dominant must maintain control. She attains psychological control by exhibiting the traits usually associated with power—by being direct, assertive, and aggressive; taking initiative; and showing confidence and assurance. And she reinforces her power and status by using various dramatic techniques (costuming, lighting, body language), verbal commands, and strategies for physical control (pain, bondage, and humiliation). She acts as though she knows exactly what she wants and does not apologize for making the submissive feel the intended discomfort. If she makes a mistake, she passes over it quickly by briefly acknowledging it or by continuing as if it never happened or was intentional. "Being dominant," Danielle once commented wryly, "is never saying you're sorry."

While some men willingly submit, since they want to be controlled or want to give up their power as a gift to a dominant woman, at times, the male will resist the dominant's exercise of power. He may hold back or rebel because he is truly afraid that she may lose self-control and really hurt him. Or he may be ambivalent about surrendering his power, finding it enticing, yet threatening to his self-image. Some men resist because they enjoy seeing a dominant get angry when her power is challenged, or they hope their resistance will provoke her to "punish" them in a way they like, or they enjoy causing trouble. Still others want to be forced to submit because that eases the guilt they feel in wanting to submit; they can claim "someone made me do it," and needn't fully recognize their own desires. Finally, some resist to test the woman's dominance. Only once she proves her power will they submit. One man explained his frequent spirited resistance this way: "Why should I give up my power? She has to be able to show me she can take it from me, and she has to make it worthwhile for me to give it up."

Such resistance may take the form of talking back, refusing or failing to follow orders, or pretending not to understand the dominant's commands. A woman's response to these challenges depends on her attitudes toward wielding power, her perception of the male's motives, and her feelings about him. She may get angry, feel threatened, or be frustrated. Or she may enjoy playing along, excited by a limited challenge to be overcome. But if the male resists too strongly, many dominants lose interest, since they would rather play with someone more compliant. And some don't want to be challenged at all; they expect the male to submit willingly. Thus, depending on the interplay of her control and his resistance, a session may resemble a hands-down conquest or, at the other extreme, a chess match with the woman playing the offensive.

For most D&Sers, the power exchange, however, is neither a rout nor a battle of wits. It is rather a game with many layers of meaning that enables them to enjoy playing with power, and the game is erotically stimulating because it is not real; for a limited period in a session or in a social interaction based on role reversal, they can assume a new fantasy role. Although the experience is real, it still has a gamelike quality, because the participants are enacting a scenario, assuming a role without the responsibility and burdens of taking on or giving up real power. Then, when it is over, they return to their usual social roles.

Some D&Sers, however, feel that the power exchange is not merely a game or a scenario—that it is authentic. These partners tend, for example, not to use safe words, lest the session seem merely like a game the submissive ultimately controls and can stop by uttering the word. In the absence of a safe word, however, the woman carefully notes the male's responses to make sure he is aroused by his submission, for if he ceases to find the session erotic, she will too.

Couples who carry this power exchange over into everyday life claim this intensifies and authenticates the exchange. Although partners may not extend the exchange into all areas of their lives, they may experiment with power outside the D&S session as a way of experiencing emotional intensity and gaining self-awareness. One woman said, "I feel a flood of feelings when we do this. I feel I'm getting in touch with a more real part of myself." Another woman discovered that "I had this mean part of me I never expressed before. It was a very profound discovery, and it felt freeing to let it out. But if we were just playing I would have never felt that kind of intensity. Instead, I feel a profoundly real release." A man discussed how his intensive exploration with power led him to ask questions like:

"Who am I? What are my boundaries? How far can I open myself up to another person? What is the nature of personal power?"

Such expression of previously repressed feelings like meanness can seem potentially dangerous, and some people would argue that certain antisocial feelings should remain repressed and that the surrender of one's personal freedom to another is distasteful or perverse. Certainly the power exchange can be abused, but in general, the D&Sers who experiment in this way are highly responsible, professional people, with a profound interest in human growth and self-knowledge. They seem able to release these feelings, yield their freedom for a time to a reasonable other, and experience this "real intensity" within safe limits. Yet their exploration raises a host of questions about how far people can safely go in exploring power. At what point does the search for intensity cease to be safe, intense, and fun, and become a personal threat? These value issues are complex, and clearly D&Sers who play this way have answered such questions for themselves, though others might disagree.

LIMITS, POWER, AND CONTROL

The issue of personal limits is a critical one both in the session and in any extensions of the power exchange. Everyone has his or her individual limits, the boundaries between what he or she likes and doesn't like, and how much physical or psychological stimulation he or she can give or take. Though D&Sers usually emphasize knowing and respecting the submissive's limits, because he is the person most vulnerable in a session, dominants have limits, too.

These limits are of two types. Both dominants and submissives have categorical limits—activities they will not perform, such as piercing or golden showers. Also they have limits involving degrees of stimulation—for example, a person may enjoy some pain, but not heavy pain, prolonged pain, or pain that produces a mark lasting more than a few minutes. However, both types of limits change with time and depend on the current situation and mood.

Since the power exchange is usually erotic or satisfying only if the activities are within the participant's limits or just slightly beyond what he or she thinks those limits are, a session can succeed only if partners are aware of one another's limits. As noted earlier, many people discuss their limits before a session, whether they know one another well or not, to learn what each is "up for" at that time.

The question of limits, in turn, raises the question of who is really in control—the submissive or the dominant—a much discussed issue in the D&S community. Theoretically, the dominant is in charge and can do what she wants; but the submissive's limits define how far she should go. Some D&Sers therefore argue that by honoring these limits, as she should, the dominant is, in effect, under the submissive's control. Other D&Sers claim the dominant still maintains control, since within these limits she does what she wants.

Yet the matter is not so simple. While some men think they have certain limits and insist these be respected, others only claim they have limits, but really—either consciously or unconsciously—want the dominant woman to ignore their protests. When she does, they respect her for doing so; but if she yields they think her weak, which undermines her ability to exert her control. Conversely, if a man wants a dominant to adhere to his limits and she does not, other difficulties arise.

Furthermore, limits change over time, sometimes by chance because a dominant pushes a submissive past what he considers a limit or because a submissive persuades a dominant to do something new. For example, Max had been to several mistresses, but had never experienced golden showers and considered the idea "sick." But when he visited a mistress who did it anyway, he found it very exciting and thereafter redefined his limits, praising his mistress who introduced him to this new activity and seeking other women to do it.

D&Sers also value the dynamic tension involved in maneuvering along the edges of a limit, and many claim the pinnacle of erotic excitement is in balancing exactly at these edges, or in trying to go beyond. On one side of the boundary, the stimulation may seem too gentle to be erotic; on the other, it becomes too intense to be pleasurable. The boundary between what is erotic and what is not is a fine line that is always changing. And to extend that boundary is exciting. For the dominant, the excitement comes from finding out how far she can go and how far the male will follow her; this gives her a surge of power. Conversely, the submissive likes testing his own limits, experiencing new sensations, and feeling even more helpless or controlled. For some, surpassing a previous limit is like breaking an athletic record: they are proud of their ability to perform better than expected, and they praise dominants who force them to undertake new personal conquests.

Yet the difference between crossing a boundary to achieve an erotic breakthrough or crossing it to produce a highly unpleasant experience can be subtle indeed. It all depends on the meaning to the participants. For example, when Marvin encouraged Natasha to play out his fantasies of public humiliation, and she enthusiastically complied by handcuffing him to a pole downtown and ordering him to sell garbage in a supermarket parking lot, he felt devastated, since he was doing something to offend the public. But another time, he found public humiliation exhilarating when he and Melody were driving along the freeway in his open sportscar. As they passed several trucks, Melody took down her pants and bent over to lick his crotch, with her bare buttocks in the air. Though this experience involved public humiliation, he found this one erotic, since he felt the truckers would enjoy what he and Melody were doing and possibly be sexually titillated themselves.

Since much of this playing with boundaries involves one person forcing another past his limits, this raises some difficult questions: *Should the dominant try to push the submissive beyond his stated or apparent limits? How far should she go? Does the male really want her to respect his limits? Does he want her to try to push him or force him? And does it matter what he wants?* D&Sers have diverse opinions. Some feel the dominant should always respect the submissive's limits. Others feel she should try to take him beyond if she feels he is willing and feels "the energy" of the session is right, using any appropriate techniques, such as manipulation, teasing, or denial. Still others claim she should satisfy her own desires without worrying about what the submissive wants, for only then will she feel truly dominant, and only then will the submissive get what he really wants and needs—a truly dominant woman. She must at some level consider the submissive's likes and needs, but she should focus on herself.

But if the dominant pushes too far, the submissive will feel his limits have been violated. The erotic excitement vanishes, and he may feel angry or resentful that she has abused his trust. If the stimulus becomes too intense—for example, if a pleasurable pain is too prolonged—or if the dominant forces the submissive to do something he truly doesn't want to do, the session may abruptly end with hostility. Thus, although the exploration of limits can open up new areas of erotic stimulation, it can backfire, as occurred when Danielle enacted a fantasy Jesse described in a fantasy class.

He fantasized having Danielle and Natasha tie up the five men in the class, and Danielle turned his fantasy into a test of limits. She and Natasha ordered the men to undress and stand in a circle, facing outward. Then, they tied them up with clothesline and asked them to sing "She'll Be Coming Round the Mountain" one word at a time as Danielle poked each man in turn with a needle. While most of the men seemed to like this, even making errors so she would "punish" them by making them start the song again, Danielle went too far with Jesse, for as she stepped up the intensity of her pricking, she drew a few drops of blood from him. Later she spoke of her actions in doing so as achieving a breakthrough of limits, since Jesse had previously said he didn't like needles. But Jesse was only playing along with what was happening, because he did not "want to disrupt the game." However, later he felt resentful about being stuck. "She went past my limits," he complained. "And that's not right."

Thus there is a fine line between pushing limits successfully and going too far, which can contribute to the excitement of playing with these edges. To some, such experimentation may seem dangerous or irresponsible, but for many D&Sers, the unknown is thrilling. They see themselves as pioneers, or as one woman commented, "We're like adventurers on a dark continent."

At the same time, there is always a dynamic tension between the formal, overt power of the dominant and the real, but often unstated, power of the submissive to set limits. Each session usually involves some mutual give and take, whereby the dominant exercises power as she wishes, yet attends to the submissive's needs by staying within his stated limits, exploring the edges of his limits, or pushing him beyond.

POWER GAMES IN THE D&S SESSION AND IN EVERYDAY LIFE

Although the session is the primary arena for the power exchange, D&Sers devise games, too, as a framework for exercising and yielding power. For example, SM Church members adapt ordinary relay games to highlight the power of the women and the submissiveness of the men. In one such game, the women give each man a cherry and watch as he bends down and pushes the cherry across the floor with his penis. In another, they divide the males into two teams and each male in turn has to waddle across the room on his knees to a woman who then whips him before he crawls back to his team.

But perhaps more than any other game, the Truth, Dare, or Fantasy game best embodies the power exchange and the rules for exchanging power. Many groups have games that seem metaphors for their lives— Synanon has the Synanon Game, Transactional Analysis has its games of personal interaction—so the D&Sers have theirs, too. In the game, as may be recalled, one player asks another to choose truth, dare, or fantasy. If truth, he or she must answer a question truthfully; if fantasy, he or she must make up a fantasy on a given theme; and if dare, he or she performs as requested, sometimes with others if they are willing to participate. Although simple in structure, the game allows players to act out their relationships, D&S interests, and attitudes toward power.

Most directly, D&Sers use the game to create situations in which they can feel free to be dominant or submissive, and they usually ask questions, suggest topics, or give instructions they think the other players will like. When a game first starts or when people don't know each other well, they usually keep their requests relatively mild and nonthreatening. As the game progresses or if players are friends, the demands are stronger and the dares riskier.

One game began with simple truth and fantasy challenges. When Bertrand chose truth, Danielle innocuously asked, "What was your first fantasy?" "Being captured by Amazon women and being eaten by them," Bertrand replied. When the first players selected "dare," their instructions were similarly mild; Bertrand told Harvey to massage and kiss Danielle's feet. However, as the game continued, the players selected dares more often, and the dare-givers gave them more difficult dares that allowed them to be more dominant or submissive. For instance, Katrina asked Danielle and Harvey to play out a scene in which Danielle, as a circus trainer, made Harvey do tricks, crawl, and stand on his head like an animal. Danielle ordered Luke to crawl after her into the bedroom and lie across the bed; then she rapped him hard with a cane. Later, Luke asked Bertrand, who long had had a fantasy about teachers disciplining him, to lie across Katrina's lap and let her hit him with a ruler. Finally, Danielle asked the three men to take off their clothes and form a pyramid. As instructed, Katrina hit them across their backsides with a crop until the pyramid fell down.

More than just a game, the play reflected the players' relationships to one another. Players generally selected those they already knew to choose one of the three categories, unless someone was obviously being neglected. Also, when a person already knew and trusted the person who selected him, he or she was more apt to take a dare, although a few players, like Harvey, who loved taking chances, almost always chose dare. And dares were usually tailored to the tastes of the players. Since everyone knew Luke liked heavy hitting, they commonly gave him dares to be hit, while they often gave Harvey, who liked showing off and performing, dares to take off his clothes and perform. The unstated rule, in effect, was to respect other players' preferences and limits.

If players do violate these rules about limits, they are typically admonished or sometimes punished later—though usually in a spirit of fun. In one game, for example, Luke dared Danielle to strike Katrina while Katrina lay on the floor. Katrina refused—her prerogative as the second party to a dare, and when Luke later chose a dare from Danielle, she punished him for suggesting that Katrina do something he should have known was unacceptable to her. Danielle ordered him to pull down his pants, and she hit him much harder than he usually liked. "That'll teach you to make suggestions like that," she announced.

D&Sers also play less-structured power games, which represent exercises in psychological one-upmanship. These may occur in a scene, but they can also spill over into everyday life. Although some D&Sers feel that any such games should be played only among consenting players, others enjoy mental power plays with unknowing outsiders. For example, one day Sarona, an occasional mistress and part-time computer student, sensed that a shoe salesman was rather enjoying serving her. As he placed a pair of shoes at her feet for her to put on, she smiled at him coyly and said: "I think I'll need help trying these on." When he bent down to help, she urged him to be more submissive. "I think you'd find it easier if you bent down even more." As he slipped the shoes on her feet, she teased: "Nice to touch, aren't they?" He nodded, so she continued. "I bet you like women's feet. You probably enjoy serving women." He became more agreeable and eager to help, and Sarona thought he was quivering a bit with sexual excitement. As he wrapped her purchases he suggested that maybe they could get together after he got off work. She quickly put him in his place: "Oh, no. I'm busy. But I liked having you *serve* me very much."

PLAYING WITH EVERYDAY SEX ROLES

The D&Sers' interest in playing with power also carries over into everyday life when they play games with conventional sex roles. They experiment both with sex-role reversal and male chivalry to play up the female's power in everyday life. For example, at times, the men show off their chivalry and take over tasks usually performed by women by serving the women with a display of drama that emphasizes their servitude and the honor their service bestows on the woman served. While some men perform such service functions, including taking care of refreshments and clean-up, quite seriously, most seem to play out this chivalrous role with a kind of verve, dramatic flair, and spirit of play, as if they were enacting a scene. In turn, whether the men are serious or playful, the women respond appreciatively and ask the men to do all sorts of tasks and chores. At D&S gatherings, the males actively beseech the women with requests: Would they like a massage? Something to drink? And some make special offers to clean a woman's apartment, do her gardening, or run her errands.

Not surprisingly, the women like this attention, and are delighted to turn over mundane chores to the men. But the men see these mundane tasks as another way of playing with power. Some simply enjoy the satisfaction that come from serving and pleasing the women. Others, at times, feel sexually aroused when they serve, as they feel when they give up power in a session. The D&S code of male chivalry thus reaffirms female power and for some men provides erotic stimulation as well.

POWER IMAGERY AND STORIES

The D&Sers' interest in power also spills over into daily life because they are extremely aware of power imagery and interested in stories about power. They pay attention to the exchange of power in daily interactions, frequently interpret everyday situations in terms of power or see D&S imagery in ordinary events. For example, a visit to a children's playground prompted Danielle to comment on its suitability for D&S play: "There are bars for people to lean over, ropes to hang them from, things to tie people up with. It would be a great place for a party." And a discussion of local politics turned into a verbal game when Lance kidded that a dominant female might make a good mayor: "She could whip the budget into shape, get on the backs of the taxpayers, strike fear into the hearts of the business community, and present a more dominant image by calling meetings of the Board of Supervisors to order with a whip instead of a hammer." In turn, Danielle suggested solving the crime problem by bringing back public flogging and stocks and recommended chain gangs.

D&Sers also look for and discuss power imagery in films, advertising, and the media. When a department store ran a one-page newspaper ad featuring a woman dressed in riding boots and holding a whip, Harvey and Marvin cut it out, passed it around at a party, and later pasted a copy on the wall of the church sanctuary. "Someone in the ad department must be into dominance," Lance kidded.

In a discussion of films, Drew remarked that he liked the scene in Fellini's *City of Women* in which the hero is trapped by hundreds of women in a large warehouse and can't get out, and Lance suggested that some scenes in *Raiders of the Lost Ark* could be viewed from a D&S perspective. "People don't like to admit it," he observed, "but S&M is everywhere. For example, in one scene, Jones takes a bullwhip and whacks his way through a crowd of Arabs; in another he pulls out a gun and quickly knocks off this Arab who has been flipping his saber around to show how tough he is. Then there's that scene where Jones gets locked in a pyramid with hundreds of asps—now that's S&M."

D&Sers similarly enjoy using common words, phrases, and expressions with a double meaning, and sometimes they make plays on words to interject D&S imagery into an otherwise ordinary conversation. For example, when Teddy Roosevelt came up in a conversation, Danielle alluded to his well-known motto but altered it to emphasize its D&S connotations: "You know, Teddy used to say: 'I speak softly and I carry a big *whip*.'" Others joke about dominants being "the cream of the crop" or pun that a friend is busy, because he's *"all tied up"*; or that a student is taking a course because he wants to "learn the ropes."

Usually, they use these expressions among themselves as signs of shared understanding and off-beat wit. But at times they toss such puns at outsiders to see if they pick up the double meaning, which might indicate that these outsiders share an interest in D&S. At the same time, they enjoy chiding and besting outsiders who are naive and do not recognize these subtle clues.

The D&Sers develop their power-related interpretation of the world through their intensive involvement in D&S. At the same time, by seeing D&S power imagery everywhere they validate their involvement. The omnipresence of power imagery suggests that even non-D&Sers are attracted by power, though they may not know it. Thus D&Sers feel they are merely acting out what everyone else is covertly concerned with. Also, by seeing D&S imagery everywhere, D&Sers can gently poke fun at the mainstream society, which frowns on their behavior. Unknowingly, those who view D&S as perverse are themselves involved in some activities— such as humiliating someone in an argument or ordering someone around. But they don't understand the real meaning of their actions and would be shocked if they did; hence they are playing a joke on themselves.

This fascination with nonsexual power is evident in conversations with power themes, too. D&Sers often recount anecdotes in which the teller bested someone who initially seemed to have more power. The women's accounts describe exercising power over both men and women, while the males talk about besting a seemingly more powerful male, or about a woman exercising power over them. The latter stories emphasize the woman's dominance, while the former seem intended to illustrate that even though the male teller is submissive to women, he is still powerful because he exercises power over other men.

In a typical woman's power story, Laura described several instances in which she bested some people at work: "They kept talking about how well they could do the job, and they treated me like I didn't know anything since I was new. But then I showed them I could do it better." And Angela talked about psychologically overpowering someone who had tried to take her parking place: "I just pulled back and glared at her until she agreed to leave." Other stories describe a woman's power over her husband or boyfriend; for instance, Katherine proudly reported that she made her husband and children cook and clean at home: "I never have to do a single thing like that. I let them do all the work."

Marvin's favorite power story concerned one-upping an initially hostile sergeant. When Marvin arrived at an army base to work as an assistant surgeon, he politely asked the sergeant how to go about getting PX and other benefits. "Why should you think you're entitled to that?" the sergeant sneered and motioned Marvin away. But when Marvin returned, now armed with the knowledge that the military rank equivalent to his civilian position was a major, the sergeant's attitude suddenly changed. He snapped to attention, saluted, and announced to Marvin, "Anything you want, sir."

Lance's power story concerned turning a brush-off into personal honor and respect. He wanted to deliver a surveying camera shaped like a blow-gun to a friend in the Coast Guard who usually stopped at a small airport to gas up his plane. To make the arrangements, Lance spoke to the owner of the airport gas station, asking if he could clear an area for the plane's expected arrival. The owner, a cantankerous and unhelpful man, brushed him away. But the following day, when Lance carried his gun-sized camera toward the two arriving Coast Guard and NASA military planes, the owner was impressed and quickly cleared the field.

The next day, Lance had to retrieve the camera and decided to play upon the owner's awe of the military, both to get his cooperation and "show that unhelpful SOB something about power." Sounding as officious as he could, Lance called the owner, announced the call was official, and told him that the Coast Guard plane would arrive at exactly 16:17. One man would bring a large object and the owner should take it, no questions asked, and place it under the counter. Then, someone would come to get it, and he should give it to him immediately. The owner followed these instructions exactly, Lance reported grinning. "He thought I was some kind of powerful official when I came to get it. So he acted with real deference. I wasn't just any Joe off the street."

12

Pain, Bondage, Humiliation, and Other Techniques of Power

M ost D&Sers are fascinated by the psychological dynamics of playing with power, and they use pain, bondage, and other techniques not merely to provide pleasurable physical sensation but also to convey messages about power and control. They are intrigued by the effects of these techniques on the submissive: What does he feel? How is pain transformed into pleasure? What roles do vulnerability and humiliation play? How does the level of communication and trust between partners affect the session? In short—what makes the session *really* work?

D&Sers discuss such topics frequently, and many workshops, classes, and programs are devoted to the psychology of pain, bondage, and humiliation; special techniques like water sports; the dynamics of asserting power; and the value of using costumes and rituals for effect. Let us consider each of these topics in turn.

THE PSYCHOLOGY OF PAIN

When they explore the psychology of pain, D&Sers are especially interested in the transformation of pain into erotic pleasure, and they make a key distinction between the *masochist*, who likes pain for its own sake, and the *submissive*, who enjoys pain because it becomes pleasure; D&Sers are mostly interested in the latter.

They are aware that this transformation is a subjective experience and depends on many factors, including how rested a person feels, whether he feels relaxed or tense, his use of alcohol or drugs, and how he feels about his partner. For example, a tense or tired submissive can't take as much pain. Likewise, teasing and fear can intensify the transformation of pain into pleasure if the teasing or fear-provoking actions are accompanied by trust. As Patricia, who has been involved with D&S for 15 years, explained at a workshop, "If you trust someone, she can make you afraid of what's happening, and that's erotic, since fear heightens the breathing and the adrenalin. But without trust, there's terror. And terror turns you off, because it freezes the adrenalin."

Good communication is also vital, particularly in a session involving pain. Each person must be able to express his or her needs, wants, and limits, and the partners must make sure they have a similar or complementary purpose in the session. "People seek pain for various reasons," Patricia said. "Service, surrender, the desire to prove oneself, punishment, catharsis, heightening sensitivity, opening up psychically. But if you have conflicting purposes—say the other person wants to experience a catharsis, and you're trying to punish him—the session is not going to work."

As noted in earlier chapters, most D&Sers informally discuss their desires, limits, and expectations before a session. Also, the dominant looks for clues to how much the submissive wants or can take. Experienced dominants notice how tense or relaxed their partners are, and some observe breathing, pulse, body temperature, and other signs. One explained: "If a man is erotically aroused, he has accelerated breathing, a faster pulse, a higher body temperature, a flushed look. And you can check these signs subtly. For example, I check the pulse points in the neck or groin as part of a caress."

D&Sers have various strategies for getting themselves or their partners in the mood for a session. For example, some dominants think about what they will do while they engage in a preparatory ritual, such as laying out restraints and putting candles around the room. Or they visualize themselves in the session as they put on their costumes. Some give their submissive partners instructions on how to get ready, such as taking a bath or undressing. And some use signals to indicate they are ready, such as putting out a collar for their partner to put on when he is ready.

As the session begins, most dominants simply increase the pain they administer, gradually arousing the submissive so he can take more intense sensations. One woman explained, "I use lots of ritual in the beginning to build up gradually. For instance, I put on the collar; I slowly put on restraints; and I verbalize the dynamic behind what's happening, such as, 'You belong to me.'" Other dominants seek feedback to understand how the submissive feels now. Some use conversation to dramatize what they are doing. As one woman observed, in a general discussion of pain techniques, "When I'm punishing them, I talk punishment. When I'm doing something to humiliate them, I talk about that." But at times, some dominants like to use silence to intensify the submissive's experience. "It can help the bottom focus," one said.

Those involved in pain are also very aware of different pain sensations—such as the steady pain of a clothespin, the intermittent pain of dripping wax, the sharp pain of a needle, and the dull pain of a strap—and further distinguish pain sensations as fast or slow, random or patterned, rhythmical or occasional, expected or surprising. They agree that pain must be controlled, for accidental, unexpected pain—such as stubbing a toe—is not erotic. Thus they try to avoid such pain in a session; stepping on a person's toe when he is in bondage or leaving him too long in one position are unexciting and unerotic. When these accidents happen, some dominants acknowledge the pain, for as one claimed, "The submissive continues to trust you, so the accidental pain doesn't kill the scene." But others ignore it, such as Bridget, who said: "I claim I did it on purpose. That way they don't think I'm clumsy and lose respect."

To control the session, some D&Sers designate "safe words" that the submissive is to use if he really wants to stop. The submissive can then plead for mercy as part of the scene, and the dominant will know if his entreaties are real or just part of the play. Otherwise, the scene may end when the submissive really doesn't want that to happen, as occurred when one mostly dominant woman was playing submissive. She hadn't checked out safe words with the man who was caning her. When they started playing a school game, she began pleading: "Oh, please, sir. No. Don't do it." Like many D&Sers, she only wanted to feign resistance, to have the dominant punish her and force her to do things. But he thought her resistance was real and stopped. However, other dominants, like Kat, don't use a safe word because it detracts from the dominant's position of power. "The dominant should be sensitive enough to feel the energy of the session," Kat said.

While more experienced dominants may develop this sensitivity about how much pain to give, many newly dominant women don't feel comfortable giving pain. They fear hurting the man and hold back or apologize when they hit him, thereby undercutting their power and making the session less erotic.

To help them, D&Sers may informally reassure them, and some D&S groups use special techniques. For example, the SM Church devised a technique called the Circle of Fear. The novice places her foot inside an imaginary circle drawn on the floor and as long as she holds it there another woman administers pain to a submissive. The rationale behind this technique, Lance explained, is that "it removes the actual act of giving pain from the dominant. Instead, someone else gives it at her command as long as she holds her foot in the circle. So the woman feels tremendous support for what she is doing and realizes she has that power."

This technique led to a breakthrough for Melody when she was first learning to be dominant. Although Melody knew Marvin liked pain, each time she hit him she wanted to apologize and often did. But her apologies undercut her dominance and destroyed the eroticism of the session. Thus Lance organized a Circle of Fear for her. As he instructed, Melody sat down and imagined a six-foot imaginary circle in front of her. Marvin lay at her feet, she put her foot in the circle, and Danielle hit him again and again. Soon Marvin began pleading, but Melody kept her foot there. Since she felt the support of the group and since Danielle was hitting him, she felt less responsible and as an observer could see that Marvin was enjoying it despite his pleas to stop. So she kept her foot firmly planted in the circle, until the doorbell rang. The technique worked, for Melody stopped apologizing, and Marvin praised her: "She can really give pain."

THE PSYCHOLOGY OF BONDAGE

D&Sers view bondage as a physical sign to the submissive that he is under the dominant's control. To the extent that he can't move or escape, he is vulnerable to the dominant's desires. D&Sers feel that bondage is an especially important means for the female dominant to experience power and for the male to feel vulnerable and helpless, because usually the male is stronger than the female. But when he is bound, the female has the physical superiority; since he can't overpower her, he might as well just relax and be receptive. Though D&Sers often use bondage in conjunction with pain to make the male even more helpless and vulnerable, they use it alone, as well, to make the submissive experience his helplessness and become more aware of physical sensations including the functions and motions of the body. They may leave the bonds on for an extended period, perhaps a few hours or more, or combine bondage with a blindfold or hood. Such sensory deprivation further intensifies the experience.

D&Sers also report a "rebound effect" when someone is released from bondage and the restricted sensations come flooding back. The submissive feels so grateful to the dominant for freeing him and giving him back his faculties that he is more willing to submit to her power just as some males feel gratefully submissive when a woman stops hitting them. Another common practice further emphasizes the dominant's power: when a group practices bondage, only the dominant who originally tied the submissive should release him.

D&Sers are concerned with specific techniques of bondage, such as various types of knots and bondage positions. Thus many D&S programs are devoted to demonstrating how to tie a square knot, granny knot, and slip knot, or novel ways to restrain a person. For example, Danielle concluded one class by tying Luke in a classic hog-tie position, with his arms and legs hooked together behind his back. But most discussions and demonstrations of bondage also deal with the psychological effects of bondage, particularly its influence on feelings of power. For instance, in the same class Danielle described how helpless Luke felt and then discussed the psychological effects of different types of materials: "Even thread can have a powerful psychological effect, because the person who's tied has to be careful, or it will break, and if it does, you can punish him. So he has to be especially cautious and still—and he's doing it to himself." And certain positions make the male feel especially helpless. "Try having him kneel down," she advised, directing Harvey to do so. "Then if you tie his hands and legs behind his back and tie a rope around his cock and up to his head, he can't lift his head. And that's a powerful reminder of your power. He has to keep his head and eyes down."

Danielle also suggested using props to increase the male's helplessness and vulnerability. As examples, she had Harvey bend over a chair and snapped some ropes around him; then she strapped him to a couch, so he couldn't move; and finally she tied his arms and feet behind his back to a broom, an especially awkward position. Bondage, she explained, could be used as a punishment or a reward: "It depends on how long you keep it on, how tight you tie it, whether the submissive likes it. And, of course, you can combine it with pleasurable and not so pleasurable pain."

This psychological component of bondage was strongly emphasized in Sharon and Lance's demonstration of using chains and iron shackles. First, Sharon showed how she usually wrapped cold metal chains around Lance's chest and waist, snapped heavy irons on his ankles, and tied thick army-style belts around his arms and chest, so he looked like a mummy. After she removed them, Lance explained that he liked "the really heavy psychological impact of the metal. They're the ultimate in bondage. You can cut ropes to get out of them. But the chains are there. They're solid and strong. There's no way to get out."

Also, they found erotic the imagery and symbolism of the chains. Besides being cold and hard, the chains had to be locked into place, which, as Sharon asserted, "is an immediate, direct statement of the dominant's power." The chains and other metal restraints evoked powerful fantasies, with handcuffs suggesting kidnap scenarios, and irons and chains prompting slavery imagery. "When you're in chains, you can identify with the absolute degradation, humiliation, vulnerability, and helplessness of the slave throughout history," Lance said. "And the dominant can imagine herself the all-powerful master," Sharon added. Also, the clanking noise intensified the experience, "because it's a mark of shame. It's a constant reminder the wearer is a slave." Sometimes Sharon punished Lance by putting the chains in the freezer before she put them on or by pretending the keys were lost. "Then he feels the harsh coldness of the metal or feels he'll never get out. Now *that* has real psychological impact." Of course, she always made sure she had the key, since losing one meant having to call a locksmith or the police.

D&Sers also find an aesthetic in bondage and in pain, and they enjoy watching experienced dominants at work. In a typical demonstration,

Diana showed how she did spider bondage; using Marvin as a volunteer, she wove a weblike interlacing of ropes around his torso. A few months later, the Society of Janus sponsored a bondage contest, in which a half-dozen contestants showed off their skill. One woman came away with the best of show for strapping a man in black leather briefs, harnessing him to a large wood rack, and weaving a spider web of ropes around him.

But perhaps the most dramatic presentation of aesthetic bondage occurred at a Janus meeting when Fakir Musafar, widely known in the D&S community for his interests in piercing, sensory deprivation, and body transformations, showed how he used bondage to create extreme sensory deprivation that resulted in an altered, trancelike, out-of-body state. He passed around photographs of people tied up in very restrictive bondage—in mummy bags, bound tightly all over with string, or wrapped up like packages—and demonstrated several blindfolds, helmets, and hoods. He then asked for a few volunteers. He wrapped a man in an ace bandage face mask and suspended a woman from a large wood frame called a "witches' cradle." While the man in the mask sat quietly, merely breathing in and out of a thin straw, Fakir turned the crank on the cradle, so that he rotated the woman in a full circle from a position prone on her back to standing upright to hanging upside down and back to her original position. To describe the sensations this extreme form of bondage could produce, he said: "A great release.... You get a feeling of surrender.... You can feel renewed at the end."

Few in the audience would use these intense techniques. Yet they found it fascinating to learn about such extremes. Fakir went much further than most community members were willing to go in exploring the ultimate in bondage and restraint. But they admired his ability to explore these psychological depths, just as any hobbyist or sportsman might admire—though not intend to duplicate—the feats of a professional or champion.

THE APPEAL OF HUMILIATION

Physical or mental humiliation appeals to many D&Sers for various reasons, though what is erotic for some is not for others. For example, some men find cross-dressing so humiliating that they won't do it; others dress because they find the humiliation erotic; and still others do not find dressing humiliating—rather they enjoy expressing their submission and femininity. But all those who like humiliation, whatever its form, find it exciting because it intensifies the power exchange by emphasizing who has the power and who must submit.

As with pain and bondage, the externals of humiliation are designed to evoke an inner experience—either feelings of power or feelings of submission. Still D&Sers frequently talk about specific techniques, which may be physical—such as performing demeaning tasks, dressing in a degrading way, or being punished by a whip—or mostly verbal, involving insults, begging, and mind games that denigrate the submissive. Some D&Sers prefer the physical approach, some like the verbal, and others enjoy both.

Submissives often enjoy swapping stories about humiliating experiences. For example, at one small informal gathering, some of the humiliating experiences different men mentioned were: "being put in restrictive bondage, licking someone's boots, being required to plead or beg, being forced to cross-dress, being chained up and made to serve everyone, having someone come over and pull down my pants." But not everyone found the same things humiliating or erotic. For example, Lance adamantly announced that he hated cross-dressing, found it humiliating, and always refused to do it. But Lester found it erotic: "I like the feminine feeling of the clothes. But I also like to be forced to wear them, and even taken out in public. So that makes it humiliating to wear them." In contrast, Baby Robin didn't find dressing-up humiliating at all. He loved to dress: "I'm an exhibitionist. I love the attention. It's fun, like part of a game."

To make the session work, the dominant has to understand the submissive's definition of what kinds of humiliation are erotic. Otherwise, the submissive may refuse to participate, dismissing the activity as foolish, or he may go along but without erotic satisfaction.

WATER SPORTS AND OTHER SPECIALTY INTERESTS

Though D&Sers are most commonly interested in pain, bondage, and humiliation, many D&Sers have special interests in other power-exchange techniques and their psychological effects. Such interests include infantilism, exhibitionism, fetishes, cross-dressing for reasons other than humiliation, among many others. These activities are not necessarily, though often, linked to dominance and submission. The most popular specialty interests related to dominance and submission are "water sports": urination ("golden showers") and enemas. Many D&Sers avoid these activities, finding them too clinical or offensive. But some find the physical sensations erotic, enjoying the warmth of the urine in a golden shower or the heavy pressure on the gut in an enema, while others are attracted by these activities' symbolic meanings. For example, a submissive may view being urinated on as the ultimate degradation, a sign of complete enslavement.

But whether primarily concerned with the physical sensation or psychological effects, participants are extremely interested in technique, and they are quite serious, though outsiders may find such activities particularly bizarre, even ridiculous and disgusting. For example, at one SM Church class, enthusiasts shared tips on effective water sport techniques: "Don't eat asparagus beforehand. It makes the urine bitter"; "Try making the urine last as long as possible by using muscle control to slow down the flow"; "Experiment with starting and stopping the flow to add an element of surprise, or direct it to different body areas." Some talked about how they liked to drink urine. "It's really very sterile because of the acidic content," Harvey said. "You can even clean surgical instruments with it." And Danielle suggested, "You can direct the flow to draw pictures on a person's body when you're good enough."

When D&Sers use golden showers in a scene they usually create a long fantasy to build up to the urination, since it is such a brief climax. Thus a dominant may threaten to do it as a punishment ("If you don't perform well, I'll piss on you") or as a reward ("If you're good, I'll give you some of my very special golden nectars"). In turn, the submissive may experience it as a punishment that humiliates and degrades him or as a reward that brings him closer to the dominant. As one male explained: "One pleasure is to hold it in my mouth as long as possible and imagine that part of my mistress is in me."

Some dominants tease or threaten, but don't actually give golden showers, since neither they nor the male likes it. But their teasing or threatening emphasizes their power and the submissive's subservience and helplessness. "I told a male I was playing with I planned to pee on him," one dominant woman said. "He wasn't into it, but I threatened him with it. Then, after I blindfolded him, I poured a glass of warm water over him. And he still thinks I peed all over him," she laughed.

Though a minority of D&Sers are aroused by enemas, they are a vocal group and swap "recipes" like gourmet cooks. The most basic liquid for an enema is plain warm water, but different ingredients produce various sensations and the amount of liquid administered can make for a pleasurable, rewarding experience or an uncomfortable, punishing one. For instance, some enema fans like coffee enemas as a stimulant and some consider beer and wine enemas very relaxing. One enthusiast favors Perrier water: "That's really fun. The water bubbles and fizzes as it goes in." But they avoid using hard liquor, which can burn the lining of the colon, though they favor glycerine for a "punishment enema," because no one can hold it in for more than a few minutes.

Since enemas require a fair amount of preparation and must be given near a bathroom, they are rarely used in impromptu scenes and are reserved for the end of a session as a punishment or reward. But occasionally they are given as a surprise show of power, as occurred at one SM Church "insane asylum" party to which the men came as inmates and the women as nurses. When Jemma, a male transvestite, arrived dressed as a nurse, Danielle and Devora decided to put "her" in her place. They invited her upstairs, locked the door, and told her: "We can't have inmates like you pretending they are nurses." Then, to "punish" her, they grappled her down on a table and gave her a wine enema. Jemma playfully resisted at first, and then relaxed to experience the brief high of the wine.

COSTUMES

D&Sers use costumes to create the appropriate atmosphere for a scene and to emphasize the power differential. Typically, the dominant woman remains dressed for most or all of the session, while the male wears little or nothing. Some dominants require the male to strip or to dress in a costume that signifies his low position, such as a maid's outfit or baby clothes.

Conversely, the woman chooses costumes to play up her power. Black leather, stockings, and heels are a standard costume, while robes and uniforms express authority, warrior costumes suggest physical superiority, fancy costumes allude to wealth and status, and sexually revealing costumes convey sexual power. Also, dominants select colors that represent strength or force (black), are aggressively stimulating (red), or suggest royalty and wealth (purple). Appropriate accessories include arm or wrist bands with studs, metal belts, small dangling chains, and necklaces with dominant symbols like high heels. Yet this tough, strong image is made seductively feminine by costumes that reveal or accentuate the woman's contours: dresses with plunging necklines, tight sweaters, clinging pants, and sheer, revealing gowns.

While some dominants confine this sort of costume to sessions, many dress this way at D&S gatherings. In response, some submissive males act especially servile to a woman dressed to look dominant, as if her dominant apparel evoked a submissive response. These males not only appreciatively compliment a dominant's apparel, but some respond with flamboyant gestures to demonstrate submission: they take her hand and engage in prolonged hand kissing; they dramatically offer to serve her, asking, "Oh, mistress, what may I get you?"; and some even drop to their knees to kiss her feet. Such responses further increase the dominant's feeling of power.

In contrast, when a dominant appears in ordinary street clothing, men generally just say hello or greet her with a brief hug or kiss of the hand. And they may urge her to dress more dominantly. But dominants don't dress up only because men like it; rather, they enjoy the symbolic power that comes with putting on the costume. As Danielle once explained it: "Suppose a woman comes to a party. She's wearing her normal straight clothes and has her costume in her bag. Then she goes into the bathroom and changes. When she comes out, she has become someone new. She can feel it. She's a new being, and others can feel it, too."

RITUALS

To D&Sers, the entire D&S scenario forms a kind of ritual, consisting of rules, techniques, and imagery, and is much like a play in which the submissive is the actor and the dominant the director. Like a play, a ritual can range from a simple, informal, often impromptu dialogue to an elaborately staged scenario with many roles, props, and a complicated script. And as actors and directors do, D&Sers frequently discuss what works or doesn't work, and why.

Rituals are often based on relationships between an authoritarian figure and a powerless one: master and slave, teacher and student, nurse and patient. For example, at one SM Church party, Winnie, age 30, a psychology graduate student who attended a few get-togethers, came dressed as a police officer, and led in Luke, dressed as a prisoner in a heavy slave collar, washed-out blue tunic, and jeans. For the first hour or so, they played guard and prisoner. Winnie ordered Luke about as if he were on the chain gang, and when he failed to comply—which was often because he enjoyed "being bad"—she thrashed him with her crop. Then, hanging onto his chain, she led him to a corner hamburger stand and joked casually with the startled patrons, assuring them: "Oh, yes, he is my prisoner." Back at the party, Winnie removed her hat and detached Luke's chain, signifying the scenario was over.

In an SM Church class on rituals, Danielle talked about how to use key ritual elements—such as candles, incense, low lighting, music, and costume—to set the mood, and how to effectively incorporate other dramatic techniques, such as gesture, sound, and body position. To illustrate, she directed a brief ceremony of submission. After setting up the room with candles and incense to give it a subdued churchlike feeling, she sat on a red velvet couch and commanded Harvey, Bertrand, and Brent, who were naked, to crawl up to the altar in turn and bring her a designated object from it—a whip, cup of wine, pipe with marijuana, and two balls of string. The men were to kneel before the altar when they picked up the object, crawl along the floor on their knees, and bow before her when they handed it over. She used each object to further emphasize their submission. For example, she tied a piece of string around each man's neck and struck each male with the whip, announcing: "I will now purify you. With this whip, I purify your body. I purify your soul." She concluded the ritual by removing the string.

Such rituals, particularly those with complex elements of drama and pageantry, serve to highlight the power exchange and thereby make it a more intense, exciting experience.

13

Eroticism and Fantasy

D&Sers are extremely interested in eroticism and fantasy, not only within the D&S encounter but in all aspects of life. They frequently discuss sexual and erotic topics, often perceive sexual themes in everyday events, and share sexual and erotic fantasies. This chapter focuses on D&Sers' predilections for eroticism and fantasy within both a session and everyday life.

SEX AND EROTICISM

Whereas most adults equate sex with sexual intercourse or consider intercourse to be the goal of sex play, D&Sers view intercourse as only one aspect of eroticism: a satisfying D&S interchange need not include sexual intercourse. Similarly, while most adults consider orgasm essential to sexual enjoyment, D&Sers feel erotic activity may be fulfilling without it—in fact, some consciously postpone or avoid orgasm to prolong their erotic arousal; one D&Ser jokingly calls orgasm "the big bang theory of American sexuality." Thus D&S activity is erotic and involves some fantasy role play or a power exchange, while straight, or "vanilla," sex does not have these elements and includes ordinary penetration or orgasm.

D&Sers carefully distinguish between these two types of sex, sometimes engaging in D&S as foreplay leading to sexual penetration or orgasm, but other times playing with D&S alone because they find it erotic and exciting in itself. One man explained: "When I engage in straight sex, that's one thing. Then, foreplay leads to intercourse. But I consider erotic dominance and submission something else—and not just foreplay. For me, it becomes the main event." Another man said: "If sex happens, fine. It can be foreplay for sex. But I enjoy S&M for itself, and I don't necessarily expect sex."

D&Sers tend to have a casual, relaxed attitude toward sex because they don't feel the pressure to perform through orgasm or intercourse, unlike many non-D&Sers who consider the sex act unsuccessful if neither occurs. Frequently, whether sexual intercourse occurs depends on the closeness of the relationship. If the partners don't have a close friendship, many men don't expect D&S play to conclude with intercourse, and many women choose not to have it. Certainly, some men may still hope for intercourse, though a minority may not want it without real intimacy. But in either case, the dominant woman sets the rules, and the male expects to follow.

Some D&Sers feel that penetration undermines the woman's dominance, by making her a submissive recipient. They hold that even if the dominant woman decides how, when, where, and if sex will happen, penetration contradicts her dominant power. For this reason, some dominant women prefer to achieve orgasm through oral satisfaction, with the male below them in a subservient position. Other women allow penetration, but only in a close relationship. Many submissive men understand this dynamic and thus don't expect sex from a dominant woman they are not close to. As one male explained it: "In a session, I see the dominant woman as far superior to me and place her on a pedestal. But if we had intercourse, that would equalize the relationship. So I don't feel it appropriate to presume that a mistress should have sex with me. I only expect it in my primary relationship."

Thus D&S activity frequently occurs apart from sexual intercourse, more so for some individuals than others. For example, one man who played around extensively said that "maybe 3 to 4 percent of the time, a session will end up in intercourse." A man living with a woman reported that "perhaps 75 percent of the time we simply play without experiencing orgasm or intercourse." Others have orgasm or intercourse more often; some prefer cunnilingus to intercourse.

As noted in earlier chapters, the range of activities that D&Sers find erotic is broad. Even imagery alone can produce erotic feelings, as one man reported: "Dominance is always sexual for me by itself. As soon as I get undressed or put on chains, it converts immediately into something erotic. I experience an erotic charge and get excited." Because the session is intended to be erotic, D&Sers attempt to prolong the plateau of excitement, and this process—rather than orgasm—is the focus. In turn, by focusing on intensifying and lengthening this process, rather than concentrating on the intense but quick orgasm, D&Sers feel they make sexual activity more exciting and creative.

Further, by differentiating between erotic play and sexual intercourse, some D&Sers feel free to play and experiment with a number of partners, while reserving intercourse for special relationships. One woman who played with many partners explained it thus: "How I play depends on how I feel personally about someone. I can play with almost anyone, because sex isn't necessarily defined by the physical orgasm. For me to want intercourse, there has to be some special sexual stimulation; I have to be turned on by some special chemistry. And in a session, I have that choice." Similarly, couples like Herman and June play with others, but reserve the intimacy of intercourse for themselves.

Some dominant women withhold sexual intimacy from certain submissives during D&S play so as to leave them highly aroused for their primary partners. One woman who played with several married men did not have intercourse with them not only because she did not feel like it but also because she wanted them to be very excited when they went home to see their wives. "It's like the session hasn't stopped," she explained. "I'll give him orders to do certain things to his wife. So he's still doing the session in his mind when he gets home. He hasn't experienced orgasm yet, so it's still going on. Then, he can reach the peak of the excitement with his wife."

Most D&Sers continue to engage in straight sex apart from their D&S activity, sometimes with the same partner, sometimes with another. But some D&Sers drop straight sex by itself, because they have grown to like D&S so much, as did one woman who said: "I can have dominance without sex, though it's not as good without it; but I can't have sex without dominance anymore. A scene without sex is still enjoyable, because it becomes a kind of mental orgasm. Then sex makes it more intense and dynamic, because it's both mental and physical. But if it's vanilla sex alone—I find that very boring."

Other D&Sers claim that the sexual release they experience through D&S is qualitatively different and more satisfying than straight sex, that D&S offers a stronger, more intense release, even without intercourse. So they feel a need for D&S at times even though they may still participate in straight sex. As one man described it: "After the intensity of D&S, I feel a satisfaction, a wholeness, a kind of relief. I can have an orgasm and an ejaculation in straight sex, and it can be just physical. And there are degrees of satisfaction. But if there is S&M play before it, afterwards, I feel more relaxed. I have a complete feeling after orgasm. With regular sex I can still be tense after ejaculation. But when it's S&M sex, there's no tension afterwards."

A woman said she felt more relaxed after D&S because "D&S is more stimulating, so it builds up more tension, which leads to a more cathartic release." This powerful cathartic effect was described thus by one man: "It involves the totality of my being. After an S&M session, I won't think about sex at all for a few days, because I have been fully satisfied. But after regular sex, I think about sex all the time."

This high level of interest in eroticism carries over into everyday life, as D&Sers frequently talk about sex-related matters, tell jokes about sex, and engage in much sexual banter in both formal and informal gatherings. This fascination with eroticism is also embodied in dominants' costumes, which emphasize the woman as a desirable sexual object. Certainly, D&Sers talk about and do ordinary things as well, such as going to movies, discussing the news, and chatting about everyday trivia. But compared to other groups of people, their focus on sexuality is especially strong.

Often, for example, they reminisce about unusual sexual experiences. At one informal gathering of several SM Church regulars, the conversation turned to childhood erotic encounters. Luke reported having sex in a pulpit after a church service. Danielle described rolling around with some friends under the pews and finding it exciting because: "You're not supposed to have forbidden thoughts at church." Brent mused about the first time he was erotically aroused climbing a pole as a child. Even conversations about current events may include a sexual or D&S interpretation. After one SM Church meeting, Lance fantasized about how Patty Hearst must have enjoyed her capture: "She was tied up in the closet and then suspended in the basement. And then she probably said: 'Oh, please, do anything to me. Tie me up, put me in the closet, suspend me. Do anything you want.' Her adventure must have been a terrific fantasy. Probably better than one could ever imagine."

They also share countless sex jokes. For instance, after Bertrand, who was in his 70s, appeared at a party with a much younger woman, Harvey told some friends this reminded him of a joke about a woman of 80 dating a man of 20. "People tell her," he said, "that it's a more unusual relationship than a man of 80 going with a woman of 20. But she says she has an easier time of it. After all," Harvey grinned, "we learned in math class that 20 goes into 80 much better than 80 goes into 20." Another time, when Harvey was kidding Marvin about being bisexual, he quipped: "You must really be trisexual. That means you'll try anything." "And if you're quad-sexual, that means you'll do it in every way," Danielle suggested. "Or do it in a wheelchair," Brent put in.

Frequently, too, D&Sers develop and talk about ideas for products and services involving D&S and sex. At one informal get-together, Drew joked about how he and Diana had an S&M doll that came with its own kit of toys. "It works like this," he said. "If you squeeze it a certain way, you can get it to grow breasts. Also, it comes with a dildo you can stick up the ass. And a rod inside makes the penis become erect."

Likewise, the D&Sers often discuss the sexuality they observe in films, books, sporting events, and the like. And commonly they tease each other with sexual byplay, usually tinged with D&S overtones. For instance, before a fantasy class, Sharon suddenly pounced on Harvey, started tickling him, and invited Marvin and Jesse to join in. Another time, at the beginning of a bondage demonstration, Jesse playfully threw a rope around Natasha and grabbed her around the neck. And when Katrina appeared at a fantasy class wearing a red jumpsuit with a long black zipper, Jesse tugged on it and pretended to pull it down.

THE PERVASIVENESS OF FANTASY

The D&S community supports and encourages members to discuss and express their fantasies. D&Sers not only share long-held fantasies—many of which have long been sources of guilt, shame, or confusion for their holders—but also create and enact others. They tend to develop a fantasy perspective for viewing the world, frequently talking about fantasies and seeing everyday events as stimuli for new fantasy scenarios. D&Sers distinguish between pure fantasy, partially realized fantasy, and reality, and recognize a continuum of fantasy and reality that allows everyday mundane existence to become the stuff of fantasy. Also, a fantasy can be so intense that it seems quite real, while a real-life experience may at times take on a dreamlike did-it-really-happen quality.

D&Sers are also sensitive to the complex relationship between fantasies and sexual feelings, whereby fantasy can generate sexual arousal and sexual interest can inspire fantasies. Sometimes enacting a fantasy destroys its original sexual allure; other times, the enactment intensifies the fantasy's erotic attraction. For some fantasies retain their power only as long as they remain fantasies; once enacted, they lose their power because the imagination has been satisfied. Other fantasies become even stronger once enacted, and the person longs to repeat the enactment. At times, a person may find his experience of the fantasy contrary to his expectations and entirely lose interest in that fantasy. Or he may continue to enjoy it as a fantasy but not want to reenact it.

D&Sers also realize that some fantasies should remain just that—a form of imaginative escape that one cannot, should not, or best not attempt to enact. Taboo or bizarre fantasies of intense pain, extremely embarrassing humiliation, or male castration may be erotic, because they are so forbidden and strange, and hence an escape from the ordinary. But they are not to be taken seriously, because of their severe consequences.

It is not always clear which fantasies fall into which categories, since tastes are so variable at different times. But most dominant women understand such distinctions and know that not all of the submissive's expressed fantasies should be enacted. So they use common sense to avoid enacting overly severe and dangerous fantasies, and they look for physical cues that indicate whether the male is aroused by enacting the fantasy and whether he has reached his limits.

Finally, D&Sers are aware that the context greatly affects how much they enjoy thinking about or enacting a fantasy. They may enjoy sharing or enacting a fantasy with one person but not with another, or at one time but not another. The power of fantasy to create an erotic experience depends on the psychological meaning each person attributes to that fantasy, which reflects his or her individual psyche, background, and experience.

Besides playing out their fantasies in sessions, some D&Sers keep fantasy journals, which they use to record ideas. And some dominant women ask their partners to keep such a journal, so they can read it to discuss their partners' fantasies and then enact them or not.

D&sers also frequently discuss fantasies they might like to stage, and often they enjoy such talks even if they have no intention of enacting the fantasy, or the fantasy would be unrealistic to stage. For instance, at several D&S parties and gatherings, Angela described her fantasy of having a nude man clean up her apartment while another was tied up under the table. Brent and Alvin repeatedly urged her to call them because they would love to do it. But she never did, since she preferred imagining the scene. Similarly, Lance often talked about his vision of a live-in community of slaves and mistresses he called Eden II, where people would come for a few days, a weekend, even several weeks or months. But it always remained just that—an enticing fantasy.

Also, at times, fantasy and reality may become so mixed that D&Sers try to actually achieve near fantasy goals. For instance, Lance and Sharon carried on a search for many months for a grand estate or abandoned factory to house the SM Church in style on the off-chance the owner might be having tax troubles and be interested in using the Church as a tax shelter. And often they fantasized about the gala parties and celebrations they would have when they moved in. But the probabilities were against them, and they finally moved into an ordinary storefront downtown.

Besides conversations and fantasy journals, many D&Sers express their fantasies through various creative forms such as poems, essays, stories, plays, and books or by devising toys, games, and rituals around D&S themes. The themes of these creative outpourings include the satisfactions of male slavery or servitude and the superiority of the powerful female. Many of these works describe the woman as a goddess or priestess whose cruel acts delight her submissive slave or teach him his proper place in the natural order. For instance, one male rhapsodized about the joy of being kept as a total slave in this poem:

> She caged him in a corner box,
> Kept him tied to a leather
> Leash attached to a bracket
> On the wall that ran firmly
> From the buttocks to the balls
> Then called him most tenderly
> Like a bird until
> He danced the dance of joy to
> Her cruel stinging whip...

Another male argued for recognizing the female sex as superior because the reign of women would bring back a Golden Age of peace, which occurred once long ago when women ruled the earth. And some women write fantasy stories about disciplining slaves or presiding over a slave community.

Other works are autobiographical writings that make a serious effort at self-analysis to explain the writer's feelings about D&S. For example, Kat wrote a book about the experiences she and Mouse had when first exploring D&S, and a man who occasionally attended SM Church services wrote a book about his 20 years of experiences with mistresses.

Other personal accounts include a large element of fantasy. Marvin wrote a one-act play that combined his confused feelings when his wife was seeing another man and his fantasies about castration. Both in reality and in the play, he encouraged his wife to see this man, because he was titillated by the humiliation of being a cuckold and found sex with his wife more exciting as a result. He concluded the play by having his wife and lover tie him up and castrate him, which gave him the most intense erection and ejaculation. But afterwards the lover-surgeon sneers at him: "That's the last orgasm you'll ever have."

Other D&Sers turn to the visual arts, drawing images of dominant females—often garbed like priestesses, goddesses, or warriors—overpowering humble submissive males. Some take photographs of themselves or others involved in D&S activity or wearing D&S costumes. Others make films or design D&S games. The elaborate rituals of the SM Church are another form of creative expression, as is the interest of D&Sers in all sorts of costuming and paraphernalia. In addition to the usual D&S garb, some D&Sers wear T-shirts with sayings like: "Never underestimate the power of a woman," and "The Goddess is coming, and man is she pissed!" Also, many collect cartoons and postcards with D&S imagery, dress and display dolls that look like dominant women and submissive men, and decorate their rooms with all sorts of D&S icons, statues, and pictures. The more daring put bumper-stickers with D&S slogans on their cars.

Fantasy is also a framework for organized activity in the D&S community, the starting point for parties, large group rituals, and games. And many of the SM Church's classes are devoted to sharing and enacting fantasies, often with sexual or D&S themes. In guided fantasy meditations, Danielle would ask participants to close their eyes and lie on the floor if they wished. Then she would guide them on a fantasy journey.

In one session, Danielle asked everyone to imagine walking through a meadow into a forest and along a path to a house. Inside was a box to be opened. Though her imagery was neutral, it evoked a D&S scene for several participants, including Harvey, who saw a small gold box and just above it some whips and chains on the wall. In another class, Danielle began an open-ended fantasy story about a man walking along a beach and encountering another person and asked each person to continue the story in turn. The others soon turned it into a D&S adventure, in which the man goes into a cave where he hears women chanting. Then they surround him, tie him up, and poke him with sticks and stones.

On other occasions, D&Sers play fantasy games. One of the most common is the Truth, Dare, and Fantasy game, but others include *Slave Community*, a board game Danielle developed. In the game, the males are slaves trying to work their way up from the field to the kitchen to the house and finally to being the women's pleasure slaves, while the women are mistresses who want to acquire more slaves to do their command. Players throw the dice to move around the board and draw "action cards" instructing them to do something, usually involving another player. For instance, a card from the slave-owner pile instructs a woman to "choose any slave and have him massage your feet," while a card from the slave pile instructs a man to: "get some ropes and tie yourself up."

Light drug use, music, and candlelight are sometimes used to help D&Sers experience fantasies, too. For instance, at one small get-together at Harvey's, several D&Sers shared a plate of psychedelic mushrooms and then spent the evening listening to a three-hour tape of music and sharing the images they experienced, while they lay on the floor surrounded by candles and incense.

While a spirit of play typically accompanies the sharing and enacting of fantasies, and D&Sers commonly experiment with fantasies just for fun, some D&Sers find certain recurrent fantasies especially compelling and use them to gain personal insights. They believe such fantasies originate in a very deep and private place within the self and view them as opportunities for self-understanding and growth. Submissive men, more so than dominant women, often decide to examine and enact a deep-seated fantasy first developed in childhood in order to learn something about themselves. (As noted earlier, dominant women are less likely than submissive men to have experienced recurrent fantasies and thus are less likely to have this concern.)

A dramatic example of this self-discovery process occurred when Marvin sought to realize a fantasy he had nurtured for many years. He had long fantasized about being in potentially embarrassing or humiliating situations in public but getting out of them by using his persuasive skills. The thought of being on the edge of potential ridicule but preventing it was erotic to him, and he felt his excitement derived from his childhood, since his parents always told him not to do anything to offend anyone publicly. He assumed that the erotic tension reflected his ambivalence—wanting to offend but not wanting to—and believed his fear of offending people represented an emotional block in his character. Over the years his urge to act out this fantasy intensified, for he was not only excited by it but also felt that enacting a fear situation would help him overcome an emotional block. The result, he imagined, would be "an intensely delicious erotic pain" and a feeling of psychic release.

He told Natasha about his long-held fantasy, and she was delighted to oblige since she enjoyed having men do outrageous things for her, enjoyed the feeling of power over them, and found their antics fun. Marvin offered one idea: she could handcuff him to a post leaving a key nearby and he would try to convince a passerby to release him. Natasha agreed and offered to come up with additional ideas.

The following Saturday morning Marvin arrived at Natasha's, and she had a set of handcuffs and keys waiting. Her two suggested tasks were that he try to persuade some women he didn't know to kiss him and sign a humorous petition and that he try to sell some garbage at a shopping center. Marvin was enthusiastic about both ideas, so Natasha typed up the petition, and Marvin helped her assemble the "garbage," which included several bowls with unusual objects: small bits of crumpled paper, bent wire hangers, and envelopes with such humorous insults as "Caveat emptor—buyer beware," and "You idiot!!!" Also, Marvin wrapped some dead flowers in newspapers, and he and Natasha made signs: "Was 25¢—now 10¢," and "Get yours, while they last."

They drove to a busy downtown mall to enact the handcuff fantasy. She positioned him so he was standing with his back to the pole, placed his hands around it, snapped the handcuffs on his wrists, and put the keys about a foot away from him on the seat of a bicycle. Then she sat down on a bench about 30 feet away to watch.

Almost immediately, Marvin was afraid—the experience wasn't at all titillating or erotic. As dozens of shoppers streamed by, he worried about encountering the police and felt embarrassed and stupid. But he was determined to try, and stoically, his stomach churning, he appealed to a few passersby who looked young or hip. But they wordlessly hurried on, and when Marvin noticed a police car stop by the corner, he desperately motioned for Natasha to release him. They hurried away—his first fantasy a totally unerotic and unnerving experience.

But Marvin still wanted to continue. They went to a busy corner near the U.C. Berkeley campus, where mostly students passed by, and Natasha gave him the petition, pen, and a clipboard. He now had to convince women to kiss him and sign his petition, which was headed: OFFICIAL KRAC KISSING CONTEST ENTRY; he was to explain that he would win an all-expenses-paid trip to Ensenada, Mexico if he could get 20 women to kiss him within three hours. Gamely, he tried approaching three women, but after asking them, "Would you sign..." and receiving only strange you-must-be-crazy looks as they hurried off, Marvin gave up and walked back to Natasha, who was observing from a nearby bench. "It's utterly hopeless," he said plaintively. "No one will sign."

For their final adventure, Natasha took him to the parking lot of a large supermarket, where she set up a bridge table with his garbage display. She told Marvin to sit down on a chair beside it, and she again retreated to the sidelines to watch. Marvin once again endured stoically though he felt, he told Natasha later, like he "wanted to die." He kept his eyes down and kept hoping people would ignore him. In a few cases, when people looked over his "merchandise," he cringed and was glad they didn't look him in the eye. After ten minutes, Marvin quit, totally devastated. "I've never done anything that made me feel so terrible," he told Natasha. "And the humiliation wasn't at all erotic—it was just pure, unadulterated agony."

These escapades ended his long-held fantasy about the excitement of public humiliation. He realized that the rules he had learned very early in life against offending people precluded such humiliation from ever being erotic. He had thought he could free himself of these restrictions by enacting his fantasy and that the experience would be erotic. But although these purposes failed, he felt the experience had been a valuable one: "I learned something new about myself. I realize better what's possible and now I know something more about my own limits, and who I am, and what I can do."

14

Toys and Techniques

Since the proper use of toys and techniques is important for both pleasure and safety, D&Sers focus a great deal of attention on learning to use toys properly. People often informally show off their toys or give suggestions on techniques, and D&S groups offer organized programs on these topics. Besides providing users with instructions, such demonstrations give them insights into the symbolism and psychological effects of the exchange of power. Such psychological insights are important, because D&Sers do not engage in bondage, whipping, and other activities for the sake of the action alone. Rather they invest these actions with symbolic meaning and view them as methods for expressing and experiencing power. Formal public demonstrations also provide further social support and validation for D&Sers; and as they improve their D&S skills, they feel more comfortable and confident.

Programs and classes are offered on almost every aspect of the scene— giving pain, tying ropes, using toys, putting on chains, wearing costumes, staging rituals, and asserting power. One lecturer even argued that handwriting analysis could reveal the writer's latent interest in S&M. Almost all of these presentations emphasize the three principles of the D&S community: consensuality, safety, and awareness of others' limits. As one speaker put it: "If you don't have consensuality and safety, you don't have S&M. You have violence."

The first half of this chapter describes some typical informal and formal demonstrations on toys and techniques; the second half concerns the psychological dynamics of D&S activities.

INFORMAL DEMONSTRATIONS

Most people active in the D&S community take great pride in their playrooms and toys, and they enjoy inviting others to at-home demonstrations. Danielle and Harvey, for example, would invite people they met at SM Church classes. While Harvey would set out some popcorn, slip a paper rose in a glass, and place incense sticks in their holders, Danielle would finish dressing in an appropriately dominant outfit—a long black dress and black heels. After a bit of socializing, the demonstrations would begin.

One night she brought out a long piece of rawhide and motioned Harvey to come over and pull down his pants. Without hesitation, he did, and she looped the piece of rawhide around his testicles. "Now, watch carefully," she said and demonstrated how to tie the rawhide to separate the two testicles and the penis. "You can also use it when you go to a restaurant," she suggested, smiling slyly. "If you wet it before you go, it will get tighter as it dries. And that's fun to watch."

Once dressed, Harvey eagerly showed his collection of S&M magazines and photographs of dominant women dressed in exotic costumes—as warriors wearing capes, in space suits holding whips, and in tight black leathers with men at their heels. He and Danielle then led their guests into the playroom-bedroom, a cocoon of mirrors and red velvet curtains surrounding a waterbed covered by a red velvet spread. Harvey pushed aside a drape to show off his extensive collection of whips, canes, paddles, and slappers hanging on the walls. He pulled out a drawer to reveal his collection of leather cuffs and nipple clamps, and he proudly pointed to the suspension wires hanging in front of a wall-length mirror. He and Danielle animatedly talked about how they used the equipment.

Later in the evening, two new guests arrived: Jeff, an older dominant male in his 50s who was a mechanic, and Lester, the computer programmer introduced earlier, who now was dressed as his feminine alter ego, Jane, in a short plaid miniskirt, orange stockings, high boots, and long blonde wig. Though Lester preferred to play with a dominant woman for his weekly evening of dressing up, he hadn't been able to find one; and since Jeff was similarly unable to find a submissive woman, they chose to play together.

An outsider might have found this couple somewhat ludicrous, for Lester was about 6'2", thin and rangy with long sinewy legs and arms, and dressed as a miniskirted hooker with his long blonde wig slightly askew. But as they entered, no one laughed. Danielle and Harvey merely greeted them casually and introduced them: "This is Jane, Jeff's TV [transvestite]." The conversation resumed as though nothing unusual had happened, and Danielle suggested various techniques to the women: "Try putting clothespins on a man's nipple," "Try scratching him lightly with a nail," "You can snap a whip a few inches from his testicles to scare him without actually hitting him," "And teasing is good, too."

She then proposed to demonstrate how to teach a "slave" to follow explicit instructions, "which is important if you want to show your control." She stood up and ordered Harvey to "walk to the wall, stand three feet away from it, turn to the left, and get a cup from the altar." As instructed, he did. "You see," she concluded, "you must leave nothing to chance."

Harvey was now eager to try out a new paddle he had recently purchased, and Danielle suggested moving to the other room. "Is your TV into pain?" she asked Jeff. He said yes and told her Lester's limits, established so that Lester's wife wouldn't know: "Any amount of pain is okay, but Jane can't have any marks." Danielle asked Jane to bend over a stool, and as Jane complied, his miniskirt shot up, revealing a garter belt and tight white women's panties with a hole in the crotch for his testicles. Danielle rubbed Jane's backside to prepare him, and then hit him with different paddles and crops, while explaining the strokes: "The last part of the crop that hits conveys the pain"; "When you use a cat, be careful not to wrap the ends of it around."

The final demonstration was performed to Ravel's "Bolero," a classical piece that begins slowly and quietly and gradually builds to a loud, intense conclusion. Danielle placed furry cuffs on Harvey's wrists and ankles, directed him to lie spread-eagled on the bed, and attached one of the four chains dangling at the sides of the bed to each cuff. "They're much faster than using ropes to tie someone up," she observed. As the rhythms of "Bolero" began to quicken, she teasingly swished the crop above Harvey's head and explained that she would show how to make pain erotic and enjoyable for the submissive by building up from a mild sensation to strong pain.

Slowly and softly, she began stroking the crop up and down his body, as if she were brushing him with a feather. She tapped it lightly along his backsides and thighs, and as the music swelled, she tapped him harder and harder. Soon he began to squirm and breathe heavily, and she hit harder. Harvey liked it, for he experienced pleasure with the pain. Finally, as the music peaked, Danielle gave him two last hard whacks, and finished by rubbing his rear gently and tickling him to show that he found tickling, but not the whipping, really unpleasurable. As she tickled him, he writhed on the bed, screaming for her to stop. "You see," she said, "he didn't scream for me to stop when I was hitting him. But he does now. Tickling can be much worse."

PUBLIC DEMONSTRATIONS

Demonstrations of toys and techniques are frequently staged by public groups, sometimes as performances, though usually as classes or displays of equipment. Whatever their format, they provide a mixture of information, personal validation, and social support.

A typical demonstration as performance was Kat's presentation at a monthly meeting of the Society of Janus. About 50 people, mostly regulars with varying D&S interests, squeezed together into the large backroom of a bookstore. Kat briefly introduced her partner, Mouse, and one of her "favorite submissives," Hank. She asked for a dominant to volunteer a submissive—a usual practice at D&S presentations, since the submissive is not supposed to volunteer himself: presumably, he has given over his will to the dominant.

Eventually, Jeff volunteered Lester, introducing him as "Slave Jane." Lester was wearing khakis and a white shirt, so he looked quite masculine, but these were actually women's clothing. Kat beckoned for Jane to come forward, and told him: "Take off your shoes, pants, and shirt." Jane did, revealing that he was wearing a collar. "Good," said Kat, "a sign of submission."

Kat told Jane to bend down and kneel like a frog, legs spread apart and rear in the air. Kat circled around him, brandishing her whip, as the audience watched expectantly. Eventually, Kat intended to hit him, but first she wanted to build up Jane's anticipation by making him feel some discomfort, intensify his experience by cutting off some senses, and graphically demonstrate his submissive subservient role.

After briefly explaining what she would be doing to the audience, Kat picked up two nipple clamps from her equipment case. "I think you'd look nice in these," she teased, and attached them to Jane's nipples. When Jane flinched, Kat tugged on the clamps and teased on: "Do you understand I like to hurt people?" Turning to the audience she explained: "You see, I like to build anticipation. That intensifies the experience."

Next, Kat picked up a black leather "cock gag," frequently used in D&S sessions. The strip of black leather had a long, thick, penis-shaped leather projection that fit into the submissive's mouth. Kat waved it in front of Jane. "And now lovely Jane, if you'll open your sweet mouth"—she fitted the gag—"and now suck this cock real good. We're going to decorate you now and show that we're using your submissiveness as a thing of beauty." She hung a chain between the two clamps, attached a small fishhook weight, and put on a blindfold. "Now think of nothing but me and my pleasure, little Jane. Then, I'll keep feeling all this heat. I'll make you my pleasure toy.... You look so pretty in all this black leather and chains.... Does it hurt? Oh, good, good. I'll make you hurt more. That's the whole idea."

Kat explained to the audience that she liked to experiment with limits, that a person's limits change as he gets more excited. Kat stroked Jane's upturned rear and removed the gag, remarking: "Well, do you like the crop? Let's find your limit." Jane was to tell Kat if the whipping hurt too much, but otherwise to remain silent. Kat ordered Jane to kiss the gag ("Now wasn't that delicious?") and began hitting him, gradually increasing the intensity of the strokes. As she did, she explained that she would increase the pain until she approached Jane's limit, because "That's when it's really hot."

During the rest of the demonstration, Kat spoke alternately to Jane and the audience: "A few tiny marks here.... Very nice.... Okay, now put your face against my crotch and breathe.... Oh, my, she's trembling.... Oh, that's wonderful.... Now, let's put some pretty marks on your ass.... This time, we'll add some more weights.... You can do it.... Oh, how lovely.... We're at an edge here." The crowd watched wordlessly, barely moving, fascinated by the intimate rapport Kat had developed between herself and Jane.

When she was done, Kat took off Jane's blindfold and clamps, cuddled his head against her thighs, and praised his performance and endurance: "Oh, you're very beautiful.... You did yourself proud." In turn, Jane nodded in agreement and enjoyment.

As Jane dressed and returned to Jeff, Kat described the energy exchange the audience had just witnessed. She didn't use signals, she said, but focused on the energy or heat she felt: "It's an electric, roaring feeling in my cunt, and I follow that. When I feel it, I have a connection with the other person. It's telepathic. And when I'm tuned in this way, the other person is loving his submission. But when it goes away, I feel I have lost that connection." The succeeding comments from the audience indicated that they, too, had felt this energy when engaged in D&S.

Representative of the classes providing instruction in the safe use of equipment and techniques was Devora's class, held at Harvey's apartment for about a dozen students, mostly members of the SM Church. About half were novices who wanted lessons; the others had been in the scene for years but, like many in the D&S community, enjoyed seeing demonstrations, much as sports fans like watching pros.

Devora laid out several dozen pieces of equipment on the floor—whips, chains, paddles, canes, hoods, blindfolds, and cuffs. She began by strapping a series of hoods and blindfolds on Harvey, having him model each one in turn, to illustrate how they deprived a submissive of his sight, hearing, or ability to communicate. She provided a running commentary— "People tend to be more silent when blindfolded.... It makes the experience more intense. Mostly, dominants use blindfolds, which can be as simple as a scarf or ace bandage. But some people like the hoods, since they give the submissive a very secure, contained feeling that shuts out the outside world. But don't keep them on too long, they can get hot."

Next came some gags—"A good way to shut the submissive up. That makes the submissive feel a loss of power, because we depend on our ability to communicate so much." Then, as she fitted a rubber-ball gag into Harvey's mouth, she cautioned: "But stay around after you put it on, and if he has any problems breathing, take it off."

As she used several whips and paddles on Harvey's backside, she offered the usual tips: "The whip can be gentle or nasty. Avoid hitting anyone on the side. Don't let the tails of the whip whip around.... It helps to work up real slow. If you build up, you can play with your victim longer.... Be careful with paddles. They can leave bruises if you use them too long.... Slappers make a nice sound. You can tease someone with just the sound or the thought of the spanking."

As Harvey displayed his shining red rear, Devora passed on advice about leaving marks. "Some people mark more easily. Some submissives like their marks to last as a reminder of their experience. It's a symbol of their endurance and their gift of pain to someone else.... But others don't want any marking, because they don't like a lot of pain or don't want anyone like their wife or lover to see." The dominant can control this, Devora explained: "You can use lighter strokes, or hit with a wider surface that won't leave a mark that endures."

To show how much control the dominant has, Danielle demonstrated how some use marks to create a kind of "S&M art." This way, she pointed out, "the dominant can make the act of hitting someone more aesthetic or poetic. You're not just hitting or hurting him, but you're glamorizing him as a sexual object. So you are a kind of erotic artist."

Danielle then directed Harvey to crouch over, backside in the air, and stood behind him thoughtfully, holding a rattan cane. She raised it, aimed for a certain spot on his backside, and whipped it down, leaving a thin red mark. She placed a dozen marks, observing, "I like to draw pictures. Sometimes I'll do cross-hatching on their ass." When she finished, Harvey circled the group, showing off the checkerboard pattern, and participants praised her handiwork: "Great," "Interesting," "What control!"

Finally, Devora illustrated how proper stroking causes different types of pain—a topic D&Sers commonly talk about, much like golfers and tennis players compare strokes. Devora swatted Harvey with several whips, canes, and crops, and he described the varying sensations. "That one stings," "That one feels sharp and flat," "Now the pain seems to radiate outwards." Then she suggested that the dominants try using the equipment on themselves, on their hands, so they could understand how it felt. Also, she urged the dominants to mix pain with tenderness and caring, as experienced D&Sers do: "That helps to turn the pain into pleasure and gives the submissive an incentive to continue to experience the pain. Also, it helps build the connection between the dominant and submissive by reminding the submissive that the person hitting him is emotionally present." Too, occasional pleasure could be used to tease: "Try to rub occasionally, since they need some tender care. Besides, that can lure them into a sense of false security. Then, when you hit again, there's that element of surprise."

Among the other suggestions Devora and Danielle made were: "Be aware of spacing, rhythm, intensity, and duration"; "Control your wrist action for the best effect"; "For variety, try pinching the nipples with your toes. Or slap someone with your foot." They concluded with a series of cautions about safety: "Don't ever kick the balls. It's only safe to slap.... Remember, you can threaten with branding. But actual branding is only for the advanced."

Public presentations of toys similarly emphasize safety as well as the unique, bizarre, and aesthetic qualities of the equipment. Usually these sessions are well attended, since D&Sers are extremely interested in learning about new items to vary their sessions. At a meeting of the Society of Janus, Mr. S., a well-known maker of leather clothes and toys—mostly for the gay community, but with a growing heterosexual clientele—came to show off his wares. Approximately 50 D&Sers attended the meeting, held in the backroom of a gay leather bar. As everyone watched, he took one toy after another from his floppy black leather bag, held it up, briefly described how to use it, and passed it around. People grabbed at and played with the toys enthusiastically.

After stressing the importance of safety ("Let me assure you, every toy has been field tested before it's marketed"), he noted the exotic, bizarre qualities of each of the items. For example, as he held up a small piece of leather, shaped like a parachute, and a thin tube of leather with lacing, he commented on the unique penile sensations these items would bring: "This is a ball stretcher; the feeling is exquisite. And we call this one a meat tenderizer. It rubs against the guy while he's screwing and produces a marvelous feeling."

As he passed around other toys, the members of the audience looked at and fingered them with relish, sometimes slapping or poking them at someone else. Mr. S. often talked about their aesthetic appeal, which D&Sers consider important, since toys not only give sensation but also serve a symbolic function and fulfill status needs. Thus, in buying equipment, many spend large sums and commonly look for high quality and select items that are attractively, or even flamboyantly, decorated with symbols of quality and style—silver studs, gold embossing, plush fur, and rich leather trim.

Mr. S.'s presentation acknowledged these needs. He held up collars of varying widths and stud designs. He demonstrated stylish ways to tie and restrain the submissive in cuffs with sheepskin linings, adjustable leather shackles, and intricate leather harnesses. For nipple-torture enthusiasts, he showed a wide range of exotic devices, many of them imports, such as alligator and crocodile clamps with adjustable screws. Finally, he described the psychological effects of different materials as he displayed several garments made of rubber and leather: "Leather is usually associated with strength, power, and pain....But rubber is more sensual and linked to bondage, because it's tight and grips the skin."

Finally, Mr. S. concluded by acknowledging the D&Sers' concern for secrecy in acquiring this equipment, leading many to shop from catalogs. "That's why we keep a low profile. . . . Some people don't want to be seen going through a leather shop. . . . Many feel buying a toy or something in leather is very personal. . . . Some are very nervous. . . . So we don't have a sign on the door."

Yet, once inside, he found, people wanted to feel free to express themselves, because they were making purchases to fulfill inner needs. "So we try to make it a safe space for them, so they can feel free to try on exotic clothing or hold erotic toys in their hand. . . . People find that exciting. . . . We want to encourage that, and let them go absolutely wild."

15

Insiders and Outsiders

Since D&S is generally considered unacceptable or perverse by those in mainstream American society, most D&Sers lead double lives. Otherwise, they are mostly middle-class people in respectable jobs; they feel they must hide their D&S activities from outsiders. With insiders, they can share their interests freely, and this intimacy leads many to feel especially close with other members of their encapsulated community. But with outsiders, they must be careful: some will understand, others may themselves be closeted or potential D&Sers, but most will be unsympathetic and judgmental. Thus most D&Sers keep their everyday lives and D&S activities largely separate, and maneuver cautiously between the two. This chapter examines the psychology of this double life—the intimacy among insiders and the difficulties of relating to outsiders.

THE SPIRIT OF CLOSENESS IN THE D&S COMMUNITY

A spirit of closeness and commitment prevails within the D&S community, although many members' nonmonogamous experimentation might initially seem incompatible with closeness and commitment. But even those who engage in a series of short-term relationships and switch partners frequently feel a loyalty to the D&S community. The private, intimate nature of D&S and the need for secrecy in relating to outsiders draw D&Sers together. Also, since those who play around strive to be nonpossessive, feelings of resentment and jealousy tend not to interfere with their sense of closeness with fellow insiders. Furthermore, most active community members see each other frequently, share their intimate fantasies and desires, openly talk about who they are seeing and what they are doing, and participate in D&S scenarios together. All these activities promote closeness, as does their shared perspective and interpretation of everyday events in terms of power, eroticism, and fantasy. Thus, even when D&Sers drift away from the community for a while to pursue other interests, when they are ready to return, other community members normally welcome them back.

This closeness, in turn, contributes to a spirit of mutual help within the community, particularly among those closest to the core, as is usually true within small intimate groups. The core of insiders tend to regard themselves as family members, and they do errands for one another; lend books, equipment, and money; assist with making and installing D&S equipment; provide child care; and even offer temporary housing for a member who needs it.

While much of such help is typical of any close group, some of it reflects dominant and submissive dynamics. A male may enjoy helping out as a way of showing his submission to a dominant woman, and she may view his help as a sign of her power. In some cases, the participants, and most particularly the males, find this service erotic, as a kind of real-life session to be played out, or they may enjoy the psychological satisfaction involved.

For example, Luke often volunteered to do tasks because he received deep pleasure from helping and being told what to do. He enjoyed doing all sorts of tasks for Kat: typing, filing, acting as a maid in preparing refreshments, and cleaning up after the dominant women's support group. When he lived in a cottage behind Diana and Drew's house, he helped Diana with various household tasks, such as painting, gardening, and clean-up, and from time to time she expressed her appreciation by dominating him in a D&S session. He later worked out a temporary slave-servant arrangement with Nina, who worked as a professional mistress. And he spent many hours doing office work for the SM Church.

RELATING TO OUTSIDERS

In contrast to the openness they show to those in the community, D&Sers are careful in how they reveal themselves to outsiders. Some tell close relatives and friends because they want to share this important part of their lives with them and think or hope they will understand. Others look for signs that an outsider might want to get involved before they mention D&S. But generally, D&Sers don't actively proselytize. They are well aware of the stigma attached to D&S and fear the real possibility of losing friends or jobs. Also, they quite naturally hesitate to discuss very intimate subjects with outsiders who may not understand even if they don't reject them socially or personally. Still, when and if they can, most hope to let important others in their lives know. Gradually and discreetly, they may reveal themselves, as they feel it is safe, sometimes looking for signals that someone else is already involved in D&S, and sometimes dropping hints or slowly leading up to a revelation if they think someone will be receptive and understanding.

To prevent inadvertent public exposure, some D&Sers use only first names or made-up names in their D&S activities, giving out their real names only when they get to know someone really well. Others use their real first and last names with those they know as friends but use a pseudonym when they go to a mistress or commercial establishment. "I use a phony name when there's a monetary exchange," Brent once explained. "But my relationships with those in the community are intimate and real, so I want them to know who I really am."

In sizing up outsiders—particularly when looking for potential partners—D&Sers commonly look for signs or signals that the person is already involved in D&S or at least receptive. An outsider's clothing is an important source of clues, although these clues may be quite subtle, since heterosexuals into D&S don't telegraph their interests like some gays who wear colored handkerchiefs or leathers to indicate their preferences. Most D&Sers dress conventionally, though some women dress with dramatic flair, and both males and females may add subtle embellishments that are signs of being dominant or submissive. For instance, a woman may wear especially high heels, often dress in black or red, or put on jewelry suggesting D&S interests, such as a necklace with a dangling high heel or a handcuffs pin. Similarly, a man may wear a chain around his neck that suggests a slave's collar.

But clothing is not a foolproof sign. As one man complained in frustration: "The media has been picking up on S&M imagery. Somebody might have the look without being into it. You can't know for sure." So D&Sers look for verbal clues and at times test a person by throwing out subtle, joking hints to see how the person responds. An innocuous but suggestive comment or an ambiguous, teasing question may provoke a telling response. If the outsider seems to pick up on the cue and appears receptive, they push on a little further; if not, they drop the subject, as Sharon did. "Sometimes at a party," she said, "I'll say something like: 'I enjoy it when men do things for me,' and see if the man responds." Likewise, Brent looked for women to drop these kinds of hints and indicated his willingness to comply when they did.

Thus D&Sers usually engage in a great deal of hedging, looking for and giving off signals to be sure the other person really means what he or she seems to mean and avoid any embarrassment resulting from a premature revelation to someone unreceptive to D&S. In turn, since they expect this coyness and caution, when they meet people who openly kid about D&S, they usually consider them outsiders. As Danielle put it: "A person who is really into dominance wouldn't want to draw attention to himself and have outsiders think that's what he's into. A real submissive would be more discreet. He wouldn't want anyone to think he was. And real S&Mers don't joke about it like that. They don't say things like: 'Whip me, whip me.' They're really serious about their interest."

Outside the D&S community, this search for signals isn't always productive, since only a small percentage of the population is openly involved in D&S. But D&Sers still enjoy looking and testing. Besides the faint hope that the search may be productive, many enjoy the process itself, especially when it leads to the edge of near exposure. Danielle explained the feeling thus: "I love to test straight people to see how they feel. I put forth a question and see their reactions. Then, if they seem interested, I go on. But if not, that doesn't matter. As long as you smile and act as if you're joking, you can get away with a lot of things."

TELLING OUTSIDERS

D&Sers tend to keep their activity secret from parents and relatives, unless they are fairly sure they will be receptive, feeling that family members are likely to be especially judgmental and critical of their activities and will be concerned about protecting the family name. Also, they tend to avoid telling anyone who is highly religious or conservative, as well as business associates, bosses, and casual friends. At work, in particular, they fear possible repercussions, such as difficulty in working with co-workers or even losing a job.

D&Sers also do not generally tell their children. They feel any explanation would be inappropriate for young children; and while older ones might understand, parents fear they may tell their friends, causing problems for themselves and their children. Those parents who engage in any D&S activity at home typically do so only when their children aren't around, hide their D&S equipment, and do not discuss it in their children's presence. A very few D&Sers who are especially active discuss the issue with their children; women who work as mistresses, for example, find their frequent activity hard to hide. But such revelations are quite rare.

D&Sers vary extensively in how much and whom they tell. While some, particularly newcomers, choose to be very private and hide their participation from anyone who is not already involved in the scene, most choose selectively among their spouses, lovers, close friends, and relatives, and tell only those who they think will be receptive. A few feel open enough to tell almost everyone.

Typically, as individuals become more involved in the scene and more comfortable with D&S, they feel freer to expand the circle of those they tell. For example, when Marvin started coming out, he used to almost slink into D&S meetings, spoke to no one, and told no one outside the scene about his D&S interests. "I was too ashamed of what I was doing, at first," he said. But as he met other D&Sers who seemed like "fine, ordinary, normal people," he felt more self-assured about his activity and freer to discuss it with others outside the scene, and he gradually told his girlfriends and a few selected friends. Similarly, at one time Harvey only told his wife and some trusted friends. But after several years in the scene, he said, "Now I could tell anyone, if I think that person might be interested."

Before they tell someone, D&Sers usually put out feelers to find out if he or she has a tolerant attitude, much as they probe carefully to learn if someone is already involved. They make casual but telling remarks alluding to female domination, such as: "Women are becoming more assertive in the office these days, don't you think?" Or they comment on some observed D&S-type behavior to see if that ignites a receptive spark, such as: "I saw this movie about some boys in an English boarding school, and were they disciplined by their teachers!"

In making any revelation, a D&Ser will be very sensitive to the other person's personality and openness to the topic. "You have to take each person's personality into consideration," said Harvey in explaining his own strategy. "You have to judge how much they can accept. I give them a little. Then, if they are receptive, I go on." D&Sers pursue a slow, gradual strategy, because they know that if they reveal themselves too quickly, the other person may be shocked or unprepared to modify his or her past negative images to continue to see the teller in a positive light.

For example, before telling a lover, Marvin would make sure his relationship with the woman was secure, that she perceived him as a "normal, good, and respectable" person. Then he would occasionally mention his interest, making it clear she didn't have to be interested for their relationship to continue. Next, if she seemed curious and receptive, he would mention some of his fantasies, usually telling his dominant male fantasies first, since he found most women more comfortable being submissive. Gradually he would tell her his submissive fantasies as well. Finally, if she was receptive, he would propose acting out the fantasy. He introduced several women into D&S this way.

In talking to outsiders, D&Sers also often use neutral terms or phrases to describe their activities. They tend to avoid emotionally loaded terms like *sadism, masochism,* or *S&M,* and use euphemisms to describe their activities, such as: "I like to explore dominance" or "I'm interested in creative, alternative types of sex."

Sometimes the recipients of these hints turn out to be more interested or involved in D&S than expected, and D&Sers enjoy talking about such incidents, for they represent another source of personal validation. Danielle had this kind of experience with her brother. She felt especially close to him and felt he had fairly liberal attitudes about social issues, but she proceeded cautiously by dropping hints. She was doing leatherwork for various customers and offered to make him a leather purse or belt for Christmas. When he said he would like that, she casually replied: "You know, people have been asking me to make the strangest things. One person wanted me to make him leather cuffs, a blindfold, and a whip." Danielle had merely hoped her brother would respond receptively to hearing about her D&S interests. But he turned out to be a secret D&S enthusiast too and had not told her because he felt she wouldn't understand. "Forget the purse and belt," he told her. "Make us some cuffs." The result was a new closeness with her brother.

Not all revelations are successful, with the results ranging from teasing to outright rejection. Travis, the biology graduate student, met with teasing when he told a few friends that he had fantasies about having a woman dominate and hit him. "Oh, yeah," his friends said, punching him playfully. "Is this what you like?" But after kidding him for several weeks about his "eccentricity," they eventually accepted it, and a few went to a D&S meeting with him.

When men tell their wives or lovers, many get the response "that's weird," or "that's sick." Possibly this occurs because they presented their case badly, but for whatever reason their partners respond negatively, they commonly drop the topic after that. Some find themselves dropped by a friend they thought would understand.

One D&Ser who unintentionally revealed himself almost lost his job. Jesse came to work wearing a pair of women's panties, as a mistress friend of his had directed, and his boss saw them in the men's room, which had open stalls. "What are you, some kind of pervert?" his boss asked. "You know I could fire you for that." However, since Jesse had been doing a good job and couldn't easily be replaced, his boss relented. "But don't let me see you wearing those again."

Despite such slips, however, D&Sers seem to be mostly successful in reading signs about outsiders' interest and sensitivity. When they do miscalculate, they usually manage to smooth over these situations by playing down their revelation or dropping the matter. Or sometimes the person who inadvertently discovers their involvement tactfully pretends not to know, as occurred when one of June and Herman's teenage sons saw one of their whips around the house. They knew he knew or suspected something, since he moved the whip, but discreetly he said nothing.

This success in smoothing over potential problems when their interest is revealed may be due in part to the fact that most D&Sers are respectable people with high status. Thus some people who are initially unreceptive tend eventually to accept or tolerate this "deviation" as a mild eccentricity, as Tom, the machine shop owner, discovered when his brother-in-law found out. "I certainly never intended to tell him," he said. "I didn't think he would understand. But when he stopped by and saw the chains on the bed, I felt I had to explain. At first, he seemed really shocked. How could we really like to do such a thing? But then, he dropped the subject and never brought it up again. It was like it hadn't happened at all."

Sometimes D&Sers enjoy almost telling someone about their activities. This is another form of playing with boundaries, creating a tension much like teetering on the border between pain and pleasure or stretching previous limits. They tease with hints about D&S but stop before an outsider really understands. The outsider may suspect but does not know. Such play is a way of both chiding outsiders with their little secret and generating an exciting dynamic tension between being safe and getting caught.

D&Sers love to share stories about such intentional or unintentional close calls. Lance described how a fire inspector arrived one day to inspect the SM Church office. Lance led him into the livingroom, one wall of which had an altar to the Goddess with several candles, cups, and incense burner, and a statue of a male kneeling before a woman. And across the room a flashy red-and-black SM Church banner hung on the wall, with the elongated letters "S" and "M" barely distinguishable. "But the inspector didn't notice a thing," Lance exulted. When the fire inspector asked, "Is this all there is?" Lance managed a "yes" that barely concealed a laugh, and the inspector left satisfied. "But," Lance grinned mischievously, "he missed the dungeon in the basement, where the Church keeps all its toys."

16

The Dark Side of D&S

Despite the public image of D&S as a form of weird, violent, even sick behavior undertaken by people who enjoy hurting or manipulating others or being hurt and controlled themselves, people in the scene typically approach D&S with a sense of playfulness, fun, imagination, and creativity. They also stress safety, consensus, and responsibility and emphasize that the dominant should be aware of the submissive's responses, so that D&S can be a joyful, fulfilling experience for both partners.

To an extent, D&Sers mock the straight establishment for being conservative and "uptight"; yet they do so in a spirit of playful fun, not in bitterness or anger. Also, when they talk about how other people don't understand, it is not with resentment, feelings of guilt, or any fervor to change others. Rather they comment on the excitement they claim others are missing.

But one cannot ignore the dark side of D&S. Some activities can be dangerous if participants are inexperienced, irresponsible, or out of control. D&Sers are aware of this possibility and constantly monitor themselves and others to make sure nothing untoward happens. Nevertheless, on rare occasions, something dangerous does happen. This chapter discusses some of these incidents, which are mainly of five types:

1. A male fantasizes about some heavy D&S activity and the woman actually does it.
2. An inexperienced dominant woman loses control.
3. A male excited by danger repeatedly puts himself into dangerous situations.
4. A "submissive" male turns against a dominant woman.
5. D&S play goes too far and leads to public embarrassment.

ENACTING SEVERE FANTASIES

Usually D&Sers appropriately distinguish between fantasy and reality and responsibly determine what fantasies can be safely and successfully enacted. But from time to time a male has a severe fantasy he wants or says he wants to act out. If the dominant thinks he really means it, she may actually enact it rather than playing it out symbolically or merely pretending she is going to do it. Not only will the male usually find such an experience unerotic, but he may be physically hurt. The pain is usually temporary—for example, welts from a whipping may last several days or weeks, though occasionally the marks may be permanent as in a piercing that goes too deep.

Most commonly, D&Sers avoid such problems by symbolically enacting fantasies of heavy D&S activity. For instance, some submissive males have castration fantasies, for they imagine giving up their manhood as the ultimate sign of submission. Some even ask a professional mistress or a girlfriend to act out this fantasy. But the male doesn't want her actually to do it, and the woman instead plays out a scene that ends short of the ultimate act. For instance, one mistress told a client, who came to her three times with a castration fantasy, that it would really happen each time. She began the scenario by leading him into a room where she had laid out some surgical instruments. She tied him up, blindfolded him, shaved his genital area, swabbed it with alcohol, and teased him about whether he could really take the pain. Then she concluded each session by telling him that he wasn't ready for the operation.

However, in some cases, a woman does carry out a severe fantasy that the man doesn't really want enacted, most usually fantasies about receiving a severe whipping. When Travis first started to act out his long-private fantasies, he told a professional mistress he "could take anything, including heavy pain." So she whipped him severely, and although he begged her to stop, she dismissed his pleas as mere play acting, which such pleas often are. But whereas an experienced dominant observes the man's body language to differentiate pretend pleas from serious ones, this woman didn't pay any attention and continued to hit him. For Travis the session was a terrible experience, and the large red welts lingered for two weeks. While some males might like lasting reminders of a whipping as a kind of "battle wound" that they think about or display, Travis did not like them at all and left the session feeling very angry. "She didn't care what I really wanted—she just creamed me," Travis said.

INEXPERIENCED DOMINANT WOMEN

Although any dominant woman might lose control or behave irresponsibly on a given occasion, dangerous situations are more likely to occur with an inexperienced professional mistress rather than an inexperienced nonprofessional, probably because the latter tends to hold back or to be overly solicitous about whether the male enjoys what she is doing. Inexperienced nonprofessionals may at times exercise poor judgment, but they usually err on the side of leniency.

In one dramatic case, Jesse was seriously hurt by a novice mistress. He saw her ad for sessions in the paper, called, and she invited him over. "Knowing what I know now," he said, "I would have been suspicious when I went to her apartment." But at the time he was a novice, and when he walked in and noticed some whips, crops, and other toys scattered around her apartment, and saw her sloppily dressed in a halter and jeans, he didn't think this unusual. "I know now she should have been better organized," he explained. "A professional mistress has to be organized about herself and her toys, since this is how she makes her living."

However, at the time, suspecting nothing, he agreeably let her tie him to the table, with his hands strapped together beneath him. She began by cropping him roughly on the thighs, which is usually not an erotic place to hit. When he didn't respond, she took a razor and drew a line across his chest. As blood flowed, Jesse practically fainted. Finally, disgusted by his continuing lack of erotic response, she went out, leaving him tied up and still bleeding, and left the door slightly ajar behind her. As he heard her footsteps fade away, Jesse began screaming, until a neighbor discovered and released him.

An inexperienced dominant may occasionally lose control at a party, carried away by the convivial atmosphere. While a party was swirling on upstairs, Harvey allowed his friend Gloria to tie him up on a massage table in the basement. Soon after, Madam Tiger, a visiting novice mistress from Nevada, dropped in to watch. A male wearing a collar was balanced on his knees beside her. The two women chatted briefly and arranged a swap. Madame Tiger would take control of Harvey, while Gloria went off with her "slave" in the collar. Such a swap is a common, quite acceptable procedure, but Madame Tiger started hitting Harvey hard with a chain— an excruciatingly painful and very unsafe activity. Harvey pleaded with her to stop, but she continued hitting. Fortunately, a few minutes later, Devora, who was patrolling the party with Danielle, appeared and rescued Harvey.

COURTING DANGER

A few males who are attracted to heavy pain occasionally find themselves in dangerous situations because they refuse to acknowledge their own limits. Such incidents are rare, but do occur. Luke, for example, now in his late 50s, has had recurrent bouts of alcoholism, and he had trouble adjusting emotionally after some serious injuries sustained during World War II. His emotional problems, in turn, led him repeatedly to surround himself with unstable characters, whom he introduced to the scene. He claims to like playing the role of a bum and associating with the down-and-out as a release from his earlier days as a "straight and narrow" businessman and worker.

Though he has recently sought to reform himself and become a more settled, stable member of the D&S community, Luke can relate a series of dangerous and painful D&S experiences. For a time, he lived with Marlene, an inexperienced and seemingly irresponsible woman of 19. Of several of their sessions, Luke says, "I thought she was going to kill me, because she didn't know what she was doing." One time they went to a party, where she tied him up, suspended him in cuffs and chains, and beat him severely with a knotted whip. Since she didn't know how to use the equipment, she left him in suspension too long, dangerously cutting off his circulation. Also, she repeatedly wrapped the whip around his body, leaving deep bruises and welts.

Despite such experiences, though, Luke continually courts danger, and he describes his brushes with mayhem with perverse pride, as if they prove how strong, courageous, and therefore worthwhile he is. Even after his doctor cautioned that his lifestyle would kill him, he continued to visit a mistress friend who at times treated him to extremely brutal sessions. In one of these, she strung him up and hit him so hard with a bullwhip that the whip snipped small pieces of flesh from his chest. But he didn't protest, because, "the woman seemed to be having so much fun. She was really getting a rush, and I didn't want to interfere with that." Other times, she whipped him nearly to unconsciousness, and he often proudly pulled down his pants to show off his latest wounds.

Given the obvious dangers, others have tried to dissuade him from seeing these women and seeking out severe pain. But he rejects their urgings, claiming that he needs this kind of experience, no matter how much he suffers. "When I don't get S&M," he said at one gathering, "I have to take Thorazine to relax. Or I get drunk. So S&M is almost like a drug to me. I need my S&M fix."

Luke's behavior is quite atypical. Though many D&Sers are excited by fantasies about danger, they don't want to enact those fantasies. What is unique about Luke is that he does.

REBELLIOUS SUBMISSIVES

Dominant women sometimes worry about the possibility of a supposedly submissive male turning on them, although such incidents seem to be rare, particularly when the partners have a good personal relationship. For example, as described earlier, Laura worried when the retired military officer she was dating insisted on teaching her self-defense; she feared that he was preparing her for a violent physical confrontation. But her fears were never realized.

But occasionally a new client will turn on a professional mistress. One novice professional, working out of her apartment, reported that a client, a big burly contractor, suddenly grabbed her whip, hit her with it, and beat her up. And two women working in a large B&D establishment described how customers turned on them. But the management monitored the rooms, and as soon as the women cried out, a staff member appeared to show the man out.

PUBLIC EMBARRASSMENT AND LEGAL PROBLEMS

While some D&Sers are titillated by flirting with publicly revealing themselves as D&Sers, such play can cause embarrassment, threaten relationships or jobs, or cause legal problems. Such incidents are rare, but they can have serious consequences, such as the case described earlier where Jesse nearly lost his job when his boss discovered him wearing women's panties. More serious are the incidents that have legal complications. One evening, for example, Luke was babysitting for a friend's nine-year-old daughter. He and the girl were kidding around and he playfully and unthinkingly pulled down his pants, much as he did in front of a group of D&Sers at a party. The little girl laughed, and everything seemed fine. But afterwards the girl mentioned something to her mother; her mother happened to tell the girl's grandmother; and when the grandmother remarked on the incident to her social worker, the social worker felt it her duty to report the matter to the police. Luke was soon hustled to jail on a child-molesting charge, though the mother had no intention of pressing charges.

When others in the D&S community learned what had happened, several rushed to Luke's aid, and after two difficult weeks, the charges were dropped and Luke released. But had the mother been vindictive or the D&S community less supportive, Luke would have faced a serious criminal charge arising out of what Luke and the D&S community viewed as harmless, good-natured public humiliation.

PART V

THE COMMERCIAL WORLD OF D&S

17

Professional Mistresses

In general, the commercial and noncommercial scenes are distinct, although some professional mistresses participate in noncommercial D&S and some women interested in dominance temporarily try out the commercial role. But in general professional dominants have different backgrounds than women involved in personal D&S. Also, the men who visit mistresses make a distinction, noting the lack of caring and sincerity in the professional scene.

The professional scene is a highly fragmented one, consisting of a heterogeneous group of free-lance dominants who advertise their services through local or national publications. Pros in the large cities with an active D&S community, such as New York, Los Angeles, or San Francisco, usually confine their advertising to a local sexually oriented newspaper, though some advertise in national magazines, too. Dominants in smaller cities and towns depend on ads in such national publications as *Kinky Contacts* or *Dominant Women,* and some even offer to travel.

Most dominants seek personal contact through a session, though some offer to make fantasy tapes, carry on sexy phone calls, or write sensual letters. Each mistress has her own style and services, as these sample ads show:

SUBMISSIVE BOYS MAY CALL ILSA for hospital discipline, cross-dressing, humiliation, teasing, and other forms of B&D therapy.

SHOW ME HOW Well You Obey or be tied and tormented 'til I have my way! TV [transvestite] training by Maya.

SUBMIT YOUR HUMBLE SELF AT THE MISTRESS' FEET.

Ads in the national publications usually include photos of mistresses looking appropriately tough and haughty. Occasionally, photos accompany ads in the local papers.

Most mistresses work out of their homes alone, some in small groups of two or three. The larger cities host a sprinkling of organized "chateaus" or "dungeons" where several women work together, supervised by a head mistress or master, who usually does not take clients. Some organized houses are well-designed and equipped clubs that resemble conventional social clubs for the well heeled, except that the rooms feature a variety of racks, bars, suspension devices, and other toys. At the other extreme are seedy, ramshackle houses that appeal to customers who have less money to spend or whose fantasies of being humiliated and degraded are served by the dilapidated premises.

An example of the former is the Chateau, with houses in Los Angeles and San Francisco. Customers in San Francisco enter a massive concrete converted warehouse at the fringes of an area of discount stores and cheap restaurants. They wind down a long corridor to a fashionably decorated suite of rooms. Here about a dozen women work in shifts as dominants, submissives, or switches. In contrast, customers of a "dungeon" located in a private lower-middle-class home are greeted at the door of a dark, musty, crowded garage by one of the half-dozen or so dominant women who work there. She leads them into a small room with a heavy iron door, or up a flight of rickety stairs to a narrow upstairs bedroom.

While these organized settings offer customers several women to choose from and more equipment than a woman working alone can afford, they cannot match the personal feeling of a session held at a mistress' home. But in either case, the client pays at least $60 to $75 for an hour's session. A solo pro, of course, keeps the entire fee; a mistress at a house usually has to give about half the fee to the house.

Most pros work at home since they make more money and like the freedom. But some—particularly novices—prefer working at houses to obtain a ready supply of customers and protection from the occasional customer who turns out to be dangerous. Women who work alone are usually strictly dominant, however, which opens them to less danger than the female submissive, except for the occasional male who fantasizes about overpowering a dominant woman.

Women working alone are usually quite cautious in screening prospective customers. Most depend on their intuitive sense of a new client during an initial phone conversation or discussion. Only if they feel comfortable with him will they arrange the session. Some have husbands or lovers nearby to monitor their sessions. Women working in the houses usually rely on the house to screen new clients. And sometimes, as at the Chateau, the staff monitors the sessions, too, for added protection.

RATES AND INCOME

Since the going rate for dominants is $60 to $75 an hour and a little more—$70 to $85—if the woman is willing to play submissive or switch, mistresses with a regular clientele can earn a relatively high income—about

$900 or $1200 a week for the woman who averages three to four clients a day five days a week, but most dominants do not work this frequently.

Generally, the women who earn the most are those who work alone, work regularly, have good skills and a good style, provide an attractive, tasteful playroom, and personally enjoy D&S. The woman who works solo keeps the full fee, has low advertising costs (a few dollars a week), and, once she has her equipment, has no major operating expenses. The nicer the neighborhood and house interior, the better the clientele and the higher her rates. In addition, a skilled professional who enjoys D&S is more likely to have repeat customers; as one professional explained: "Most clients can tell if a pro doesn't know what she is doing or is only in it for the money, and this usually results in an unsatisfying session, so they don't come back. Besides, if a pro isn't into D&S personally, she is apt to 'burn out' soon and quit."

Though some women do quite well, most average about $100 to $125 a day. The typical pro spends a great deal of time waiting for the phone to ring, screening new clients, and setting up appointments. Unless she has repeat customers, who almost always appear for appointments, she is likely to have a large number of no-shows, for only about 10 to 20 percent of a pro's first-time customers show up. "When I worked as a mistress," one former mistress said, "I spent a few hours a day on the phone screening clients to weed out the phone freaks and crazies, and, at most, I only saw one or two clients a day. Generally, I averaged about 15 calls for each appointment I made. And then perhaps only 3 out of every 5 men showed up." Other women choose to see only two or three customers a day because each session is emotionally and physically draining.

While women with regular customers who are making a good income may stay in business for several years or more, the field is characterized by a high rate of turnover. Many women drop out if their income doesn't match their expectations. Some turn pro only temporarily, when they are between jobs or want to pick up some extra money. And some burn-out quickly because they don't personally enjoy D&S or let their customers persuade them to act out fantasies they find distasteful.

THE MISTRESS-CLIENT RELATIONSHIP

Although each mistress has her own style of dominance and D&S preferences, her business success depends on her customers' satisfaction. Thus she must consider client's wants and needs while at the same time retaining power and control, so that each man will have a submissive experience. She must therefore maintain a fine balance between giving the submissive what he wants, showing that she is still in charge, and satisfying her own dominant persona. Achieving this balance is further complicated as the male's erotic satisfaction may depend on her pushing him to his perceived limits or slightly beyond.

Most mistresses acquaint themselves with a customer's wants during a brief conversation before the session. A mistress will ask her customer about his fantasies and desires: What does he consider erotic? What has he liked in previous sessions? Some mistresses even review a customer's written instructions. A mistress can then plan a session that will give the customer what he says he wants, though in her own style.

In general, mistresses feel they should cater to the customer because he is paying them. One pro reasoned pragmatically: "I'm willing to do anything a client wants as long as it doesn't disgust me. Since he's paying, he should go away satisfied. Besides, if he's satisfied, he'll come back." Even though responding to a man's desires, they feel they still retain the power. "It's okay to take his money and give him the kind of session he wants," one explained, "as long as you don't see it as your giving him power over you. It doesn't have to deaden your dominant energy."

A few professionals, however, do insist on doing things their own way, though this approach puts off some clients. These women believe that the most powerful erotic arousal for the submissive male comes when he is truly out of control; he must truly surrender to the dominant's power. As one former mistress explained: "I wanted their total submission. I wanted it left up to me. Otherwise, the session isn't real. They're just pretending. And that isn't pleasurable for me." Yet, even so, she was sensitive and empathetic to her clients, and observed their responses to her so the session would be pleasurable for both.

In short, though the male is paying to be submissive and wants the woman to take control, it is not always clear who is really in control of the session—the mistress or the male who has his likes and limits . . . and pays.

IS IT PROSTITUTION?

Since mistresses receive payment for an erotically stimulating service, some clients and non-D&Sers think of professional dominance as a form of prostitution. But mistresses and others in the scene make a clear distinction between professional dominants and prostitutes, arguing that the mistress doesn't provide sex (defined as intercourse, fellatio, cunnilingus, or hand manipulation to orgasm). "It's not prostitution," one mistress asserted. "I don't have sex. If the man has an orgasm, it's because he causes it; I don't do that."

Others distinguish between mistresses and prostitutes in terms of power, since the mistress has the power to decide whether the customer will achieve sexual release and in what way. As one professional argued: "A prostitute has sex with anyone. I only do it with special customers, and then

I decide if they can have sex with me or not. A prostitute has no choice." Still another stated that: "When a woman is a prostitute, she has no control. The customer pays her, and she does what he wants. But when I have a customer, he is not buying a sexual object. He is the object, and I do what I want; I have the power and control."

Other mistresses emphasize the skills or special services the dominant offers: "The client is paying you for your skills, knowledge, and an equipped place to do a session," one mistress said. "He's not paying for your time or your body. He's paying the dominant just as he would pay a lawyer or doctor for his skills. So the dominant is like a professional who offers special skills."

A few view the mistress as offering a form of sex therapy. "She's not just offering the male a sexual encounter, though sexual feelings are part of it," claimed an occasional mistress who worked as a sex surrogate, "She is fulfilling his needs and providing him with sexual therapy." And a mistress who worked as a part-time nurse saw both her jobs as helping men in need: "I feel I share my love and care with each client. So I see it as another kind of nursing."

Even mistresses who have sex with some customers distinguish their work from prostitution on the grounds that the male's primary interest is in D&S, rather than in sex, and they have the choice of whether to offer sex. As one mistress with a steady clientele explained: "Prostitutes may engage in B&D or S&M with their clients, but sex is usually the main reason the client visits the lady. In the case of the professional mistress, the client's main reason in going to the session is for S&M, not for sex. However, since S&M can be arousing, as well as being emotionally and intellectually stimulating, most clients want some sexual release. Then, it's up to the pro to decide what form of sexual release she allows the client to have. The prostitute usually doesn't have that kind of choice."

Typically, the dominant allows some form of sexual release at the end of the session, though most only permit the client to masturbate or stimulate him manually or with a piece of equipment. These restrictions emphasize her dominant power and provide some protection against legal problems, because allowing a client to masturbate is the least incriminating form of sexual activity should a new customer be a police officer. Some mistresses do offer oral or genital sex to favored regular customers, and a few advertise that they like oral sex—usually described as "oral worship" or "oral satisfaction." But others make it clear from the first that they are not offering any sexual contact, and the larger, more established B&D houses require their dominants to take this approach.

Satisfied male customers also distinguish dominance from prostitution. "Though I'm buying sexual services," one explained, "I'm also giving my power to the mistress, and she has the choice of whether to give me sexual satisfaction or not. Sure, I'd like it. And maybe I even expect it, since I'm paying. But in the fantasy game we play, I don't have that right to demand it. My fulfillment is up to her." But dissatisfied customers may see dominants as merely specialized prostitutes. "She's just giving the male what he wants," one commented. "He's paying for it and she's giving. So what's the difference?" said another. And people outside the scene often consider mistresses in a similarly uncharitable way. "They're prostitutes," one female word processor remarked with finality. "They sell sexual service."

OCCUPATIONAL HAZARDS

Besides the potential danger from the rare unruly customer, professional mistresses have two large problems nonprofessionals don't have—no-shows and the possibility of arrest.

The no-shows—about 80 to 90 percent of the men who arrange their first appointment—are men who find their excitement and release in simply fantasizing about the session or who are ambivalent about seeing a mistress. A mistress tries to identify the fantasizers on the phone by keeping the conversations brief enough to discourage "phone freaks" who just like to talk. At the same time, the initial conversation must be long enough for her to clearly indicate the kinds of services she offers ("You understand there will be no sex") and set some safety guidelines ("I don't switch and I'm not into heavy pain").

If the mistress and man agree to a session, she may have him phone a few hours or minutes before the appointment to reconfirm. For example, at the dungeon, the women have the prospective client call from a gas station about five minutes from the house for the final directions. Only after he calls does the dominant prepare for the session.

Some mistresses, particularly those who work in groups, handle the no-show problem by double-booking first-time customers—a strategy not normally needed with regulars, who are usually reliable. They schedule two appointments at the same time, guessing that one may not show, to make it more likely they will actually have a session. Should both customers show up, the mistress coyly tells the second arrival her first appointment is running a little longer than expected and asks him to wait; if she is working in a house, another woman may take the appointment, a ploy that usually works, since the first-timer has not met the woman he has come to see.

Though rare, the mistress must consider the possibility that a new client is a law enforcement official. Mistresses try to discourage policemen from showing up by telling new prospects on the phone that they offer no sex. When they meet the customer, they tell him again, and unless they know and like the customer, they permit no sexual contact. And some mistresses, including those in the more established houses, like the Chateau, never allow any sex. Yet, even without offering sex, mistresses do risk a charge of lewd and lascivious behavior. One mistress was convicted of performing a lewd act because a client masturbated himself to orgasm and she urinated on him. Thus, when a new client calls, the mistress usually encourages him to describe his fantasies, since the more he says, the less likely he is to be a police officer. At the first meeting some dominants ask the client directly if he is a policeman, since an officer is supposed to identify himself if asked. Or they maneuver him into a compromising position; for example, a mistress may make a new client take off his pants before any money changes hands, assuming that a police officer would hesitate to do so.

Even so, there are occasional arrests, mostly of women working as a group in small private houses. Generally, the police ignore the women who work alone at home; they don't have the time or inclination to pursue them. And the bigger more established houses, like the Chateau, seem to have worked out some modus vivendi with law enforcement. Since they make it clear they provide no sex, and perhaps because they have some powerful customers, their operations seem protected.

MISTRESSES AND CLIENTS: WHO ARE THEY?

Mistresses and clients are in many respects like those involved in the noncommercial D&S scene, and there is much overlap. Some women who enjoy dominance, such as Sharon and Kat, experiment as pros for a few weeks or months, and a few, such as Devora, make it a regular occupation. Correspondingly, some men who go to D&S groups or have D&S relationships go to mistresses. Yet many mistresses don't socialize in the scene, and some men only visit mistresses discreetly.

Clients are much like men in the noncommercial scene, though perhaps a little more successful and affluent, since they can afford the high fees. Typically, these clients are high-level business and professional men who are strong, powerful, and successful in their daily lives. They express a strong need for submission as a counterbalance to their everyday stresses or, in some cases, as a punishment or penitence for manipulating others and wielding power.

Generally, the more affluent clients tend to visit mistresses in better neighborhoods or at houses with a more luxurious decor. But mistresses in both the upscale and the less posh setting have clients from all walks of life: students, engineers, computer programmers, teachers, doctors, lawyers, bricklayers, truck drivers, accountants, salesmen, and so on. Some clients are shy, unaggressive types, but most are the more dynamic, assertive males who want a brief submissive experience. Most clients are white, too, possibly because the rates are high and minority group members tend to have less income.

Mistresses report that their clients differ significantly based on age. The older ones, they claim, are generally more reliable, easier to satisfy, and more amenable to control. "The older clients are easier to work with," one mistress asserted. "They're more likely to show up when they call, and they're less demanding. They're more realistic in what they expect. And they tend to be more relaxed and let me do what I want. By contrast, I find the younger ones in their 20s all kinds of trouble. Some come without any money. And they're the ones that give me a hard time trying to resist in a session." Another said older clients were more willing to let her take control whereas the younger clients were more cynical, suspicious, and rebellious: "They're more likely to be concerned if they're getting their money's worth and complain if they think they are not. And when I have hassles about sex, it's always from the younger ones. The older ones know I mean it when I say no sex, but the young ones often try to test me. Or they complain that I said I might when I did not."

While male clients and males in the noncommercial scene are quite similar, professional women fall into two distinct groups. Mistresses in the first group resemble women in the noncommercial scene; those in the second group do not. In this first group—about half the mistresses I met—are dominants who previously worked at high-status or middle-level white-collar jobs (such as nurse, secretary, or teacher), much like the non-pros. Their main motivation for becoming a mistress was that it offered an opportunity to do something unique, interesting, and fun. The prospect of good pay was an incentive, but they also valued the chance to meet new people with novel, intriguing sexual preferences and to learn more about themselves. They were bored with their previous jobs and viewed being a mistress as a temporary or part-time fling that would allow them to explore their own sexuality, get rid of traditional inhibitions, and discover a new, exciting lifestyle. Eventually, they planned to do something else; but for a time, they wanted to explore.

For example, Kat, a former social agency director, became a mistress for a few months after she discovered D&S to be intensely erotic with her lover Mouse. Deena, a graduate student studying to become a sex therapist, spent three months as a mistress to expand her understanding in working with clients. Devora, once a secretary, turned to mistressing full-time after she and her husband, Ken, found they enjoyed D&S, and she felt she could make more money more easily as a mistress than as a secretary.

In contrast, the other group of mistresses I met are generally not involved in the noncommercial scene, come from a lower-status background, and previously worked as hookers, waitresses, go-go dancers, or in other marginal or dead-end jobs. For these women, being a mistress is much like being a prostitute except that it pays better and doesn't require them to have sex with the clients. They don't particularly care for their customers, and they see their role as one of putting on a good act for the client and giving him what he wants for his money. Some view mistressing merely as a way of putting their dominant personality to use for good money.

For example, Glenda, a 40-year-old mistress, operates a small house of dominatrixes from her private home. She worked as a hooker for several years, was arrested, and decided to try something new. "Since I have a strong personality, I thought I would be a good mistress," she explained. She mentioned the new venture to her boyfriend, he encouraged her, and she began advertising, with immediate results. In a few weeks, she had a half-dozen women working for her on several shifts and had a rapidly growing clientele. But, ironically, though dominant professionally, she is submissive to her boyfriend, "because I love him," she said.

Inge, a mistress in her late 30s, has worked as a go-go dancer and stripper, but finds being a mistress an easier way to make money. "Besides," she added, "since I'm a lesbian and don't like men very much, I love the opportunity to humiliate them. And I get paid for it, too." To play up her tough image, she calls herself Inge, the name of a popular S&M star who played a tough Nazi commander in one of her films, and advertises accordingly: "Dare to step into the power of the terrifying Mistress Inge. Experience the sadistic dangers she offers. She loves to torment and punish her slaves."

Regardless of their background or motives for turning professional, women find being a mistress an easy business to enter. They can do so without acquiring extensive skills, though they need to learn about techniques and safety precautions. Once they advertise, their ads soon bring results since so many submissive men are looking for mistresses. Bella, the former nurse, simply put an ad in the paper and within a few days began seeing clients even though she had little practical experience or knowledge of dominance. She read a few magazines and books for ideas to supplement the D&S activities she enjoyed with Benji, but learned most of her skills on the job. Women who have more extensive experience can merely begin asking for money for what they already know.

Typically, novice mistresses join an organized house or small group of women to gain experience and assurance. As they learn the business and acquire a stable of regular clients, some gradually branch out on their own.

Though they expect more risks in working independently, the freedom and money are much better.

THE INTERSECTION OF THE TWO LIVES

While some mistresses and clients try to keep their commercial and noncommercial lives distinct, for others, the boundary is blurred. For example, Brent not only keeps his D&S life separate from his home life with his wife, but he distinguishes between his commercial relationships with mistresses and his personal relationships with D&S friends by using a made-up name when he visits mistresses or goes to the Chateau. But with others in the D&S community, he uses his real name.

Other clients keep their relationships with mistresses strictly commercial, even though strong personal ties develop, to alleviate their guilt about having an extramarital relationship. Paying a mistress indicates that the relationship is a commercial one that they can set apart from their personal lives. For example, Danielle, who once worked regularly as a mistress, continued to see two married clients after she returned to school to study real estate. She told them they didn't have to pay anymore, since she was leaving the business and considered them friends. But they insisted on paying. "They wanted to pay," she explained, "so they could feel the relationship was not a threat to their marriage."

Similarly, some mistresses keep their work separate from both their everyday public lives and their noncommercial D&S activities. They try to keep contacts from overlapping to reduce possible embarrassment should they encounter someone out of the usual context. For example, Briget was working as a secretary while mistressing on the side. At an office party, she ran into one of her former clients. She said hello quickly, then vanished, as soon as she could into the crowd. "I was a little embarrassed," she admitted, "though he was much more embarrassed than I was." Similarly, at a Society of Janus party, Briget was nervous about encountering some of her clients, who she knew would be there, for she was afraid her professional activities would contaminate her social relationships. "I don't want to feel toward my personal friends as I do to my clients," she said. But she managed the encounter successfully: "I just said hello to my clients as if they were my friends, and they were comfortable with that."

Some mistresses also try to keep their business and personal lives apart by resisting clients' overtures to become friends apart from the commercial session. Women who do this tend to be those who see dominance as a job and have a background of lower-class work, including hooking. Their rationale for resisting is that the client who wants to see them outside of work just wants a free session and isn't really interested in them personally. "It tends not to work out when you see a client outside of work," one explained. "It's likely he wants a freebie. And he gets riled if you don't come across, for he really only wants your body."

By the same token, some women who work as submissives and dominants try to keep these roles distinct by using different names to express the two sides of their nature. Though many women readily switch in noncommercial relationships without using two identities, professionals usually find that customers want to relate to them in a particular way— knowing that the mistress plays different roles can spoil a client's fantasy. Thus when Briget worked in a house as a dominant, she called herself Big Bad Annie; when she played submissive, she was Sondra; and when she switched, she became Madame Fanny. "I even have a different personality that goes with each of these names," she said.

Quite often, though, these lives and roles do come together. Many mistresses attend noncommercial D&S groups and private D&S parties, and they often encounter their clients in these settings. Sometimes, they continue to see these clients for money; but often, after meeting in a noncommercial setting, they become friends and may begin dating. Or sometimes a commercial relationship turns into a personal one. For example, Dorothy began dating a few men who paid for a few sessions; Danielle sees some former clients as friends; and Sarona married a former client after dating him for about a year. When a mistress marries or gets serious with someone, she may retire but stay active in the noncommercial scene. Others drop out entirely. Generally, the mistresses who get involved with clients are from middle- or upper-class social backgrounds, since they already share similar lifestyles and values and their common interest in dominance draws them together.

Finally, commercial and personal lives may overlap if the dominant specifically orchestrates some carryover. She may instruct the male to do humiliating, or otherwise titillating, erotic acts between sessions such as wearing women's panties to work so he feels her continuing power and his submissiveness to it.

ORIENTATION TO DOMINANCE AND SEXUAL PREFERENCES

Characteristically, mistresses or former mistresses play around extensively, whether involved in a serious relationship or not, but their orientations to dominance or submission and their sexual preferences vary. A few of the mistresses I met saw themselves as completely or almost exclusively heterosexual. But most were exploring bisexuality, though they considered themselves primarily either heterosexual or gay.

Some mistresses who are exclusively dominant at work are mostly dominant in their personal relationships with males, females, or both. Others adopt the dominant role only for customers, while some switch in both settings. Several women who began working commercially as submissives learned dominance, and subsequently only or primarily played dominant.

For example, Kat worked first as a submissive and then as a dominant for several months, while experimenting with both sides of D&S with Mouse and other men, though being primarily dominant with women. Briget began working as a submissive for her dominant female lover, and after learning to be dominant on the job, she continued to play both roles with men and women. Andrea, who worked at a B&D house one summer as both a dominant and submissive—to take a break from the staid world of elementary school teaching—was almost exclusively submissive in her personal relationships with men, though she experimented with being dominant with a few men she dated. Celia, a publisher who considered herself primarily gay and bisexual, was dominant with male customers and friends. But with female lovers, she played all the roles—dominant, submissive, and switch. And others work out still other combinations, depending on whether they are playing for money or for fun, or whether with a woman or a man.

EVERYDAY EFFECTS

Mistresses find that their jobs influence their outlook and everyday life, sometimes from the very first day. Some of these changes are similar to those reported by newcomers to the noncommercial D&S scene. For example, after a day of working professionally, mistresses often want to play the opposite role at home, much like many who use D&S to counterbalance their roles in the workplace. When Sharon worked as a dominant for a few weeks, she had little energy left for being dominant at home, even though Lance urged her to do so. Conversely, mistresses who have several submissive sessions often return home wanting to be dominant. "It's a question of balancing the energy," one woman said.

Some notice that their attitudes to men change after they turn professional, for they begin to think about the men they meet as though they were clients. Some women find this experience exhilarating, feeling powerful as they imagine the man desiring submission so much that he would pay for it, and they enjoy picturing themselves putting him through his paces. "I do this all the time and I love it," one mistress said, "because I love to see men crawl."

But others find it unnerving when they discover themselves perceiving males in everyday life as sex objects to be controlled or humiliated. Jan, who worked as a professional for a few days explained: "I saw my attitudes begin changing a few days after I started learning how to be a mistress. I was having lunch with a man who was interviewing me for a job and I imagined him crawling on the floor. And that really bothered me, because I felt if I worked as a mistress on the side, it might make it difficult for me to relate to men in the business world as equals. And I was afraid that might create problems since I also want regular work." The next day she quit.

Some women who work as mistresses for an extended time report developing difficulties in confining their dominant role to their work. Instead, it may carry over into their lives at inappropriate times, as happened to Suzanne. She had worked as a mistress regularly for four years, seeing about four to five clients a day four days a week and lived in a house with two women who worked as mistresses and a third who did not. Continually, she found she had to struggle to keep her dominant persona from interfering with her being her normal self with friends. Sometimes, she recalled, she would suddenly assume her dominant persona in social situations and act forceful and severe, unnerving her friends. She would quickly catch herself and go back to being Suzanne; however, she said: "It makes me feel a little schizophrenic, and sometimes it makes me wonder who I really am—the mistress role I assume, or the person I once thought I used to be. It's sometimes confusing, and my friends think it's weird."

On the other hand, some women like the carryover, because they find they are more confident and assertive in everyday life. "I feel more powerful and sure of myself generally, after working as a mistress," one woman said. "After spending several months telling men what to do in a session, I feel better able to tell people what I think in the real world, too."

18

The Professional Session

Because each customer has different interests and each mistress has her own style, every professional session is different. Almost all sessions, however, begin with similar preliminaries: (1) The mistress talks to the customer for a few minutes to put him at ease and learn what he expects; (2) she agrees to fulfill his request or refuses if it seems too difficult or degrading—or if she suspects he's a policeman; (3) she collects the money as quickly and tactfully as possible, to downplay the commercial aspect of the session; (4) she announces the rules for the session and gives a safe word; (5) she and her client enter the fantasy world by assuming the new personas of mistress and slave or servant.

Likewise, most sessions end with closing rituals. Toward the end, the mistress uses some signal to let the man know the session is ending and it is time to return to the real world, much as a hypnotist gently helps his or her subject come back. Some mistresses coyly set the stage for a subsequent session or assign a task to be done before the next session: "Well, the next time you come, we'll see if you're still such a bad little boy"; or "Now, I want you to keep a fantasy journal for me and wear your cockring next week when you go to work, so you'll remember me." And some remind the client of the time by saying, "Our half hour is almost up. Do you want to stop now, or go on for another half hour?" But most mistresses are subtle in letting the customer know they are done. When the customer is dressed, the fantasy is over, and he re-enters the everyday world.

To give the flavor of a professional session, this chapter describes several sessions at two very different B&D houses—a down-at-the-heels private residence called The Dungeon and the well-equipped Chateau.

A DAY AT THE DUNGEON

The half-dozen women working at The Dungeon learned about it through an ad in the *Spectator*, a local sex newspaper: "Work as a mistress in a private house. No experience necessary. Will train." Lady Rosa, the head mistress, screens all phone applicants briefly, asking why they want to work as mistresses. If satisfied with their sincerity, she invites them over for an interview.

The prospective mistress arrives at The Dungeon, an ordinary white stucco row house that needs a paint job, and is greeted by Margaritta, a short busty Latin woman, who doubles as Lady Rosa's secretary and a mistress. The living room is filled with several overstuffed armchairs, a long sagging couch, and hanging plants. Lady Rosa, a tall commanding woman in a deep purple gown, conducts all the interviews. These brief chats seem intended largely to assess the applicant's sincerity. Rosa also describes her background: "I used to work as a cocktail waitress, bartender, and occasional hooker.... Then, since I had a dominant personality and my boyfriend encouraged me, I thought I could make money this way. I read a few books on what to do, worked on my own for a few months, and decided to expand." The interviews end with her discussing fees—$75 an hour, to be split between the mistress and the house.

If a deal is struck, Rosa shows the newcomer the basement dungeon— they go through a narrow kitchen, with dishes piled high in the sink, down a flight of rickety stairs alongside the back of the house, and through a creaky wooden door with peeling paint into the garage. At the far end is a heavy black metal door with bars on the small window. Behind it is the dungeon— a dank musty room about the size of a large storage closet. It contains several dangling hooks; a table with incense, candles, and bowls; and crops, whips, paddles, and other S&M paraphernalia. "This is where we see most of our clients," she explains. The tour concludes in an upstairs bedroom equipped with a massage table: "For special clients, or to use in a pinch if the other room is busy and the client can't wait."

New mistresses are offered either the noon-to-5 p.m. or 5 p.m.-to-10 p.m. shift, and make an appointment for training—Rosa prefers to train her own women. "Also, there's no sex," she concludes, "so everything's perfectly legal." However, if a woman wishes and is discreet, she hints, sex is possible, too. "If you know a customer really well and are sure he isn't a cop, then, that's up to you."

The training session begins with Lady Rosa explaining her procedures for learning the customer's wants, collecting the fees, minimizing no-shows and no-pays, and avoiding busts: "They'll call to set up appointments with Margaritta or the mistress whose ad they answer. Before they arrive, they have to call from a gas station about 10 blocks away to confirm. That way, the mistress knows they are really coming and can get dressed." The mistress is to greet her customer at the garage door, lead him to the dungeon, and ask him to very briefly describe his past likes and dislikes and any limits: "Don't ask them to be specific about what they want. It's psychologically stronger to ask what they don't want or if they have limits. It emphasizes that you're in control. And point out that once the session starts, you're in charge."

Next the mistress is to tell him the house safe word, *Camelot,* remind him there will be no sex, ask him to take off his pants, and ask if he is a police officer. "Do this before you ask for any money," she advises. The mistress is to be subtle in asking for her fee: "Ask them: 'Do you have something for me?'" Once she has the money, she is to handcuff the customer with his hands behind his back ("So he won't take off with the equipment"), tell him not to move, explain she will be right back, and take the money to the head mistress for the day—there is always at least one other woman in the house to make it safer for the dominant with new customers. Of course, this also ensures that mistresses turn over a share of the money: "It's too easy for a mistress to say the customer didn't show up if she's here alone, so she doesn't have to split the fee. I want to avoid the temptation."

Finally, Lady Rosa offers some tips on running the session. "Someone will call down from the kitchen five minutes before the session ends. If the customer wants to go longer, get more money.... Though there's no sex, you can always offer customers the option of jacking themselves off.... It's good to think up reasons to punish them.... Make sure they show respect for their mistress.... If they like humiliation, you can insult them. Tell them: 'I don't know why I bother with you'; make them act like a pig or sing songs; crush potato chips on the rug and ask them to eat it. But if they aren't into this, avoid it; it's a turn off.... And you can ask if they've done any of these things with a girlfriend, but stay away from their wife.

The novice is then invited to join an experienced mistress in several sessions and act as her assistant. And if she isn't dressed appropriately, Lady Rosa finds her something suitable.

When Barbara arrived for her day of training, wearing ordinary street clothes, Lady Rosa led her to a closet with her transvestite wardrobe—for males who like to dress up—and pulled out some garments—a pair of spindly heels and fish net stockings, a garter belt, and a faded blue maid's dress with frilly white cuffs. Then after dressing, Barbara joined Margaritta in the bathroom where she was giving Henry, a new customer, a golden shower. The bathroom was a tiny cramped room with a narrow aisle between the bathtub, toilet, and shower. As Barbara entered, she saw Henry, who looked like a young math student with acne, completely nude in front of a large baroque mirror. He rubbed and tugged on his penis while he watched himself in the mirror. Margaritta stood towering above him, taking frequent gulps from a can of beer, so she could build up enough fluid to give him a golden shower. Normally, she would have drunk a huge quantity of something about an hour before he arrived. But Henry had suddenly appeared at the door desperately asking for someone to do something immediately. Since the day was slow, she had made another unusual concession. Normally, any customer would pay the full $75 for a 50-minute session, or $50 for 30 minutes. But Henry said he had only $25. Could he come for a shorter time? Margaritta had agreed to 15 minutes. However, since he paid for a golden shower, she had to give him that even if the session went longer, which it did. By the time Barbara appeared, they had been in the bathroom 20 minutes.

For a few minutes, Margaritta continued to guzzle the beer. Then, she suggested that Barbara get the letter Henry wrote describing his fantasies and read it aloud, since she only had time to glance at it when he arrived. Barbara began reading, while Henry continued massaging his penis, and Margaritta drank more beer. The letter listed about 20 things he liked: "I love to have a woman sit on my head"; "I love golden showers, particularly when the woman pees into my mouth"; "I like it when a woman puts her shoe into my back"; "I find it very exciting to know a woman has given golden showers to hundreds of other men."

Margaritta sought to comply. She lifted her heel and ran it along his shoulder, straddled his back, and acknowledged she had done countless sessions with other men, although in truth she had been a professional for only three weeks. But Henry believed her. "So you've given hundreds of golden showers," he gushed, tugging even more furiously on his penis. "It makes me excited just to think about it."

When Margaritta finished the beer, she sent Barbara out for a cup of water. Meanwhile, Lady Rosa called out impatiently that the session had already gone on over 30 minutes. But Henry still hadn't gotten his shower, so Margaritta persisted, and when Henry asked her to dip hot wax on his back, she sent Barbara out for a candle and complied. However, she refused his request for brown showers: "That's too heavy for me. Besides golden showers are sterile. Brown showers aren't." When Margaritta finally said she was ready, Henry had one last request: "I'd really like it if I could put my head in the toilet and hold open my mouth."

After she agreed, he backed over to the toilet, leaning on his buttocks and arms like a crab, and let the back of his head dangle into the bowl. As he continued to tug on his penis, Margaritta straddled him, gave him the shower, and when she finished, told him the session was over. Though it had been far longer than 15 minutes, Henry was disappointed. "Isn't there anymore?" he asked.

Margaritta grimaced at him. "No. . . . It's time to go. . . . Get dressed," she hurried him. "And next time," she added, as he scurried out, "give me more warning, so I can be prepared."

Margaritta and Barbara then joined Lady Rosa and Inge in the livingroom, where they waited for customers to arrive. As mistresses often do during their frequent waits, they compared notes on customers, commented on unusual requests, and talked about recent personal events.

Inge mentioned that her regular customer, Danny, who liked to pretend to be a dog, was arriving soon: "He's really an ordinary sales executive and his wife knows nothing of his dog behavior." Lady Rosa said she was trying to launch a troop of women wrestlers. Inge said she was thinking of branching out on her own and seeing some private customers in her home.

When Danny arrived, Inge asked if he felt comfortable having a mistress-in-training observe. He consented, so Barbara joined them downstairs after Inge came back to give Rosa the money. When they returned, Danny was kneeling on the floor beside his clothes, his hands cuffed behind his back, per Lady Rosa's instructions. Inge uncuffed him and ordered him to put his clothes neatly on a chair. She drew her black cape around her with a flourish to emphasize her authority and stood behind him, brandishing a whip menacingly as he crawled to the chair with his clothes.

He put them down, but Inge snarled at him, since he liked humiliation: "No, that's not neat enough. I want to see you do it better." Obediently, he refolded them carefully. Then, she gave him her usual dog instructions. "Now, I want you to get on your hands and knees like a dog, and I'm going to give you some instruction. First, you can only speak in dog language unless I tell you otherwise, and that means one bark for 'yes,' and two barks for 'no.' Then, when I give you permission to talk as a human, you will always preface each statement with 'Mistress.' Now is that clear?"

Danny crouched on the floor, nodded, and gave a "woof."

"Then, let's see you walk around the room on your hands and feet like a dog."

Again, Danny complied. Inge then attached the cock ring to his penis and led him around by that. She asked him to sit up and bark. Once she tugged on his cock leash, and it fell off. She slapped him across his face for this indiscretion. "Can't you even keep it on," she yelled, snapping it on again.

Next, she took a handful of crackers from a box, telling him "these are dog biscuits," and she ordered him to eat them off the floor. When he finished, she put a bowl of water on the floor and said, "now drink from this." Afterwards she ordered him to parade around in front of Barbara. Inge petted him and asked him to sit up, beg, and roll over like a dog. He complied, but she alternated grimaces, the comment: "not good enough," and slaps, with strokes of praise on his back or head.

After awhile, she wanted him to be a human again. "You can now speak in human language," she said. But when she asked him if he understood, he answered with a bark. "You stupid idiot," she said derisively, "I'll have to discipline you for that." She ordered him to stand up and put his hands in two leather cuffs dangling from the ceiling. Then, she removed his cock leash, dripped hot candle wax on his back, and lashed him several times with the whip. Afterwards, she seductively danced around him, squeezing and jiggling her breasts with her hands and popping them in and out of her bra. She had once worked as a stripper, and now she played the tempting, but unavailable, stripper for him.

"You'd like to have these, wouldn't you?" she teased, "—but you can't." She pushed one breast up to her face and sucked on it. "You're wishing you could do this, aren't you? But no. It's not for you." She sucked again, as he gazed at her longingly. "However," she teased, rubbing her body up against his, "maybe if you're good I'll let you come at the end of the session. But only if you're good."

He nodded eagerly, assuring her he would behave, and she released him and ordered him to "lie on the floor like a dead bug." But when he curled over in a fetal position, she whacked him sternly with her crop. "No. Not like that. On your back. With your hands and feet in the air." After he did so, she directed him to lie down flat. "Now you have till the count of 10 to come. Can you do that for us? Since you've been ccoperative, I'll let you do it." He sprawled out, and she placed a vibrator against the base of his penis, and began counting slowly... 1 ... 2 ... 3. His whole body began shaking. "Now come," she ordered, and he had an orgasm.

After he left, she explained that Barbara's presence made the session more exciting for him, since she had been one more woman to see his humiliation. "He comes back every month and we do exactly this. Nothing else. He just likes to be a dog."

However, not all sessions work. If a mistress does something her client doesn't like or fails to distinguish his real objections from his play-session protests, she soon loses her control over him, and the session may end abruptly. For example, later that day, Frank, a building contractor in his late 40s, arrived for his first session with Inge. She was behind schedule because her earlier client had requested an extension. Rather than keep Frank waiting, Lady Rosa asked him if he would like to participate in a training session with herself and two novice mistresses. Frank, who had been to many previous mistresses, agreed.

After the usual preliminaries, Lady Rosa put leather cuffs on Frank's wrists and ankles, and chained them to hooks in the wall, since he said he liked light bondage. She ordered him: "Face the wall and keep your cock pressed against it." She began to hit him, while the novices watched. He flinched silently with each stroke. "Now I think I'll put you in hobbles." Lady Rosa released him from the wall, snapped a metal contraption around his ankles, strapped a nipple shield made of two leather circles around his chest, and hung two nipple clamps on his nipples. Frank quivered as she put them on, yet despite any pain, Lady Rosa pointed out that he was enjoying what was happening: "You see. His cock is erect. You can always tell if a man is enjoying what you are doing if you look at his cock."

But, in moments, the tenor of the session changed. Inge suddenly arrived, her black cape fluttering behind her, and immediately acted as though she were in charge of the session, though Lady Rosa had not told Frank that Inge would take over control.

Inge pushed in front of the group, scanned Frank's body quickly, noticed he had tied a leather thong around his scrotum before coming to the session, and began mocking him: "So you've tied up your own cock. Now who told you to do this? Couldn't you even wait to come here? We're the ones who give the orders. So for that, I want you to get down on your knees. I'll show you who's boss."

Uncertainly, Frank bent down, while looking up at Lady Rosa for reassurance. "Yes, go ahead," Lady Rosa said. As he crouched over on the floor like a frog, Inge hit him a dozen times with a cat and dripped candle wax on his back. She ordered him to stand up, and when she noticed his penis was not erect, she began teasing and insulting him. This turned out to be a major mistake. Although Frank had told her on the phone that he liked humiliation, he had meant only physical humiliation, such as being tied up or put in hobbles. Verbal humiliation and insults turned him off.

But Inge did not know this and blithely proceeded: "Come on now. Pull in your stomach. You're really fat. And why isn't your cock up? And it's so small. So puny.... Why aren't you excited by this? I feel it's an insult to me you aren't excited. Why not? Aren't you man enough?"

Frank said nothing, and Lady Rosa remained silent, too, though she later commented: "Unless you know a man likes it, you don't undermine his virility. That's sure to turn him off."

Next Inge tried the same teasing she used successfully with Danny. She jiggled her breasts and sucked them. She brushed against Frank seductively and teased: "But you can't have them. You can only look." Even Lady Rosa joined in, pushing her breasts out of her dress. But though Frank watched intently, he didn't become sexually aroused. Then Inge put the vibrator against Frank's cock—usually a sure way to arouse a man. But Frank didn't respond.

"Well, we'll have to do something else," Inge remarked. She released him from the hobbles and ordered him to roll around on the floor and act like a dead bug. Although Danny had found this activity exciting, Frank merely rolled about half-heartedly and then lay flat on the floor on his back.

"Now that's not right," Inge chided. "Can't you do anything right? Now, come over to me and beg like a dog." When he cupped his hands together without much enthusiasm, she teased: "Well, this is the first time I've seen a dog pray." Again, as the women laughed, and Inge explained how to do it, he meekly complied.

Had Inge been more sensitive, she might have still salvaged the session by recognizing that Frank didn't enjoy humiliation. Under some circumstances, a man does not perform correctly because he wants more humiliation and punishment. But for Frank, this wasn't the case. Also, Frank had been confused by Inge's sudden entrance, since he thought Lady

Rosa was his mistress. But Lady Rosa did not follow the usual procedure for one mistress turning her slave over to another. So he wasn't sure who was his mistress.

Then, Inge committed the final gaffe. "You know," she said in exasperation, "I don't think you can do anything right. I think you've been trying to make a monkey out of me. But that's not something for me to do. So now you're going to be a monkey instead. I want you to scratch yourself to amuse me. Maybe you can do this right."

She sat down in the chair, with her arms crossed in front of her and glared at him. "And now you can begin." But Frank would have none of this. Playing a monkey was just too ridiculous. He stood up and began tearing off his nipple shields. "Oh, just forget it," he said.

"That's Camelot," Lady Rosa announced, recognizing Frank's meaning, "that means he wants to stop the session." Frank nodded and began to dress, explaining why the session hadn't worked and describing what he really liked—light bondage, light whipping, and being teased by sexual talk. But, like most men who experience a bad session, he didn't ask for his money back. Not every session works, they know, and they view a bad one as "just one of those things." He felt the women had tried to give him a good session: "That's all you can expect.... I've been to dozens of mistresses before and I've dated a mistress for several months. Since she's leaving the area in a few weeks, I was hoping to find someone new. Now I'll just keep looking."

After he left, the women had a brief discussion of the failed session. Lady Rosa said he hadn't been clear enough in explaining the kind of humiliation he wanted, and she felt Inge had been too pushy. Margaritta suggested there was no need to feel upset "Since he only paid $55 for a half-hour session and had four mistresses, he shouldn't complain." And Lady Rosa concluded the discussion on a pragmatic note: "I don't want a client who is so picky about what he wants and then isn't clear when he asks for it. Besides, there are plenty of other clients. So there's no point wasting all this time talking about Frank."

A NIGHT AND THE CHATEAU

In contrast to the air of disrepair and distrust surrounding The Dungeon, the Chateau, one of a small chain of three B&D houses, resembles an upscale social club, with a waiting room like that in a doctor's office. On a typical evening, nine or ten men sit in the waiting room, silently flipping through magazines about sex or motorcycles, gazing down at the floor, or glancing anxiously around the room. In the adjoining room, women are fixing punch and dip for a party, scheduled to start at 6:30 p.m.

Though most customers, as in any B&D house, come for their session and leave, the Chateau organizes these parties to create a somewhat more social ambiance. But even so, the waiting men don't seem to want to talk very much. They are interested in relating to women, not other men. And some feel reticent, even embarrassed, about being at a B&D house in the first place. A few of the women occasionally drift into the waiting room to perk up the silent men.

On one such evening, Lorelei, a short woman with a pert elfin look appears and asks: "Would anyone like to hit me?" She has a thin riding crop in her hand and looks around the room for takers. A few men glance about, looking to the others to do something first. But no one moves. Lorelei tries again, dropping down onto her hands and knees, her rear in the air, and crawling around the room, the whip in her mouth. Tentatively, one man puts his magazine aside, takes the whip, and whacks her lightly. She smiles, and with the ice broken, another man follows suit. But then no one else takes up her offer, and she leaves the men to their silence.

A few minutes later, Sir James Hillyer, the owner, who looks like a cross between a jovial English lord and a pirate in tweeds, arrives with his two women "slaves," Gen, a submissive, and Shara, a switch; they live with him and work in the show. Shara prances into the waiting room to try to liven things up. She is wearing a studded gold collar, signifying she is an experienced switch, and she slithers about in her thin white sheath, fur wrap, and high stiletto heels, announcing: "The show will be starting soon. In the meantime, come join the party and talk to each other." But when no one budges, she gives up, too. "So don't talk to each other," she says and returns to the office.

But once the show begins, the place comes alive. A dozen or so customers follow Shara into a large unfurnished room, and they spread out in front of a large platform at one end. Then, Sir James begins the show, which is staged like an overdramatized 1920s silent movie, stylized like a fantasy. "We've just discovered some jewelry is missing," he announces. "And I've learned that one of my slaves has taken it. But no one will talk. Well, we'll just have to make them." He calls five of the women working at the Chateau to come forward, and they line up before him. He asks, "Who did it?" But no one will confess. He will have Shara whip them until they do. He begins with Gen, and with mock roughness pulls her from the line and pushes her toward the two cuffs dangling from the ceiling. "No, no," she protests dramaticially, as he tugs off her dress, revealing her frilly black underwear, and snaps her in. Shara approaches her with the whip, and strikes her across the buttocks, while her pleading continues: "No, no, I didn't do it.... Please, please, let me go."

Afterwards, he drags Lorelei and Alta to the cuffs and has them whipped in a similar way, as they protest their innocence. The audience, which has now grown to about two dozen males, watches raptly. The brief mystery soon comes to a close. Gen whispers to Sir James, and he announces that Gen has just named Shara as the thief. To punish her, he strings her up in the cuffs, strips off her dress, and whips her like the others. The case solved, it is time to party or attend sessions.

Most of the men remain, chatting with the women. A few disappear into one of three rooms for sessions. Victor, a Chateau regular, goes to have a session with Vickie, a switch he has visited before. She asks him to lie across the stool and strikes him a few times on the buttocks with the paddle.

"Act like you're my school mistress," he asks—for this is his favorite fantasy. Immediately, she slides into the role. "So you've been bad again. Well, take this. And this. You've been a bad, bad boy." After about five minutes, he asks to switch, and she lies across the stool, just as he did, and he paddles her. He likes both roles since, he explains: "I not only liked being paddled myself, but I liked watching the other boys in school get paddled, too. It was a great sport. We'd huddle around the door and peer in through the window." They switch several times, giving one another suggestions along the way. For example, Victor advises: "You can hit me harder.... Too much on that cheek for now; try the other.... Can you try the cane?"

A few minutes before the session is to end, Vickie stops caning him and offers him his usual reward. "If you want to conclude the session now by masturbating to climax, go ahead." Although the Chateau, like most B&D houses, doesn't allow its dominants to engage in intercourse and, stricter than most, doesn't allow them to touch the customer, the women may allow the customer to stimulate himself if he wants. Victor masturbates to orgasm, and then thanks Vickie for an enjoyable session, saying he will see her again.

Once he is gone, Vickie completes the usual record of a session for the house files: name of client, length of session, and his sexual preferences. The file will refresh her memory if he returns or will be a useful introduction if another woman in the house sees him next time. Few mistresses or houses have such an organized system, however. And although customers may not like to think of their visit being recorded like a clinical case, the Chateau finds that the files systematize and professionalize what is usually an ad hoc business.

19

Mistresses by Mail: Fantasy Tapes and Letters

S ome men have their encounters with mistresses through the mail. They carry on a correspondence, or they order a tape on which the mistress talks to them as though in a session, or she plays out a scene with a "slave," so they feel they are overhearing a session. When a man who enjoys submission writes to a mistress, reads her letter, or hears her tape, he gets aroused and typically masturbates. Many review these letters or tapes again and again.

Men learn about these services through ads in D&S and other sex-oriented publications. These tapes and letters cater to all sorts of sexual preferences; perhaps 5 to 10 percent are for men who like female dominance. The most popular tapes describe common D&S practices, like whipping, bondage, and humiliation. And an array of special fantasy tapes are available too, including tapes on cross-dressing, golden showers, and less usual themes, such as a female military officer who torments a male soldier or a guard who mistreats a prisoner. Also, customers can order custom-made tapes to enact their own fantasies. Some of the ads are run by working mistresses who make letters and tapes as a sideline activity. Others are run by letter writing and tape businesses, such as Nancy Andrews Tapes, run by Frank, a sprightly man in his 50s. Because men prefer to share their fantasies with a woman, Frank uses the name "Nancy Andrews," and during his five years in the business he has sold nearly 100 different tapes. Most are standards, which sell on the average several dozen to a few hundred copies, but he fills custom orders too. A tape featuring two half-hour sessions with different mistresses or a single one-hour session costs about $10. For a custom tape, which cost about $50–$80, the buyer writes out his fantasy, and the mistress makes a tape using his ideas and speaking directly to him. The women earn about $50 per hour of tape.

Much like the men who go to mistresses, men who request mail-order mistresses come from a variety of backgrounds. Some are happily married, others single. Some go to regular mistresses, others do not. And their occupations vary widely, from professional jobs to blue-collar positions.

However, generally, these males share one characteristic: they are very secretive about their D&S interests, keeping their desires hidden from wives and girlfriends. Hence they seek to fulfill their D&S desires through a faraway mistress, who writes to them or sends them tapes.

The women, most of whom are or have been pros, assume a special persona, such as Mistress Lydia, Velvet, or Crystal, just like a regular mistress, and they usually use the same name when making similar tapes, so repeat customers will ask for them. However, they frequently change names when they change roles, just as regular mistresses do. For example, when Paula makes dominant tapes, she is Mistress Majors. But when she plays the submissive, she becomes Ruby Ann.

Customers relate to these women as if they are quite real and sometimes write to them accordingly, as did a Florida surgeon who wrote enthusiastically: "My dear Mistress Majors, I just loved your tape. I do hope we can meet sometime. In the meantime, I thought I'd write to let you know a little about me, and I do hope you'll tell me a little bit about you, too. I hope that's not too much to hope.... Ever, your humble slave."

The women usually don't want to meet their customers, so they reply briefly, if at all. But Frank nurtures a man's desire to feel a personal relationship with his mistress by inviting him to purchase detailed letters or photographs of her. Occasionally, these photos are of the claimed mistress, but usually other women pose for them. Typically, the male gets a set of 10 to 20 poses of a woman lounging about in revealing or exotic attire, holding a crop or whip, or posed beside some D&S toys. These are not slick professional shots; rather, they are small snapshots featuring the woman in a homey, nonprofessional setting, so the male can better visualize his mistress and feel some personal contact with her—and, of course, order more tapes and letters.

The following excerpts from a tape called *Domination* by Mistress Cindy typify tapes in which the mistress describes what she is doing in the session. The purchaser can listen, imagine himself as her slave, and masturbate to orgasm.

> I see that you are here again, slave. I'm going to own you. Dominate you. You must understand that you are only here for my pleasure and that my pleasure comes first above all other things.
>
> You are to refer to me as Mistress. Any disobedience will be taken care of very quickly like so. (The sound of a slap.)
>
> Now kiss my boot, and do it well. Use your tongue...Lick, suck. Can't you do any better than that?
>
> Do you see what I'm holding in my hands? I'm holding a whip. If I have to use this on you I will.
>
> What a miserable little slave you are. A little pipsqueak...That is lousy. I have never seen a worse job. But then, what can you expect from a slave?
>
> Now stand up. Spread your legs. Put your arms out. Lower your

head. Don't look at me in the face. Who do you think You are? An equal?

Now, slave, unbutton your pants. Take off everything else. I want you completely nude.

Very good...Now that you are totally naked, totally humbled before me, I will require you to please me if you are worthy. Crawl on your hands and knees over to my chair.

Now remove my boots. Gaze upon my legs as you remove them.

Now tell me, slave, what do you see before you?

I have the most beautiful black silk stockings on, attached to a garter belt. It's quite sexy.

Massage my foot. Not too hard or you'll be punished....That's enough. I see you're getting too turned on. Just because I turn you on is no reason to be playing with yourself. I did not give you permission.

I see that you will need to be severely punished....Shut up. (Whack.) I said to be quiet. Stop playing with yourself. (Whack.)

I can see that the only way to get you to stop playing with yourself is to chain your hands behind your back. Are the chains cold? Do they bite into your flesh? I'm terribly sorry. (Whack.)

Now, roll over on your back. I don't care if your arms get in the way. I want you to suffer. What do you think I care about you? You're just a slave.

So there you are on your back, with your hard-on sticking out. I think I know what I'll do. (Laughs.) I have just the cure for hard-ons...I'm going to put on my boot and kick it to death...

I can hear you screaming. You must be in terrible pain.

Are you begging for my mercy already? I haven't even stuck the pin in yet. Now I'm just teasing your cock with this pin. You know how much it will hurt.

Now get up. On your knees. You've already had your punishment for the time being. Let me remove the chains and give you some pleasure. I'll lift up my dress for you. Let me pull down my stocking a bit, so you can see what beauty lies under my stocking. You can see my little garters dangling.

Now lower my stockings inch by inch. Now take this stocking all the way off. Stroke my leg, lick my ankle, suck on my toes, worship my leg.

Stand up on your two feet, put your arms out to your side. It's obvious you have a hard-on again. I thought I warned you about that. No problem. I'm simply going to tie it up and lead you by it to the rack.

Come with me. Get on the rack on your back, face up, keep your eyes closed. Stretch out, put your hands above your head, unbend your knees. You understand, of course, that you're going to have to be punished again.

You are a joke, slave. Oh, how stupid you look. You're dust under my feet. You're scum. You're nothing. Just a stupid, whimpering, sick slave. You're ugly...a jerk...a nobody. A nobody but my slave and you're here for my pleasure. (Laugh.) I have you helplessly tied up. You're totally under my power. You can't escape. There is nothing you can do. I've got you right where I want you.

As this tape illustrates, a common theme is putting the male down and playing up the female's power, while offering him occasional pleasure and perhaps eventual sexual satisfaction.

Frequently, as the tape nears its end, the mistress describes even more exotic torments. In *Dominance,* Cindy invites the customer to smell and suck her panties and watch her urinate in a glass. She orders him to drink it and then to bend over so she can insert a dildo up his ass. After she ties him up with more chains, she permits him to satisfy her orally. Finally, just as she might do at a regular session, she compliments him on his performance and urges him to come again:

> Very good, slave. You've been a good slave. You've pleased me so well. You're so obedient. You've paid so much attention to my pleasure. I hope we do it again.

Custom tapes are as specific as the male orders, and some customers supply a detailed script or list the events they want included. For example, Paul, a stockbroker, 40, included several nude close-ups of himself and a woman holding their legs in the air to show off their backsides, along with a graphic description of the female victim he wanted tormented. He outlined an elaborate plot for her torment, which began:

> *Subject:* Brenda, 5'4", dark long hair, 33 years old, 36–22–36, white skin, big ass, large nipples, very hairy crotch...big feet, long toes.

He explained that Brenda, a counselor at a girl's camp, had humiliated, tormented, and spanked Alice, a disobedient camper, and "for the final humiliation, she makes Alice suck her toes." On returning home, Alice complains to her mother, Ann, about her ordeal, and Ann decides to subject Brenda to similar torments. Paul wanted the mistress to play Ann and described exactly what she should do: rig the rec-room with various instruments, including feathers, paddles, brushes, clothespins, and dildos; set up a table with a red velvet cover; and invite over some friends to make Brenda's experience even more humiliating. Further, he asked: "A great deal of this tape should pertain to tormenting Brenda's feet to get even with her for making Alice suck her toes."

And he suggested specific torments:

> "Brenda is placed on the red velvet table on her back, arms tied straight back over her head, legs spread extremely far apart, and bent and tied at the knees...so her legs can't move. This position exposes her ass, pussy, and bottom of her feet to her audience.
>
> Ann removes Brenda's high heel shoe and runs her fingernails over the bottom of her foot. She cuts a hole in the bottom of the nylon and

torments her foot through the hole. Then she slowly cuts away the toe portion of the nylon, exposing the toes one at a time. Then, she tickles and torments the toes as Brenda pleads for mercy."

Finally, in his scenario, Ann tears the nylons off completely, torments Brenda's entire foot, invites the audience to join in, "screws" Brenda with a strapped-on dildo, and makes Brenda satisfy her orally, while the female audience cheers them on.

When a woman receives such a script, her job is to dramatize it. In another representative custom request, Dave, a business executive, asked for a tape in which a male boss is humiliated by his secretary, who forces him to cross-dress and follow her orders. This scenario is exciting, Dave explains in his letter, because the male is shamed and degraded by the female whom he normally treats as an inferior: "Let the punishment fit the crime. The executive becomes the secretary, the college stud ends up as a cheerleader... the once haughty husband shamefully plays the maid. For every male-chauvinist dominated role, there is an appropriate feminized punishment."

Dave requests that the tape include four key events. First, the boss discovers that some documents he signed without reading turned the whole business over to his secretary and authorized her to fire all the important male employees. When he tries to destroy the documents, his secretary "quickly defeats him and beats him unconscious."

Second, the boss wakes up to find he is nude, shaved, and has signed an application to work as a secretary-trainee. His secretary, now his boss, describes his duties, and when he balks, she punishes him with a whip. She shames him by asking him how he can support himself and his wife on such low pay and berates him for having a secret extramarital affair. His wife appears and volunteers to help the secretary humiliate him.

Third, the women decide he must become the perfect secretary. They give him a female name, dress him, and require him to perform to their satisfaction, while they insult him and all males in general. Finally, his wife orders him to change into a French maid's suit, so she can train and torment him at home. His wife and secretary announce that they have been secret lovers for months. They will live in a lesbian marriage in his home, while he serves them as the maid, and they insult him about his inferiority and that of all men.

Thus, in his fantasy, Dave has become a degraded caricature of the women he usually controls everyday.

Some customers take this role reversal even further and fantasize about the most humiliating, degrading experiences possible. For example, Andy, a 27-year-old civil engineer whose hobbies include swimming, pool, ping pong, reading, and movies, wanted a tape of a mistress treating him

like "absolute garbage": "She should be a real harridan, who's always
yelling and abusing me." He explained that one day, when he breaks her
favorite ashtray, she decides to use him as a replacement. She dumps ashes
in his mouth and stubs her cigarettes out on his tongue. Next, she makes him
serve as her "garbage can and toilet": "She makes me swallow everything
from food scraps, grease, coffee grounds, to snotty Kleenex, etc. Just
anything that goes in a garbage can, as well as her shit and piss, of course."

Should he resist, she manhandles him physically until he accepts.
Then, she gives him horrible concoctions and shoves his face into it. "And
now for the *horrible part*," he writes, making his fantasy as disgusting and
degrading as he can: "She doesn't know when to quit. She's driving along a
road and sees a dead dog that's been hit by a car. She scoops it up with a
shovel and brings it home. She beats me up until I eat it, and if I throw up,
which is up to you, I'm made to lick it up."

Finally, he asked his mail-order mistress to give him orders to carry out
in real life: "You can ask me to eat horrible concoctions, and I love to drink a
lot of water at the order of or looking at the picture of a dominant woman,
so don't hold back." He also urged her to suggest various tortures or
exercises.

In turn, like many customers making such requests, Andy planned to
carry out these orders. In her reply tape, Barbara told him to cook together
a box of jello, a can of sauerkraut, 1/4 lb. of cheese, a container of Cool
Whip, an egg, and a hamburger patty. Also, she told him to drink a quart of
water every 2 hours and to do 10 push-ups after each drink. When Andy
wrote back, he complimented Barbara on her "fabulous" tape and assured
her he followed her directions, though he asked for a modification, writing
in the pleading style of the submissive:

> What I'm about to ask may be a bending of the rules, but I beg you to
> consider it. The menu…was superb in imagination, but bad in taste.
> Thank you. I have eaten it for two days and will eat it for five more. Also,
> the quart every two hours with 10 push-ups is being followed. But every
> two hours is causing problems. I drink 4 quarts in the 2 or 3 hours before I
> go to bed and 3 or 4 quarts after I get home from work. Otherwise it's like
> clockwork. I do have quite a gut-ache and am costantly aroused.
>
> Anyway, could you write a little note with a new recipe you want me
> to try and the quantity and timing of water you demand I drink.

In short, through these tapes and letters, males seeking submission
privately and safely let their fantasies go into far-out, forbidden realms,
even beyond what they might like to experience. Indeed, the very
bizarreness of these fantasies seems to be a source of erotic arousal.

20

Magazines and Books

There is an abundance of magazines and books—not to mention films, photographs, and art—on D&S themes. D&Sers tend to be avid readers, looking for new ideas on sexual positions, equipment, and scenarios. Also, the literature helps D&Sers define "the scene" by presenting models of behavior and style, gives additional validation for D&S in that others are doing it, and provides source material on D&S equipment, costumes, organizations, and personal contacts. Also, males and occasionally women use this literature to stimulate masturbatory fantasies.

BOOKS AND FICTION

Relevant books fall into five major categories. First are the how-to books, with names like: *A Beginner's Guide to S&M* or *An Introduction to Bondage*. These are written primarily to instruct dominants, though submissives read them, too. Second are the psychological case studies by psychiatrists and therapists, such as Krafft-Ebing, Albert Ellis, R.E.L. Masters, and W. Stekel. Many D&Sers read these to better understand their own psyches. Third are the fantasy and quasi-historical or anthropological accounts of ancient goddess worship and matriarchal societies. Some of these books glorify famous queens like Cleopatra and Nefertiti or relate myths about pagan goddesses from Greece, Egypt, and other early societies. Most of these freely mix romantic speculation and fact. A fourth category includes a smattering of literary or classic works of S&M fiction, such as *The Story of O*, by Pauline Reage, and *Venus in Furs*, by L. von Sacher-Masoch, which describe the experience of a female and male submissive, respectively, in sensitive, literary terms.

The fifth category, however, is by far the largest—a vast outpouring of purely prurient schlock, sold in adult book stores or advertised in sexually oriented magazines. These feature one sexual encounter after another grafted onto the barest of a plot and characters whose feelings or motivations are of little concern. The emphasis is on pure action and sensational thrills, as the titles suggest: *Sadistic Schoolmarm, Prisoner of Pain, Torture Island,* and *House of Horror.*

MAGAZINES AND NEWSPAPERS

A vast array of specialty newspapers and magazines is devoted to a variety of D&S and other sexual activities. Most are sold in adult bookstores or by mail. The major D&S newspapers—*Female Domination, Dominant Mystique, S&M Express, Fetish Times, Corporal,* and *Ouch**—feature articles, fantasy stories, and ads for making contacts. Most are published regularly, and D&Sers can subscribe. In contrast, most of the magazines, selling for around $6, highlight sexy photographs and ads presented in slick, glossy formats. They are frequently undated and marketed as single issues— many are labeled Vol. 1, No. 1.

Newspapers and magazines cater to virtually every D&S fantasy, with the name and look of each indicating whether it is designed to appeal to heterosexual or gay readers. Typically, gay male publications feature strong macho males wearing leathers, riding motorcycles, or looking otherwise aggressive and tough. In contrast, the publications for heterosexuals highlight the sexuality of the female, whether dressed in D&S finery or nude. For instance, one *Woman in Command* featured a cover photo of a busty woman whose cop's uniform is pulled open to show her cleavage. An issue of *Pussy Power* featured a man with his wrists bound behind him, groveling on his knees while he licks the crotch of a beautiful blonde wearing only a corset and heels.

Titles coyly allude to the type of fantasy featured. Bondage enthusiasts can buy the *B&D Quarterly, Tied Up,* or *Bound and Gagged*; those who like their bondage tinged with S&M can read *Bound and Spanked*; and cross-dressers have *Transvestites in Bondage. Slave Exchange* and *Enslaved* focus on male slavery, while *Discipline Classes for Unruly Slaves* emphasizes slave training and discipline. There are magazines on spanking *(English Tanning)*, kidnap fantasies *(Abduction)*, fetishes *(Fetish Fantasies)*, Nazi imagery *(Fascist Femmes)*, and on women in positions of authority *(Ladies in Uniform)*.

In some magazines, women fight it out with each other or with men *(Battling Bitches)*; or they are evil, sinister, sexually insatiable creatures, as

---

*These are published by the following publishers:
Female Domination and the S&M Express, Nubon Publishing Company, New York, New York.
Ouch, Matriarch Productions, New York, New York.
Corporal and *Dominant Mystique,* Esoteric Press, Great Neck, New York.
Fetish Times, the B&D Company, Van Nuys, California.

in *Wicked Women* or *Satan in Heels*, *Waterworks* and *Watersports* feature women giving enemas or golden showers, while *Petticoat Power*, *Mistress Amazon*, *Bitch Goddesses*, or *Dominatrix Domain* treat more general dominant themes. Should the male want to imagine himself dominated by an Oriental woman, he can read *Oriental Dominatrixes*. For those interested in all sorts of bizarre sex, *Kinky World*, *Bizarre Stars*, and *Kinque* are available. Other publications list only contact ads, such as *Kinky Contacts* and *Aggressive Women*. Most of these magazines feature pictures and ads and keep copy to a minimum. Still, a few like *Lashes I*, which focuses on female domination, and *Reflections*, *Expose*, and *Variations*, which treat sexual alternatives of all types, have thoughtful articles, besides other features, like advice columns, letters, and ads.

D&Sers turn to these publications for four main reasons: to learn about the scene and get turned on; to obtain D&S merchandise and equipment; to make contact with others; and to learn new techniques. Let us briefly examine how the D&S literature serves these needs.

Getting Information and Turning On

The stylized imagery of the dominant female and submissive male in these publications presents role models for some readers, as well as giving them ideas for new activities or positions, and is sometimes arousing in itself. The dominant female image consistently combines signs of authority and seductive sexuality. Typically, the dominant woman wears high boots or heels—the pointier and higher the better—which she can use to step on or kick the submissive male. Or she can present her feet for his worshipful caresses and kisses. Capes typically give women a powerful, sinister look, and some wear decorations or accessories that suggest power or pain, such as boots with spurs or belts and leather cuffs with studs. At the same time the women's sexuality is emphasized by feminine garments that show off their legs, buttocks, or breasts, such as stockings, garters, corsets, miniskirts, long slinky gowns, tight-fitting body suits, or bras with holes in them.

The color and material of these garments also play up the woman's power. Typically, the photographs show women in black, a color associated with evil, power, and strength, or in strong forceful colors, most notably red. Most also wear leather, which suggests a strong commanding look. Appropriate equipment completes the dominant look: whips, crops, paddles, belts, and chains.

Similarly, the poses convey both power and sexuality. For example, a woman is shown wearing only a black leather corset, stockings, and long gloves, making the usually submissive gesture of presenting her naked rear to a man. But he, also naked, is bending over to lick her rectum and his hands are bound tightly behind him.

The only major variations from the usual dominant imagery are photographs of women depicted in a particular authority role, such as an officer, teacher, or nurse. Yet, even when a woman dons the appropriate costume, such as a Nazi uniform or police officer blues, she still displays her sexual attributes. One cover shows a woman wearing a police jacket and cap, looking sternly ahead and firmly gripping a billy club—but her open jacket reveals her cleavage, and she squats so that her stockinged legs and thighs peek out over her calf-high boots.

The males, of course, are depicted as helpless and without power. They are usually naked or in briefs, and many wear the appurtenances of submission: gags, ankle or wrist cuffs, slave collars and leashes, ropes, and chains. Typically, they are kneeling, lying down, crawling, or defensively waiting to be struck. Some are tied in contorted positions, begging, crying out in agony, or dangling from ceiling hooks.

Most readers look at these pictures and fantasize being in the scene depicted. Some use them as cues for new scenes, such as one cross-dressing and bondage enthusiast who saw a picture of a dominant woman towering over a miniskirted male who is lying on his belly with his hands, feet, and neck tied to a pole. After he fantasized about the scene for a while, he asked his lover to try it. Having enjoyed his fantasy, he now wanted to experience it, too.

Obtaining D&S Merchandise and Equipment

The magazines, newspapers, and catalogs that offer D&S merchandise serve an important function for D&Sers, since most items are not sold in ordinary stores and few specialty stores cater to erotic tastes. These publications also allow readers to shop in the privacy of their homes and to order custom-made equipment. The amount of variety is tremendous since the products are designed for an audience that wants something unique, different, and perhaps outrageously bizarre.

Most of the clothing items advertised are designed to make the woman more sexually alluring: fancy corsets, revealing bras, flamboyant capes, decorated garter belts, string bikinis, tightly clinging body suits, and panties with a slit crotch. Other items play up the woman's ability to administer pain, such as a pair of black deerskin gloves covered with needle points.

Much equipment is designed to emphasize the submissive's lowliness and helplessness: slave collars, leather cuffs with rings for attaching ropes and chains, various leather and metal restraints, and harnesses. The catalogs feature all sorts of hoods, blindfolds, and gags, including simple slipover hoods, hoods with removable mouthpieces, and specialty gags shaped like penises. Hardware to produce pressure or pain includes "cock rings" and "testicle trainers" that fit around the penis or testicles and tighten up as the mistress adds weights, penis sheaths with studs that dig in as the male gets excited, and clamps the mistress can attach to all parts of the body. Besides their physical effect, such as giving pain or cutting off sound, light, or communication, these gadgets have symbolic meaning as symbols of submission.

All this variety for a special interest audience does not come cheap, however. Customers must pay fairly stiff prices, particularly when they purchase hand-made or special-order merchandise. For example, leather cuffs average about $40 to $50, thigh high boots with long spiked heels and four inch platforms about $300 to $400.

D&S and sex-oriented publications also carry ads for D&S novels, films, photographs, tapes, and magazine subscriptions. Video enthusiasts can order full-length feature movies for about $100 a film, like *Dominatrix Without Mercy*, about a woman who is trained by a madame to make men "crawl, beg, and suffer, while they love every painful moment."

Making Contact

Most of the contact ads in magazines and newspapers are placed by professional mistresses, single men, and couples, although single nonprofessional women sometimes advertise, too. Correspondingly, most of the respondents are men and couples. To preserve anonymity most magazines use coded ads, and respondents include a forwarding fee with their letter. But advertisers in local publications generally use their own address, post office box, or phone number. Advertisers are often quite specific about their interests and some include photos that play up their sex appeal, usually close-ups of their bodies or shots of mistress-slave sessions. Publishers encourage using photos since they attract more correspondence.

The mistresses who "dominate" this advertising usually present themselves as tough, cruel, and powerful, though occasionally as an understanding mistress of the humble slave. For instance, in a typical *Reflections* ad a mistress stands, feet akimbo, wearing a black corset, garter belt, and studded collar, and glares out at the reader as she brandishes a whip. She describes herself as a "Creative dominant, tall, blonde mistress, now recruiting males and females into my web of slaves. I have a few openings for true submissives. I want and expect slaves for my pleasure, with unquestionable adoration. Will answer all. Send S.A.S.E."

Other mistresses offer specific types of dominance: enemas ("Wet dreams? Cum get a Bardex enema from busty Leona"); spankings ("Tall English Lady will give and take spankings"); foot worship ("Foot fetishists rejoice. California's premier foot Mistress will accept only a few foot slaves"); heavy pain ("Princess Regina will whip you till you bleed or plead"); and other specialties ("Slaves wanted for Golden Showers," "Strict but gentle Mistress Sirena wants generous submissives at her feet for oral satisfaction," "B&D shows with my female slave").

Nonprofessionals also place ads to contact other nonprofessionals for both casual encounters or a long-term D&S relationship. One Southern Californian, with the tanned look of a sales manager relaxing after a golf game, advertised for women to play: "Gentleman of leisure seeking female, dominant or submissive, for fun and games in the sun. I enjoy B&D, water sports, cross-dressing, etc. I am not a newcomer to this realm of wonderful fantasy." Another submissive, photographed in a rubber suit, mask, and hip hugging boots, asks: "How would you like a new kinky friend? Sincere young male, submissive and inventive, makes his own equipment; has a dungeon. Into rubber, leather, TV, and whatever. Seeks females and couples for a venture into the bizarre."

Some males are even willing to travel, such as a Texas male who was eager to "Travel Midwest and West Coast....I enjoy all cultures (except extreme pain)... and enjoy meeting and serving people with like interests." And some are seeking a serious relationship, such as one male who advertised: "I seek a sexually and emotionally secure woman who would enjoy exploring with me the delicious eroticism of dominance and submission in a loving caring relationship."

Couples who advertise commonly want to play on occasional meetings— and are not interested in long-term relationships. Some include pictures of themselves participating in some favored type of play. One such ad read: "We're a couple experienced in all degrees of Bondage and Discipline and we wish to have 'face-to-face' meetings with SINCERE people. Our 'playroom' is equipped to handle most scenes, including TV slaves." Their photograph showed the wife wearing a corset standing beside her naked husband who was wrapped about with seven belts and suspended arms outstretched from a wall. Other couples are very specific: "ATTRACTIVE COUPLE, she tall and totally dominant. Our interests are maid training, petticoat punishment, over the knee spanking, and other forms of corporal punishment. Wish to trade photos, home movies, cassettes, etc., with other couples."

When nonprofessional single women do advertise, they usually have a unique long-term arrangement in mind, such as a business venture or live-in situation. For instance: "EX-PROFESSIONAL Dominant Woman seeks submissive or willing man with house or apartment and small space to hold psychosexual awareness sessions....Opportunity for personal relationship with a lovely woman." Another sought a "male slave" to share her house and cook and clean.

In some cases, these "non-professional" advertisers—both women and couples—turn out to be pros. So seasoned readers respond accordingly—

hopeful they may meet others who genuinely enjoy playing with D&S, yet aware they may be contacting yet another pro.

Learning New Techniques

D&Sers also look to the how-to articles in these publications. They can find articles on the more typical D&S practices (knot tying and whipping) and more unusual techniques (giving enemas or experimenting with sensory deprivation). Commonly, both safety and technique are stressed.

For example, in a waterworks article, an enema enthusiast describes do's and don'ts and recommends effective procedures ("Try giving a preliminary enema, so the recipient can take more water."). In *Variations*, a bondage afficionado offers tying strategies ("You can attach screw eyes to the walls or floors or posts of the bed"), recommends a few unusual settings ("You might enjoy locking a light chain around your partner's waist and taking them out to dinner"), and cautions about safety ("Do not interfere with circulation. Either pad the wrists and ankles by wrapping a washcloth around them and tying on top of the cloth, or obtain padded leather cuffs.") An *Expose* writer outlines tattooing and piercing techniques; and in *Reflections*, an expert on the subject, Fakir Musafar, explains how to use sensory deprivation and various restraints—helmets, masks, hoods, cages, boxes, and mummy bags—to create a "glorious, trancey, spacey state" in which the submissive floats in "an indescribable high."

Certaintly, some D&Sers read these articles simply to learn about others' fantasies and do not plan to use the described techniques. But others do experiment, and they consider these articles a major source, along with meetings and informal conversation with D&S friends, for expanding their repertoire.

D&S Tales

Tales of erotic encounters, sometimes illustrated with photos, liberally dot D&S newpapers and are featured in some magazines. Many tales are presented as though they are true, but most are fantasies of extreme, intense, or uniquely bizarre sessions and situations. The typical story is written from the perspective of a male protagonist—since most readers are male—although sometimes a professional mistress or a woman in a D&S couple describes her experience. The underlying message in all these stories is the power and superiority of the woman, the weakness and inferiority of the male.

Readers look to these stories both for erotic arousal and for new scenarios and techniques. Among the most common situations and themes are the following:

● A session with a mistress: Some of these tales are fairly realistic depictions, but many feature extremes of pain and humiliation, unusual combinations of mistresses and slaves, and other improbable variations on the basic session.

● Complete enslavement: In these tales the male protagonist willingly becomes his mistress's full-time slave—or one of her cadre of slaves—or he may be sold into bondage. After describing the abject humiliation of his position, he may boast of how much torment he can endure, describe his fears of being punished for insubordination, and rhapsodize about the wondrous powers of his owner.

● D&S groups and communities: These tales describe further unusual (and usually improbable) activities among large groups or communities of dominants and submissives.

● Recognition tales: These tales describe chance encounters in which either the male discovers a woman is a dominant or meets a woman who helps him discover his true submissive nature.

● D&S with family members: Although almost all D&Sers hide their activities from their children, parents, and relatives, in these tales family members become eager, active participants.

● The ultimate fantasy—castration: These tales appear somewhat less frequently, but are usually presented as truthful accounts.

● Ambivalence and resistance: These tales describe the ambivalence the male protagonist initially feels in submitting to a dominant woman. Although the situations are quite exaggerated, the feelings described are fairly realistic.

● The superiority of the women, the inferiority of the male: This theme runs through all the literature, but in some articles it is featured.

To illustrate the nature of these stories, let us consider typical examples of each of these categories.

The Session with the Mistress

In these stories, the male is usually strictly submissive, though sometimes he has the opportunity to switch with the mistress or take out his dominant urges on a submissive woman. In one representative story in *Corporal*, a traveling salesman answers an ad of a dominant seeking slaves. Mistress Tina arrives at his hotel room, orders him to undress and to stand in the corner, snaps handcuffs on him, pulls a latex-hood over his eyes, and jams a penis-shaped gag into his mouth. Then, after she dresses up like a typical mistress in tight black leathers, she asks him to kiss her feet, crawl on his belly, dress up like a French maid, serve her some champagne, and kneel on the floor like a human foot stool. Then she whips him and gags him, orders him to "worship her orally," inserts a fat rubber dildo into his rectum, makes him drink a golden shower and perform other "outrageous, atrocious acts."

Sometimes these sessions go on for days, and may involve several mistresses. For example, in an account of a slave-training weekend in *Ouch*, a man describes how one mistress, Aradia, lends him to several friends, who put him through his paces at a private beach house. He licks their shoes clean, prepares their meals, eats dog food from a bowl, and when he doesn't satisfy them, they call him names. One mistress orders him to act like a horse and dog and takes him out for a walk on a leash. Another mistress ties him up and keeps him blindfolded and gagged for several hours. A third dresses him as a woman and forces him to make love to her girlfriend. When he subsequently tells Aradia that he learned from his training that all women are mistresses, derive pleasure in different ways, and that he must serve all women and return their love, Aradia is so pleased, she decides to keep him as a slave forever.

In these mistress stories, males also emphasize how much pain they suffer, and they seem to glow with pride at the amount of forcefulness, discipline, and pain the woman can offer. It is as if their level of endurance or suffering demonstrates some manly pride that expands as the woman's power over them increases and they are able to "take more."

A typical example of this outlook appears in "The Whipping," a poem which appeared in the *SM Express*. Here, one man ecstatically describes a whipping from a girl he belongs to.

> ...Why will she hurt me and mark me once again?
> Because I *belong* to the girl, Karen. I am hers. She
> receives pleasure from whipping me. She gets wet.
> Thus I am hers to whip. Simple enough...
> I *am* a slave. Circa 1977...
> Swishing burning whip of leather...
> Squeals. Cries. But I do not beg...
> Buttocks ignited. Whip marks for days...
> I am aflame...Now I make no sounds. I have reached zenith...
> She can whip me now till dawn. Forever...
> I am *yours* to whip, Karen. For always and always.

In another representative poem from *Ouch*, a man talks about how he wants women to be forceful and cruel, because males need to be punished. Also, he claims that when a woman shows she is strong and in command, the male will want to serve and worship her. He writes:

> Women, be forceful, demanding and strict!
> Use your males! Punish! They need to be kicked.
> Pay them a hundredfold; even be cruel!!
> Manhood is out. It's your turn to rule.

Males, beg your Mistress to never forgive!
Learn how to serve her as long as you live.
Crawl at her heel, touch her toe with your lip!
Praise her grand beauty and worship her whip!

Complete Enslavement

In these tales, the writer typically claims to have found true happiness in living a 24-hour-a-day female dominance lifestyle. Frequently, the male boasts of how much torment he can take, fantasizes about being punished or dismissed if he doesn't please, or rhapsodizes about the wondrous powers of the female in charge.

In one representative story, James meets a woman at an S&M club who is looking for "a permanent live-in domestic." Since her present slave is leaving due to a long illness, she is looking for a substitute. He arranges to have her move in with him and agrees to pay the rent and all expenses, plus give her his monthly check.

When she arrives a few days later, she places a collar around his neck, asks him to crawl ahead to lead her to her room, puts on some sexy clothing—black bikinis, bra, and stockings, and places a hard leather chastity belt on him, so she can exercise her control over him in two main ways—rewarding him or denying him sexual release. She whips him hard to show him what he must try to avoid by serving her well, and during the eight years he serves her, he takes care of all domestic duties and carries out her every command.

In another account a reader reports that he was constantly in bondage and reminded of his slave status in various ways. "My nipples and penis are pierced and I wear rings through these piercings. At night, I am required to sleep in slave chains, and my wife owns a nice collection of whips which she particularly likes to use. I am her slave and either I please her or I suffer. Sometimes I suffer just because that gives her pleasure."

D&S Groups and Communities

These tales help readers feel more secure, since they are about a large network of D&Sers who know each other. Also, some find it titillating to think about participating in a large group.

In a representative letter to *Fetish Times*, a New Jersey "slave" claims he is one of seven males who meet weekly with "eighteen wonderful women," who are primarily businesswomen from about 40 to 50. They meet in a townhouse of one of the women, and at each meeting, the women give them 30 lashes with a cat-of-nine-tails, and order them to lick their boots and satisfy them orally. Another male in a series of *Corporal* articles describes the ongoing adventures of a network of 14 couples who have banded together to promote female dominance in erotic play and everyday life.

Recognition Tales

In many stories a discovery occurs—the male unexpectedly encounters a woman who turns out to be dominant, or a woman recognizes his true submissive nature and forces him to submit. In either case, he is ultimately made powerless by a strong, commanding woman.

In one such story, "Room Service," from *English Tanning*, a doctor is relaxing in his hotel room after a dull conference, when the chambermaid, a "statuesque beauty," pops in with clean linen. She starts to clean the room, sees him reading a spanking magazine, scolds him for reading such "nasty" literature, and suggests he should have a good spanking, because "then you wouldn't have to read about it." He removes his pants, lies across her lap, and she proceeds to spank him, ignoring his cries to stop, because she tells him, "I always spank children until they cry." The next night, she returns, giving him more of the same, and in the end, he clings to her, whispering softly: "Mama, I love you."

In another story, a reader relates in a long rambling letter to the editor of *Female Dominance* how he was transformed from a "macho" to a slave. As a senior at college, he dates a beautiful young blonde. She alternately leads him on and rejects his advances, until he kneels before her, begging for favors. She pulls his face to her boot and promises him a reward for licking it clean with his tongue; he does so, feeling an inexplicable thrill. After two weeks of additional humiliation, "She had me trained to the point that She just had to phone at any hour, and I'd rush to Her apartment, ring the bell on my knees, and crawl in when She opened the door."

Eventually, she drops him, but the encounter teaches him about his true inner nature, and he is now another woman's devoted slave.

D&S with Family Members

In these fantasy tales, the male discovers that family members are secretly D&S enthusiasts or entices them into performing D&S activities. Some readers find such stories especially titillating because they challenge social taboos or depict the introduction of once-disapproving family members into the scene.

In a representative tale, presented as a real-life experience in *Fetish Times*, a mistress, Erika, discovers that her 11-year-old niece, Gretchen, has become interested in sex. Gretchen, already showing her proclivities towards dominance, urges Erika to give her a "boy" she can whip. Erika offers her Barney, a 30-year-old lawyer, who is excited at the prospect of being punished by a young girl. When Barney arrives Gretchen instinctively expresses the dominant spirit. She tells him to strip, puts handcuffs on his wrists, slaps him for being late, hits him several times with a rubber-covered truncheon, and has him kneel and lick her shoes. After a lengthy and exciting session, Barney promises to appear before her weekly for discipline and to "be respectful of all women from now on." As the story illustrates, even a "mere child" can make him obey.

In *Corporal*, an L.A. male describes how his wife included his son, 16, and two daughters, 12 and 18, in his discipline sessions, thus adding to his humiliation. She usually disciplined him in private, but one evening, she announces at dinner that she is going to have the whole family watch. To make his humiliation even greater, she asks the youngest daughter to undress him; when she giggles he finds this especially humiliating, yet thrilling. His wife then ties him in a spread-eagled position, so he will be as exposed as possible, and spanks him while the others watch and enjoy his punishment.

THE ULTIMATE FANTASY: CASTRATION

Tales of castration, the ultimate fantasy of submission for some males, appear from time to time. In an "autobiographical" account in *Female Domination*, a lifelong submissive explains that after two year of marriage, his wife informed him she could no longer tolerate him as a man, so he could become her slave or leave. When he opts for slavery, she puts a chain dog collar around his testicles and padlocks it and does not remove it for twenty years. During this time, she tortures him, brands him on his buttocks to remind him he belongs to her, and puts him in his cage or makes him watch when she dates other men. After 20 years, she decides to castrate him and leave him with a single testicle so he would keep wanting to achieve an orgasm. "That way," he writes, "she knew I would have no relief from desire.... But from time to time, she goes into gales of laughter and gives me the only relief I can know—a severe whipping."

Some readers find such stories exciting, titillated by the perversity of the punishment and the exquisite pain of the male's everlasting frustration. But, as the editor observes in a note accompanying the story, "as a fantasy, it's quite a turn-on... but as a reality, it turns cruel." Doubtless, men excited by such imagery would agree.

AMBIVALENCE AND RESISTANCE

Tales that describe the male protagonist's ambivalence in submitting to a dominant woman are unusual in that they tend to depict recognizable emotions, not just exaggerated activities. The male sees the dominant's power as both intriguing, yet frightening, and he thus experiences both fear and desire—an intermingling of emotions that contribute to his excitement. He may doubt both his own ability to satisfy the dominant woman and the acceptability of his desires to submit, but ultimately he overcomes his resistance and ambivalence.

One such story reports a male's ambivalence when he decides to become a live-in, full-time slave to a "cruel, strict, affectionate Mistress." His inner nature is "craving the ecstasies of a Mistress' whip and discipline," but he believes it is wrong to feel this way. He also describes the difficulties of being a nameless slave and sacrificing his family, friends, and work to devote his life solely to a mistress who will "whip, torture, and humiliate me continuously for no reason except for her pleasure." He escapes, but after two "horrible" months alone, he calls his mistress, begs to return, and signs a contract for lifetime slavery, in blood. He is finally gloriously happy in this relationship that goes "far beyond the word 'love.'"

Madame Wanda, a mistress, deals with male resistance in an *Ouch* article, "Why Some Men Are Afraid of Their Mistresses." She notes that many males "dream of beautiful, dominant women," but in a session they become "wary, edgy, a little fearful, sometimes a bit hostile." The male may fear he is unworthy of his mistress, that he may compare unfavorably with other slaves. Thus he both "desires and dreads" her sexual charm. "The greater the Mistress, the greater the dread. Her power is 'ravishing'—it appeals but also threatens." Madame Wanda's advice? The male should overcome his resistance and accept his submission—by concentrating on making the dominant woman happy. He should send her gifts, listen to her, let her know she is appreciated: "Treat her like a Queen...and she will be yours to worship. I assure you that a dominant woman will appreciate the slave that appreciates her. Given some genuine adoration, a Mistress will spin her silky web of control over you. And if you make her happy, not only will she want the title to your soul, but your cock as well."

The Theme of Female Superiority, Male Inferiority

While the theme of female superiority and male inferiority pervades these stories, sometimes stated explicitly, often implicitly, many articles and letters dramatically underline this theme by glorifying the female and putting down the male in no uncertain terms.

For instance, a woman reader writes to *Fetish Times*:

> I sincerely believe in the mastery of women over boys, and the time is
> rapidly approaching when it will no longer be 'unusual' for the woman to
> be in charge, to get the check in an elegant restaurant, and to make the
> important career decisions. The males have been allowed to sit in the

driver's seat by tradition, not by any accomplishment, or because of any superlative ability. It is well known that women are physically superior... and are vastly superior sexually. One woman can take on any number of men....Can the reverse be said? It is a fortunate man that can satisfy one woman.

In some cases, the woman is presented as a supreme goddess and the male as a lowly unworthy being. For example, a "slave" from Texas rhapsodizes to the editor of *Fetish Times* about his relationship with his "TRUE GODDESS AND OWNER." He reports he is kneeling on the floor naked wearing only a dog collar as he writes, and at the command of his goddess and owner who has ordered him to do so, is writing to "proclaim HER Imperial Divine Majesty...HER Incomparable Beauty, Wisdom, and Authority."

He submits willingly to her numerous demands, because "I have gained a feeling of purpose and meaning to existence through submitting to my DIVINE DEITY, putting HER Will, HER Pleasure above all."

Other males underline their low degraded position, sometimes using the lower case "i" to emphasize this. For example, in an *Ouch* article, slave benji describes himself as a lowly insect or toy. As he puts it:

> i am one of these insects buzzing around her feet, obediently laboring for her glory, her realm, and her pleasure....i had to work hard for the privilege and beg for it.

In turn, his mistress treats him disdainfully "like a simple toy which she might or might not have any use for," and reminds him of his low position in numerous humiliating ways, such as tying two bells to his penis around Christmas and requiring him to praise Her Supreme Highness every time they jingle. But he concludes these are perfectly appropriate given his "worthless position," and he wears her leather cockstrap as a symbol of his "unconditional submission" and seeks to show her complete obedience. Why? He explains:

> I am seeking total loss of human dignity and my own will. My mind will eventually only function under her orders and as required for my duties to Her Majesty....Some of us are born to rule, some are made to obey and serve....To worship and serve her is the only pleasure left in my otherwise worthless life.

21

Erotic Power in the '90s

Today, the D&S scene is much more open and mainstream than when I first wrote about it in *Erotic Power,* in the early 1980s. At that time it was even difficult to get the original hard copy version of the book into major bookstores, since many buyers refused to carry it. Then, the *San Francisco Chronicle* covered the opening launch party for the book with a half-page article and photo spread. The party made the 11:00 P.M. KGO news. Other appearances on major TV talk shows followed, including *Phil Donahue* and *Sally.* Soon the bookstores followed, too. Since then, Madonna's *Sex* book, films like *East of Eden* with Rosie O'Donnell, trendy leather fashions, songs about power on MTV, and even the account of Dick Morris, President Clinton's political guru, barking like a dog for his $200 an hour hooker have all have made D&S very mainstream.

With that in mind, in 1996 I revisited the scene I had written about in the early 1980s, asking the questions: "What's new?" and "What's changed?"

REVISITING THE SERVICE OF MANKIND CHURCH (OR SMC)

To start off I contacted "Lance" and "Sharon," who were heading up a group called the Service of Mankind Church (or sometimes the Essemian Sanctuary of the Darkside Goddess or SMC) back in the early 1980s and are still in charge today. As a sign of the times, the group even has its own Web page—at http://www.darkside-goddess.org—and it has grown to about 1,000 members, with about 700 outside of the San Francisco Bay area, where the group is still centered, and has monthly functions and a regular newsletter with articles about the spiritual aspects of female domination and male submission.

When I called, the group was having a party through one of its offshoots, La Madrona, which is mainly for couples only, although a few single men or women were permitted to come as special guests. "Why don't you come?" said Lance, and so, in mid-September, I found my way to an old house near Twin Peaks in San Francisco, which had been turned into a kind of D&S fantasy world and dungeon by its owner, Mistress Sondra, a long-

time D&S practioner in her 40s, who worked part-time as a mistress when
not running her freelance marketing business.

I arrived early, just as the doors were open for arrivals from 8:00 to 10:00
P.M., and was greeted by Sharon at the door, and then introduced to the
hostess Sondra. Like other women I later met at the party, they were dressed
in stylish D&S scene attire suggesting female dominance—Sharon in a
sparkling gold lame dress and white bowler hat, Sondra in a slinky, skin-
tight black sheath, most of the other women in tight-fitting short black
dresses and heels. The men were dressed casually in sports attire or jeans;
however, as the party progressed, most of them stripped to their briefs or
nothing at all, though some wore collars, handcuffs, and chains—all
symbols of the submissive male, while the women remained dressed
throughout.

But first, as I and others arrived, an assistant wearing a T-shirt and
chains handed out hot pink "Party Orientation" flyers with a list of cautions.
It was a list of rules similar to that handed out at many such parties—or
known generally—rules that were quite common in the scene when I first
wrote about it, and are still in practice today. Some of these rules include the
following:

• All play must be safe and consensual. We don't allow... play involving games that one of the partners sincerely does not want to be involved in.

• Party etiquette clearly requires you to ask before touching, playing,
or joining in someone else's play. Further, a NO should be respected, and
should be given and accepted politely.

• Drinking, drugs, and play parties are incompatible.

But there was one new consideration—the incorporation of more high-
tech play than was common in the 1980s, as reflected by this rule:
"Electrical play has been found to cause severe feedback on the stereo.
Please ask the host before doing electrical play."

After this brief orientation, Sondra began leading tours of the house,
and many arrivals wandered about by themselves. Apart from the large
kitchen and living room, a large family room on the main floor and several
rooms on the lower level were all designed for D&S play. There were
dangling hooks and pulleys from the ceiling in most of the rooms; several
racks, massage-style tables, and mattresses in a room downstairs. A small
dark alcove illuminated by a blue light had a rubber floor and bars, which
gave it the appearance of a medieval dungeon. Down the hall from this was a
room that looked like a doctor's examination room, with a proctologist's
examination table that featured several straps and a strange beeping
electrical device for bondage and electrical play. It was quite a bit more

high-tech than the typically smaller and more informal setups I had seen in the early 1980s.

After the tour, I joined the early arrivals in the kitchen, where there were mostly nonalcholic drinks like fruit sodas and Cokes, plus some beer, and a simple spread of chips, vegetables, dips, and cookies. A few people were some of the old-timers, still active in the scene 15 years later, and there were many newcomers, with most of the attendees in their late 20s, 30s, and 40s.

"So what's new or changed?" I asked, and people were soon eagerly filling me in on the scene today. As new people arrived, they joined the conversation and offered their opinions too.

THE SCENE TODAY

One of the first key differences today is the role of the Internet—there are news groups and World Wide Web sites on the topic. Among the news groups there are at the time I checked: "alt.sex.bondage; alt.sex.femdom; alt.sex.spanking; alt.personals.bondage, and alt.personals.spanking," while some of the major D&S organizations and publications have their own Web site. Besides the SMC site, there is also a site for Janus, another group I wrote about at www.blackiris.com/SFLeatherMC/janus/Janus.html; www.qualitysm.com for QSM, a bookstore and mail-order business specializing in D&S information and erotica; www.fantasies.com for a club in Mountain View called Backdrop; and sites for other groups. Then, too, there are forums and bulletin boards on online services, like America Online, where people can make contact as well.

Not only do people use these sites as a place to read and post information, but they are a way for newcomers to get into the scene if they live or travel to certain areas. For example, in some areas, people have started what they call "munches"—gatherings in public places which occur every week or so, where a few regulars can meet newcomers and then refer them to other activities in the scene. One 40-something woman named "Ruth" (not her real name), who works as a computer professional in the Silicon Valley and who has been in the scene with her husband for about 10 years, both in the New York–Boston area and on the West Coast, told me how she sponsored one each Wednesday. Another woman, "Denise," in the Palo Alto area, had a similar munch on Thursday.

Typically, the members of these groups met in the same local coffee house each week, pulled together a few tables to accommodate the people who showed up, and then anyone who came could join in the conversation or just listen. Generally, each group averaged about a half dozen to a dozen people each week. While a few of the people were part of a core group of regulars, others were new. Ruth felt the setting made the gathering especially comfortable for newcomers. As she explained:

"When people first come, we're in a public place, and they can see we're a group of very ordinary people, not a bunch of weirdos. We're also in a place where people ordinarily sit down at tables with others to have coffee, so they can freely join us or leave, and contribute to the conversation or not, as they want. Then, if they feel comfortable, they can introduce themselves, and if they want to get more involved, we'll refer them to one of the organized groups like Janus or the SMC."

But she wouldn't, as she pointed out, refer newcomers to one of the more private parties that are put on around the Bay area. The newcomers had to first gain acceptance through these more public groups or through personal friends. Then they could be invited to these more private events—about several hundred of them each week around the Bay area, generally on Friday and Saturday nights (as in many other major cities, such as New York and L.A., where there are also active D&S scenes). But first newcomers have to go through a gradual introduction and screening process—to make sure they understand and would follow the rules, such as those given out at this party I attended. Then, too, the screening was to make sure the newcomers would be responsible members of the community committed to safe and consensual play, and not expose participants in the scene to undesired public attention.

In fact, one East Bay group, which held a more private munch in the form of an informal dinner for newcomers, went through a more intensive screening process on the phone. In this case, after learning about the group on the Internet, or perhaps through an ad in a local publication, people would first call. Then, the person who answered would put the caller through a detailed screening interview to learn more about him or her and make sure he or she was serious about participating and willing to abide by the rules. Only then would the caller be invited to attend and contribute a small fee towards the dinner. Afterwards, if everything clicked, the newcomers would then be referred on to other groups and activities.

Besides the Internet and some commercial services, there are some weekly adult publications in major cities, like the *Spectator* in the San Francisco Bay area, which provide entry to the scene. In fact, the *Spectator* is now published by Kat Sunlove, the woman I wrote about in *Erotic Power* who first acquainted me with the scene when she was teaching classes on D&S and working as a mistress in the early 1980s. Today there are also more organized orientation programs through various groups. While some of these groups existed then and still do, like the SMC, Janus, and the Eulenspiegel Society in New York, there are new organizations devoted to giving classes, like QSM in San Francisco. And many of these groups now have their own bookstores, selling books via direct mail or to participants in their classes. So generally, the whole scene seems much larger and more organized now than in the early 1980s.

Another big difference is that women are taking the initiative to seek out the scene themselves. Fifteen years ago, it was extremely rare for a woman to participate independently. There were many more men in the scene than women, and most of the women who came to public events were introduced by their husbands, significant others, or the men they were dating. Subsequently, if they developed an interest themselves, they generally stayed active only as long as their partners did. Only a few stayed on if their relationship broke up or if their partner lost interest in the scene. The small number of women in the scene on their own were commonly working full or part-time as mistresses, and had a personal interest as well.

Today many women are actively seeking out the scene themselves, and typically make their first contact through the Internet, online chat rooms, ads in publications like the *Spectator*, and books on the subject (such as *Erotic Power*). They feel the desire to be dominant or submissive themselves, are curious about the scene, or see it as a chance to meet a partner who shares their interests.

For example, at the La Madrona party I attended, there were five women in their 30s and early 40s, who had come on their own. One was a woman I'll call Trudy who worked as a successful professional in a bank, and wanted to transfer the sense of command she felt at work into a personal relationship. She had started off about two years earlier by placing an ad in one of the adult magazines, *Encore*, describing her desires, and had gotten responses from about 200 men. After screening the calls, she met several of them, dated a few, and eventually found herself falling in love with one of them. But after they broke up about a month before this party, she called the SMC's number, which she had previously gotten from one of the men she met through the ad, and after she described her situation, Sharon invited her to the La Madrona party.

As for the other four women, three were friends who worked in the computer field and found they shared a curiousity about D&S. Then, after one of them, who I'll call Maria, a feisty Latin American woman, heard about the SMC in an Internet chat group, she called, left her number, and got a call from the group's membership chair, Paul, a computer professional himself, who invited her to come to the party as his guest. "Can I bring my friends?" she asked, and when he said yes, they all first attended a general SMC orientation during the week to let them know about the scene and party etiquette. The fourth was a graduate student in English, Nancy, who had started taking creative writing courses and writing about female

domination fantasies, when she heard about the SMC through the Internet
and went to an orientation, too. Then on Saturday, they all turned up at the
La Madrona party.

A TYPICAL PLAY PARTY: REVISITING THE SMC

Apart from the addition of some more high-tech toys and equipment, the
SMC party was very much like the parties that I attended in the 1980s. It
was as if nothing really essential had changed. While there were about two
dozen new people, some of the old timers were still core participants, such
as Lance and Sharon and a few men still in the scene 15 years later. Also,
among the old-timers was a couple that switched top and bottom roles, and
when they weren't engaging in female dominance play, like tonight, they
were running a club for couples in which the men were dominant and the
women submissive, called Gemini, that had started in the early 1980s. They
had taken over the group after the original organizers had broken up and
dropped out of the scene.

The party's atmosphere and activities were very much like any typical
party—from the 1980s or now. During the early evening when the doors
were still open for arrivals—from 8:00 P.M. &10:00 P.M. at this event;
sometimes from about 9:00 P.M.–11:00 P.M. at other parties—the atmosphere
was generally like an ordinary social get-together. Initially, most people
gathered in the kitchen, with a few people going off from time to time to
tour the house, and everyone just talked. The conversation touched on
everyday activities, D&S interests, attendance at other events in the scene,
and a little of what people did in the real world—though not too specific,
since most participants wanted to keep this other part of their life private.

For example, the woman banker never mentioned what bank she
worked at, nor did the people working with computers name the company
where they worked, and no one asked. And when one man began talking
about studying science in graduate school and someone wondered what
science field, his partner suddenly joined the circle and told him firmly: "All
right, that's enough. I just thought I'd better cut in before you reveal too
much." So he immediately shifted back to talking about generalities.

Then, a little after 9:00 P.M., a few of the couples began drifting off to
the family room or to the rooms downstairs to start playing—mostly in quiet
one-on-one scenes, while a few people stayed on the sidelines to watch. But
in keeping with the party guidelines, no one tried to join these private
scenes.

The scene in the living room was typical. One woman stood poised
with a small black leather whip with several strands, while her husband

undressed down to a small black thong and jock strap and leaned over a large leather gym horse. Then, she began whipping him, alternately increasing the force of the whip, and stopping for a few moments to brush his reddening buttocks with her hands.

Meanwhile, downstairs, another woman had strung up her partner on a large iron frame so his hands were tied above his head while his feet were spread out and cuffed to the bottom of the frame. Then, she similarly began whipping him, while in another room down the hall, a man was lying down on a mattress, as his partner bound his hands. And still another man, Lance, was quietly lying on his side in the dungeon, where he had been left as a "punishment" by Nancy, the graduate student in English, after he had asked her to be his mistress and said he would be her slave for the night.

For the most part, the scenes were fairly quiet and were between pairs, reflecting the focus of the partners on one another. In turn, this was different from many of the parties I had attended in the early 1980s, where there was more of a spirit of informal group play, with many participants moving in and out of different scenes with different people acting as submissive or tops, and often multiple tops changing roles in scenes. Also, back then, the scenes seemed to have more of a sense of drama and performance, with more play-acting and verbal interchange. But now the partners seemed to be more serious in relating intimately as a couple, and they combined their play with a great deal of gentleness, say by pausing during a whipping to use gentle caressing strokes. Meanwhile, anyone who watched did so quietly, unobtrusively, without asking to join a scene, since these scenes were more like private conversations one could listen in on, as long as one kept a quiet distance; and any distracting side conversations were promptly shushed.

The one exception was the brief period when Paul, the membership director, and Ralph, an older man of about 60 who had also come unattached, invited the three new women who had come with Paul to experience an introductory S&M lesson. Both Paul and Ralph stripped down to their collars, and Paul showed one of the women, Julie, how to put his legs in stirrups and hoist them up, so he was balanced on his shoulders. Then, as he instructed, she began whipping his bare backside. Occasionally the other two women took the whip from her and joined in, and from time to time, Paul added some suggestions, like: "Hit a little harder... More to the right... You can lower my legs a little now. They're getting numb... You don't want to leave someone in this position more than fifteen or twenty minutes."

Meanwhile, a small crowd gathered, and accompanied the whipping with light insults and teasing, suggesting that maybe it was time for Paul to shut up and let the women take charge. Finally, one of the observers stuck an apple in his mouth, prompting remarks like: "Hmmm. Now doesn't he look like a succulent pig," . . . "Yeah, an obnoxious one at that. But at least he'll be quiet for now."

At the same time, the three women, though new to the scene, seemed to become totally involved in the experience, liking the sense of power. As Maria, the Latin American woman commented later: "I like being able to tell guys what to do now . . . Ever since I got rid of my husband, I've wanted to do that."

After this scene broke up, the other quieter scenes with couples continued on a little longer until about midnight, when people began to pack up the toys they had brought and head home, or in a few cases, went to still other parties. Meanwhile, those who stayed gathered in the living room and kitchen to continue talking.

In sum, it was a quiet, more serious and sober atmosphere than I remembered from the 1980s. Perhaps a reason is that there is more concern now with safe sex, family values, and monogamy. Perhaps this atmosphere was more in keeping with the times than the wilder and crazier late-night bashes I remembered from the 1980s.

Just before I left, since the clubs were now a big part of the scene, I spoke to Trudy, who worked in the bank, and Nancy, the graduate student, who had both come on their own, about going to the clubs together. Both were eager to go, and so we talked about going to several of the clubs. Finally, as I said my goodbyes, Ruth told me she would send me the addresses of several sites on the Internet. I would have to check on these, too.

REVISITING THE SOCIETY OF JANUS

Another big part of the scene in the early 1980s was the Society of Janus, only a few years old at the time, having been founded in 1974. It was set up originally as an educational and support organization for individuals interested in a range of sexual exploration involving a power exchange— including S&M, bondage and discipline, and dominance and submission. An underlying premise was that any exploration would be based on "a safe, consensual, non-exploitive transfer of power between partners," to quote the group's newsletter.

Today the organization is still growing strong. In fact, it is larger than ever. Back in the 1980s, there were about 200 members. Now it is up to around 650, with about 125 members outside of the San Francisco Bay area, and it has also inspired a few spin-off groups in other parts of the country, most notably Threshhold, a similar organization in Los Angeles, with about

500 members. This group had once been considered the Society's L.A. chapter when it first started in the early 1980s. Then in the mid-1990s, it became independent, though closely tied with Janus. In addition, Janus was closely affiliated with many other active organizations in the scene, including the SMC and its La Madrona group which I had just attended a few weeks before. As I looked through the latest newsletter, I noticed the board had just passed a reciprocal agreement to allow La Madrona members to attend Janus functions and vice versa and list La Madrona activities in its newsletter. Also, Janus was an organized presence in many alternative lifestyle fairs, from Support AIDS parades to the Folsom Street Fair.

I decided to attend one of the group's monthly programs in late September—a program of "Domination Techniques" by Mistress Katrine. It was one of a series of regular programs dealing with a range of topics on exploring a power exchange, including playing with leather toys, a history of the D&S community, and a bondage beauty competition, featuring different styles of bondage.

As it turned out, this particular program was being led by the same woman who was an active member of the SMC, reflecting the close and overlapping ties between members of this community. The meeting was held at The Power Exchange, located in a plain brick building in San Francisco's SOMA (or South of Market) District—a meeting center for a variety of groups interested in playing with power—both gay and straight, with some events for men or women only.

As I walked in, I picked up some flyers, colorful postcards, and brochures describing the Power Exchange and some of the groups that met there. One card described the setting: "4,000 square feet, including Fantasy Rooms, Bondage Equipment, Voyeur Rooms, and a Fantastic Juice Bar!... So unleash your Wildest Fantasies and take a step beyond!" Another, featuring a hunky guy in cutoff jeans, described one weekly event at the center as being "the world's largest high voltage sex multiplex for men." And lest women be forgotten, another card, which featured the picture of a thin voluptuous woman in a firehat, red corset, and black stockings, announced the opening of its "raging new Fantasy Club exclusively for women" on Sunday nights. And nearby were brochures about Basic Safe Sex Guidelines, erotic photo processing, and new books and magazines on erotic topics.

Then, since I still had about 20 minutes before the 8:00 P.M. program, I explored the area. As I passed through the main reception section, where Janus coordinators were greeting attendees and collecting the small admission fee (just $2 for members), I passed by a kind of medieval bedroom and throne room, featuring a down-covered king-sized bed. Around it were shields of medieval knights, and a table with platters of food reminiscent of a

Henry VIII feast—including a "stuffed" ceramic pig in the middle. A little further down the hall, two men were finishing the construction of some dungeons for a dungeon room, which consisted of a half-dozen empty cells, with ropes and pulleys hanging from the ceiling.

If this had been a party, participants might have used these rooms for assorted fantasy play. But this was just an ordinary meeting where the presenter put on the program on a raised stage, while attendees took seats to listen classroom style. So despite the erotic topic, the atmosphere was more like that of a local PTA or community meeting, with people quietly talking or just sitting and waiting until the program began. It was much like a similar program in the 1980s, though I noticed one immediate difference— there were far more women in the audience—about 40 percent of the group, whereas back in the early 1980s, there were much fewer women in the scene. It was more like about 25 percent. Another difference was that most of the faces were new—only a few old-timers were there, and most of these were now club officers. But the age mix was roughly about the same—about a mid-20s to mid-40s crowd, with a sprinkling of older members.

Finally, shortly after 8:00 P.M., with about 60 people in the audience, the program coordinator Steve began the session by making general announcements of activities of interest to the D&S community—some sponsored by Janus, others by other affiliated groups. In a few cases, program leaders were seeking volunteers for future programs, such as for one event led by a noted member of the community who specialized in body piercings—Fakir Mustafer. I had attended a couple of his programs almost 20 years before, and this time he would be talking about "Branding and Burning Your Slave." The announcement brought appreciative laughter from the audience, who knew that the controversial title was somewhat wilder than the program itself which would deal with doing body art on a willing submissive—not quite the image of mayhem the title suggested.

Then, Steve took a quick survey for a future program. "What kind of piercing would you prefer to learn about—common or uncommon?" Immediately, it was clear as hands went up that common piercing evoked little interest; everyone wanted to know about "uncommon" techniques. "Well, it's clear this is an uncommon audience interested in uncommon things," Steve commented, reinforcing the group's image of itself, as everyone laughed again.

Next, a member visiting from L.A. announced an upcoming exotic fashion show featuring D&S fashions, explaining it was called a "Bizarre Bazaar" at the Hollywood Palace, and many thousands were expected. It was another sign of the mainstreaming of the D&S movement.

Finally, members were invited to start thinking about the group's annual Bondage Beauty Contest, which typically drew about 150 participants. As Steve explained, "There are about seven or eight categories—like 'Best Knot,' 'Best Rope,' and 'Funniest Bondage.' Come with your partner and create whatever bondage fantasy you want. Then everyone there will judge who's the best in each of these categories."

With that, the regular program was ready to begin and Mistress Katrine, introduced as the founder of one of San Francisco's foremost salons of dominance, took the stage. She was a tall, strong-looking woman, in her early 40s, who looked a little like a nurse, which she was on a part-time basis. She was dressed in a tight black corset with red lace trim and wore a long white scarf, giving her a kind of tough but gentle look, which is exactly the style of D&S she practiced. As she explained, she liked to combine strong play, which included a wide range of activities from spanking, whipping, and caning, with the tender touching and teasing of a playful nurse.

"It's a unique style," she began. "It combines B&D, S&M, D&S, fantasy and role playing, fetishes, corporal punishment, and other activities—but all combined with a warm, loving, caring, yet dominant style of play."

So what exactly did Katrine mean by this? She went on to explain. As she did, she might have been giving a talk in the early 1980s. Perhaps some of the terminology was different; perhaps some of the toys might be a little more high-tech. But otherwise, the kind of activities and approach she talked about were very much the same as almost 20 years before.

Perhaps the one major difference was how Katrine had gotten drawn into the lifestyle herself. In the early 1980s, most of the women were drawn in because a partner attracted to D&S took the lead; few had their own fantasies that triggered their interest. By contrast, Katrine did have early fantasies. As she explained:

"My earliest fantasies were of D&S and S&M. When I was 6 or 7, I imagined being submissive, being tied up in bondage. But I couldn't explore as a child."

When she started dating, she couldn't explore either, because the guys she met didn't really understand what to do. Even if she gave them handcuffs or a rope to tie her with, they were basically going through the motions, following her instructions. But afterward, they didn't know what to do next. Then, in her early 30s, about 10 years ago, she met Carl, a man who had fantasies too. After about one month of dating, they decided to live together, joined Janus, and soon everything opened up. She answered an ad to work as a professional dominatrix and began to work professionally on a part-time basis, while still working on-call for a local hospital as a nurse. Meanwhile, she explored being a full-time submissive with Carl at home. But soon, though she had fantasies about submissiveness, she wasn't very submissive. She often rebelled when Carl was in charge. And so they soon began to experiment with switch roles, which worked well. At times, she would be dominant, and at other times he would.

Eventually, all of this exploration led her to decide to work as a dominant on her own, so she set up her own house of domination at her home in San Francisco that she called the Salon of Domination. It was both her own home and a place for personal and professional play, with virtually every room either a dungeon or playroom. Though she and Carl continued to be monagamous and switch roles with one another, they each had one or more play partners who took the submissive role. Back in the 1980s, I had met a few couples who pursued such a way of life, some of them still together and still living this lifestyle, and just as it was uncommon then, it was still unusual now. But otherwise, the lifestyle was much the same, reflecting again how little had changed.

Katrine then went on to explain just how her interest in many styles of domination influenced her play. Basically, she liked using a wide variety of toys to stimulate different senses to heighten the erotic experience. She also liked it when the submissive would give up more power and take more of whatever she as the dominant wanted to give—subject, of course, to a pre-session discussion or negotiation so she knew what kind of activities the submissive liked.

To demonstrate, she invited Nadia, a woman in her 20s who had participated in sessions with both her and Carl, to be her submissive. After blindfolding Nadia with a white executioner's wrap—"to take away vision, which is the strongest sensation; the second is speech"—Katrine stripped Nadia down to her black bra, panties, and garter belt. Then, as Nadia stood meekly on the stage waiting, Katrine explained how her best toys included the imagination, voice, and parts of her body, like her arms, hands, fingernails, even her butt for rubbing erotically against her submissive. Though she had a whole tool kit of objects from whips and canes to soft rabbit fur and feathers, she pointed out the many ways the body could be used to sensitize and arouse a submissive, such as scratching with the nails, biting with the teeth ("the back of the neck's especially good"), holding the submissive like a puppy, and wrapping her body around his. "Plus you can use your hair, feet, breath, even moisture and sweat. Once you take away the person's sight and speech, they are left with their receptive senses—hearing, taste, smell, and touch. They're more sensitive to those things."

Then, after inviting Nadia to lie over her lap, Katrine demonstrated by giving Nadia a spanking, describing how she intensified the experience by techniques such as conflict and resolution. "You aren't just hitting the person, but you are creating a painful sensation and then replacing it with pleasure. For example, you stop spanking, then combine it with some tenderness. And you're in control." Then, with another series of slaps she talked about how she liked to work with energy, gathering it by striking the person so the energy would be drawn to that spot, then diffusing it by stroking or striking the person in motions to draw attention from that area. "By gradually building up the energy," she added, "you can make the person you are working with even more sensitive and break down their inhibitions, so they can experience even light touching more intensely—and take more of pain or other sensations as well."

Then, as Nadia continued to lie in her lap, Katrine emphasized the importance of negotiating with the submissive before a session. "Then, you have an idea what they want. But most will describe what they know before. So you can try exploring. If you find the person responds erotically when you do something, you can do more of that." And as she emphasized, it was the submissive's response that helped to turn her on, too. "I only enjoy playing if the person is responsive," she said.

Meanwhile, as she spoke, I thought about how much her comments reminded me of hearing Kat and several other mistresses talk about what they did almost 20 years before. They, too, spoke about working with energy, alternating pleasure and pain, using sensitizing techniques to up the arousal level, using teasing and seduction techniques to manipulate, and wanting a responsive partner to make the session exciting and fun. While Katrine brought her own personality and style to the mix, in many ways her talk could have been one I heard 20 years before. So in many respects little had changed; the basic dynamics of the power exchange that attracted people to the scene were still the same, though each participant brought his or her own uniqueness and flair.

Then, after asking Nadia to bend over the chair, so her bare butt was facing the audience, Katrine demonstrated some basic whipping techniques, using a long leather cat with many strands. "I like to build up tension by playing with the whip," she began. "I start off by touching the submissive gently, working up the intensity, so they can take more. And then..." she hit the whip along Nadia's backside a little harder, "...I like to spice it up with a little sting now and then." Then, after weaving a few verbal word pictures—"I'd like to take you up to the mountains and tie you up...I'd like to do this and that to you...Just imagine what we might do if we went to the beach,"—Katrine noted that "I like to verbally fantasize during the session. It's like thinking out loud...Though I may whisper it to the person, too."

Her discussion now brought back memories of classes on fantasy I had long ago attended, taught by Sharon, Danielle, and others from the SMC. Nearly 20 years ago, they had talked about both enacting and talking about various fantasy scenes, using the imagination to step into other worlds.

Similarly, Katrine was using that techinque now, using her soft, silky voice to describe that world.

Then, like years before, Katrine spoke about making sure everything was consensual and safe, and using safe words or signals to limit or stop the scene if necessary. "You need to find out, especially when you play with someone for the first time, what they think. You need to ask at times—'Do you like this? Did this feel good? Do you want more?' or 'Are you sure?' Or if the person doesn't want to talk because they are in a trance, give them something they can use, like a bell. Then, they can use that to signal you when they want you to stop." Such signals could be particularly important when part of a scene included pretending to resist, when in fact one really wanted the scene to continue or intensify. The word or action could signal when the desire to turn down the intensity or stop was for real.

When I had first encountered the scene about 20 years ago, these notions of safety and consensuality had been bedrock principles, much in contrast to the images of S&M and D&S that sometimes hit the evening news when some angry or mentally unbalanced person really does torture another person. And now here Katrine was emphasizing them once again.

Finally, after a short break for soft drinks and socializing, Katrine demonstrated the art of sensual caning, using Tommy, a man she had played with in many scenes before. He was someone who especially liked heavy intense caning, and he had brought along his own collection of canes of different lengths, thicknesses, and tips—carried in what looked like a bag for archery arrows. When he spoke, his English accent reminded me of Victor, the English surgeon, who I had met years before, who told me how many English boys first learned to appreciate the erotic power of caning at the hands of the boarding school teachers.

After Tommy undressed and bent down over the same chair, his butt in the air, Katrine began sensitizing his backside using a black rubber paddle. As she continued slapping him firmly for about 5 minutes as his backside reddened, she explained some of the techniques she was using. "As you hit harder, slow down. It gives them a chance to recover from each blow."

Then, after testing a few canes by slapping them in the air and selecting one, Katrine began to whip the cane in the air over Tommy, as if to tease him with the pain that was to come. After pointing out that what helped to make this erotic is the payoff of erotic arousal associated with each stroke or the inner burning sensation that follows, she began to strike Tommy, pausing or bending over to stroke and rub him gently between blows. Meanwhile, Tommy breathed deeply between blows, obviously aroused, despite the bright lights and audience of about 40 people left over after the break and still watching. In turn, Katrine explained some of the dynamics of what were going on: "He's high off the pain, and I feel high giving it to him. At first I didn't like giving pain because I didn't like it myself. But then when I was playing with a person who wanted it harder, I saw how he responded with a pleasure response. So, I came to realize it was okay, and I found I got turned on by hitting a person who liked it." Also, I found I was turned on by raising someone's pain threshhold—getting him to take something he didn't initially want. But he did it for me, and he liked it, too. The experience gave me a sense of my own power."

Finally, Katrine concluded by talking a little about playing at the edge—something I had heard people in the scene talk about again and again years before. It was that appeal of doing things differently, of breaking through barriers, of exploring new ground—much like a mountain climber wants to take on a still higher mountain because of the thrill of meeting the challenge. As Katrine commented: "I need that psychic hook. The submissives I like playing with are giving to me, trusting me, even letting me do things with them they haven't done before. So I'm getting them to push through these barriers—and that's what's exciting for me."

So what about Tommy? After he got dressed again, he briefly commented on why he responded as he did, echoing the comments I had heard from many men and women I met in the scene many years before. "For me the pain is weird," he began. "I love it, while I hate it. I'm attracted to it though it hurts because it turns me on. And what does it for me is that while I'm being caned, I feel like I'm in this intense energy bubble, and I like being there. I feel contained, like I'm inside her energy. And I like that feeling. So each time I'm hit, I feel that rush of energy too, and that feels good. Very good. That's what keeps me wanting more, until the energy builds to a climax, and then there's a final release."

And with that, after a few more final questions, the evening ended, and I left thinking how much things were still the same. There was something very '90s about the way Katrine and Tommy talked more explicitly about energy, as if it were some high-tech force that helped infuse the scene. And of course Katrine added her own unique style to the mix. But otherwise, the talk about safety, consensuality, sensitivity, fantasy, and the techniques of mixing pleasure with pain were much the same. And I kept thinking of that old adage: "The more things change, the more they remain the same." In this case, that certainly seemed true.

VISITING THE INTERNET

What *is* new today, however, is the Internet, which, has through its newsgroups, become for some a virtual community, and for others a kind of online magazine or smorgasbord of personal and commercial ads for partners, services, and events, and occasional postings of fantasy stories. Also, there are numerous organizations and individuals who now have Web sites to promote their activities and services, and assorted forums and support groups on commercial services like AOL and CompuServe.

Although some of these postings still cater to local interests—such as notices about local events and parties, like "munches" to bring those in an area together in a nearby restaurant, and ads to meet partners or clients who live nearby—a major change is that D&S has gone global, with postings from people all over the world. A few are even in other languages, most notably German. And while many of these posts from all over are for mail-order products—most notably books, tapes, videos, and photos—many people are posting their own fantasy stories, comments and questions about the scene, or looking for e-mail correspondences which may or may not lead to a meeting. For some people, just the e-mail contact itself is enough.

I spent a couple of days exploring this world, downloading a sampling of messages from the major Internet newsgroups devoted to various D&S activities—alt.bondage; alt.sex.bondage; alt.personals.bondage; alt.sex.spanking; alt.personals.spanking; alt.personals.spanking.punishment; and alt.sex.femdom—seven in all, each with thousands of messages in about 2 weeks—an average of about 2,000 to 4,000 messages from about October 20 to November 4. And these figures don't include the many thousands more people who are presumably just visiting the site to read these messages—or "surfing and lurking," to use the current Internet lingo. And then I checked out a few of the Web sites mentioned in these newsgroups.

EXPLORING THE NEWSGROUPS

While there are some regulars who communicate back and forth within these newsgroups, sharing ideas in cyberspace rather than, say, at a face-to-face meeting or a local group event—most notably on alt.sex.spanking and alt.sex.femdom—these groups are mostly dominated by commercial announcements about sex toys and literature, dominatrixes seeking clients, women offering fantasy phone sex, and invitations to visit assorted Web sites, mostly with more commercial announcements. And many of the same ads appear from site to site.

Here's a sampling of typical announcements:

FREE! PORN PICS AND SEX STORIES

HOT LIVE SEXXXXX CUM AND PLAY NOWXXX

Horny Girls Sex Site

But then if you wade through all the commercial announcements, there
are the more personal notices and occasional virtual conversations or fantasy
stories about the topic. More generally, the posters seem to be males,
looking variously to play the submissive/slave or master/top role; professional
mistresses seeking males who would like to be paying clients either in
person or through a cybercorrespondence; some couples seeking other
couples or an additional woman (generally submissive) to join them in their
play; and a few nonprofessional women.

For example, here are a few typical ads (I've changed e-mail names for
the sake privacy):

From alt.bondage:

A few submissive males seeking dominant women—either professionals
or nonprofessionals for play:

> Male 45, 160 lbs 5'10:, brown hair and eyes, seeks Domme Female to use
> bondage, leather and toys to make me obey. Prefer tall, slender, high heels,
> leather bra with breasts exposed...I will serve you well Mistress!!!!!!

> Thank you for reading this message! I am a 25-year-old, handsome,
> physically fit, lifestyles submissive male in search of a Beautiful Mistress or
> couple. I am into B&D, S&M, serious role-playing, corporeal punishment,
> dressing for pleasure, and all fetishism. I believe in quality not quantity,
> and expect safe, sane, and consenting adult fun...Please e-mail if inter-
> ested in a real meeting. I promise you will not be disappointed!...Thank
> you for your time. (TNServant)

A couple of couples seeking women or couples:

> We are an attractive, business professional couple into B&D. My subfem is
> VERY HOT, and bi. We seek bifems and select couples into Bondage and
> role-play for meeting. We are REAL, and SERIOUS...please be the same.
> (MasterRJNY)

> We are an experienced R/T and a switch Mistress interviewing for the right
> bifem or the right couple to be our subs. Let's talk about the adventures we
> could share in sensual magic. (PowrLA)

A few queries and answers:

Do you know a mistress that can help me? (Motorman)

I know someone who may be able to teach you the "Ropes." (Tony)

I just may be the person you're looking for. (Terri)

And then, some of the postings may sound fairly explicit, though many of these turn out to be for commercial services—or involve some kind of exchange for pay, such as this one:

Hi, my name is Jeremy and I LOVE phone sex. My girlfriend Tammy and I are horny all the time and we need red hot lovers to tame our flame. Fuck my tits and slide your hard rod up my ass till we both cream. Tie me up and spank me and I'll cum all over your face. Almost ANYTHING goes with us. I'm rubbing my hot wet pussy now waiting for your call.

And then after Jeremy and Tammy offer their phone number, they advise that the cost is $15 per call, with MC, Visa, or a Phone Check accepted, and there are special club rates and a hot e-mail club too. And then they also have a Web page which includes original erotic stories to excite readers to call.

Still, some ads for personal relationships can be pretty explicit too, such as this one from a man in the San Francisco Bay area:

Muscular, short frisko boy likes girls who like to play. I am a good looking, strong, short-haired, drug-free man. I like to pass control back and forth, the way two puppies play. I look as good in pumps as you do. I will hold you down, kiss you crazy and pet your kitty. I will peel your petals back and lick under your soul, and even take walks around Nob Hill and look at stuff with you, if you want. I know a girl that might be our pet, or just you and I is cool.

And some posters become quite specific about exactly the kind of scene they want—whether it's just a fantasy or they want to trade experiences through e-mail or actually meet if that should be possible. For instance:

Looking for a submissive female in the area that truly loves very hard bondage. Must be able to handle suspension and long periods of bondage.

Hi. I'm a kinky slave with a fetish to wear plastic and would love to be in training. Have many other kinky fetishes. Please write. I'm a kinky slave male.

Hi. I never got spanked or got hit with a dildo by a girl. But I always wanted to be raped and humiliated by a girl, till I couldn't stand it and even then have her still going. I'm a nice soft little male bitch who cries and gets beat up alot. Please call and hurt me.

Hi. I am a very submissve white slave—28 year, blond, blue eyes, 5½ feet, 163 pound, circumcised, no tattoos, no piercing, clean... By order from my master I seek a free-thinking FAMILY who wants to kick this white ass. My master will give me away for 30 days. Everything you will can be done... Only permanent diseases like blinding, castration are not allowed. My master has learned me to accept every one of his wishes. So if you are interested... Please only FAMILIES. NO SINGLES.

And occasionally, posters may seek some advice, such as this woman who reported some problems in her bondage play with her husband, and got this response:

My husband and I just started bondage play and we are having trouble with my breathing when we use duck tape to cover my mouth. Does anyone have any suggestions?

Hi there. First off I would not use duct tape! I would find a gag that fits while allowing you to breathe, such as a hard ball gag or a breather gag... I can provide any of the above designs, as I am a leather worker with 5 years experience making items for the scene. Please feel free to e-mail me with any questions. I also do a lot of custom work. Take care and play safe.

Or in some case, the request for advice may itself be part of a scene that now includes the internet, like this one:

My Dom has me on my knees and is forcing me to type this. I am instructed to tell you that she intends to flog me unless someone responds with a suggestion for a task for me to perform which she will find amusing. She is already slowly beginning. Please help.

In other cases, the global possibilities are reflected in requests based on people traveling to meet from one country to another, such as in these messages:

Italian master is looking for very sub girl interested to come in Rome, Italy. (Francisco)

I am a 34-year-old dominant male presently located in Germany. I will be in the London area during November and am looking for submissive females (maybe couples where either both or just she is submissive) in the London area. Sessions to be held at her/their place. Preferred are blond females, not too tall, with medium to large breasts. Must be very submissive. Write!

And then many mistresses from all over are offering their services for males who want to visit their area or want to be dominated via e-mail. For example, here's one from LA, another from Hawaii:

> TV mistress in Hawaii looking for male slaves, playthings, or submissives for consensual fun. I prefer to play the dom, but a little role-switching might be interesting also. If you are interested, living in Hawaii, and would like to experience a tv mistress, please e-mail me...Those with gifs attached and detailed letters describing themselves, their limits, and preferences will get first reply.

> Come on...all you naughty boys. This Hollywood mistress knows you have been *VERY* bad and need her most strict discipline!! I am going to turn you over my knee and not stop until my razor strop leaves your insolent little ass cherry red! My domination is TOTAL...but my fee is *very* tiny...so e-mail me, and let me show you the error of your naughty ways...I accept e-mail and phone naughty boys as well as local Southern California naughty boys...so WRITE ME NOW!!! Your spanking is waiting!!

The other newsgroups, had similar, and in many cases, the same announcements. So just in case you didn't see the post in one place you would in another.

Yet, ironically, while the reach of these notices might be global, many of them still were for local events or individuals seeking to meet others within the area, such as these from alt.personals.bondage.

> Seeking a very Dominant, experienced SF Bay area bondage mistress to serve in a DS LTR. I am interested in submission, discipline, training, collaring, male chastity, intricate bondage and suspension...I have many skills and am very handy. Move in, rule my roost, and live rent free with me catering to your every need if things work out.

> Female & submissive?...Need more rough sex in your life?...Live within 50 miles of Philadelphia?...E-mail this man...Plan on a prompt response. Plan on being treated with respect. Plan on being abused.

And then there were several ads for local get-togethers, such as an East San Francisco Bay Munch at a brew house in Alameda ("at the door or bar ask for 'Sarah's Munch'"), with an explanation of just what is a "munch"— basically a social gathering for anyone with an interest in B&D, S&M, or D&S; requests for places to go for those living in a particular area, such as this post: "I live in the Sacramento area and I was wondering if there was a place for me to go to have some fun"; or referrals to specific activities or services in an area, such as this one headed: "NJ well-equipped dungeon sought... I am seeking to find a well-equipped, clean dungeon to rent. Not kidding, very serious. Please only serious replies." Or if someone was traveling, an announcement on the newsgroup provided a way to plan ahead, such as one alt.personals.bondage man who announced: "I will be in Nashville from November 14 to 17 with my female sub... and am interested in BDSM clubs or bars... or any good shopping spots. Might be interested in meeting with f subs or other D/S couples."

At the same time, many postings in these groups reflected an interest in practicing D&S through cyberspace—and in finding ways to do so discreetly and privately. For example, one entrepreneur who advertised on many of these news groups announced that he had started a "Female Domination by Audio Cassette Hypnosis Program" and he was looking for submissive male volunteers to help in developing the program which would involve visualizing in trancelike state things like obedience, humiliation, doggy training, and adult baby activities. As he explained: "You will listen to the tape as often as possible, both during the day and at bedtime. You will keep a log detailing the circumstances of listening to the tape and any effects it has on you. I will want to know what works and what doesn't work." And another poster described a new anon remail service, explaining that a lifestyle friend had started this anonymous remail service and "offers a FREE 24-36 hour trial. Check it out and sign up at..." Then, anyone interested could go to the indicated Web site to sign up.

In some cases, I found fantasy stories, often followed by requests for comments, such as one man who posted a rape fantasy about a male slave captured after the collapse of society and repeatedly subjected to sodomy by his new master. In other cases, a woman was the dominant partner, tying up, spanking, and otherwise dominating her slave.

Frequently, there were requests for pictures or tapes—or offers to sell them, such as this sampling from alt.sex.bondage:

Listen to Me Scream in Ecstasy! I love to masturbate when you're listening... Take a listen! (followed by an 809 number, which has been linked to high-price phone numbers in the Caribbean)

I have pictures of my girlfriend that I'm willing to trade for Bondage pictures. These Pics are of Susie in a teddy, and tied. E-mail if you're interested.

Again and again, there were references to Web sites with erotic materials, such as the following alt.sex.bondage postings:

An all Adult Web Directory... This directory will change the way you find sex on the net! (followed by a www address)

Fetish-House... Visit our site at http://.... The oldest Fetish-house world-wide, with its own production. Rubber, latex, leather, pvc, textile, adult baby's, bizarre, toys, videos, magazines, and more.

LIST OF HARDCORE & FETISH SITES! This site has links to tons of free porn sites! (followed by a www address)

And from time to time there were some extended discussions about activities and philosophies of play, though this was rare. But primarily they appeared in the alt.sex categories, like alt.sex.bondage, alt.sex.spanking, and alt.sex.femdom, rather than in the groups that started off with alt.personals, that tended to be more devoted to emphasizing personal ads and announcements. For example, some excerpts from a typical exchange between a few submissive males and a lifestyle dominant:

> Mistress Alicia wrote: 'My requirement is honesty... If you wish to retain the right to negotiate, to ask me for specific things to be done to you and to essentially tell me what to do, kindly do not tell me that you are submitting to me. You're not. You're bottoming. There is a difference.'
> I agree with this completely, Mistress Alicia. When I'm subbing I want what happens to happen because the Domme wants it, not me. I don't like to suggest things at all. I even have a tendency to not want to be honest when someone asks me what I like or what I'm into, because I've found that even though I may love doing something with one Domme, that is usually because she enjoys it and shows how much she likes it to me.

And another male commented on her comment as follows:

> I haven't been in the 'scene' very long... though I practice the art for years... But I have gotten the strong impression that the words 'bottom, top, sub and dom' are going through a change in definition. That not too long ago the terms were interchangeable... but now you will get a lot of argument about it. Perhaps it is asking too much to expect that potential playmates understand all the connotations that you put on words. Even with a lot of explanation, I would expect there be confusion... From what I've experienced myself, after you relax, being more 'subly' gets easier, because that experience is more long-range and takes longer to work into.

When I checked out the spanking posts on alt.sex.spanking, alt.personals.spanking, and alt.personals.spanking punishment, many posts were the same or similar as on the various alt.bondage newsgroups (alt.bondage, alt.sex.bondage, and alt.personals.bondage), with the added interest in spanking, paddling, caning, whipping, and other play with pain. In fact, some posters referred to the news groups as a kind of cybercommunity focused around this interest which they playfully called "assville." And some posts featured the theme of punishment or recalled memories of childhood punishment scenes, like trips to the woodshed to be punished by Dad or discipline from English boarding school days. And here there appeared to be a somewhat more even mix of submissive men seeking "strict" women and masters seeking women wanting to be spanked, in contrast to the bondage category that seemed to attract more dominant men who wanted to tie up their submissive partners.

For example, here's a representative ad on alt.personals.spanking from a New York male seeking to be "punished" in the course of serving and being obedient to a woman:

> I'm a 39-year-old submissive white male that is seeking to serve a female as houseboy. I'm 6'0, 185 lbs, attractive, but most important, experienced at housework with a strong desire to clean under the supervision of a lady. Scrubbing floors, laundry, cleaning bathrooms are my skills...You are a dominant female between 30–45, would enjoy having a man clean your home, and would feel completely at ease using a crop or paddle to show your displeasure at unsatisfactory work...I ask to be treated as a servant and disciplined for work not meeting your expectation. I'm very discreet, and hope for the same from you. My obedience will be unquestioned.

And here's another from a man in Washington State:

> Male, late 40s looking for a female to administer a hard spanking and enema...I live in east Washington State and can travel during the day for your enjoyment. I have a very nice selection of enema equipment and a willing bottom that needs to be reddened with a firm hand and hairbrush.

And as for dominant men seeking women, well, here's a sampling—and in some cases, their ads seemed much more sexually explicit than the ones posted by submissive men seeking women. For example, here's one man offering graphic pictures of his wife, with this explanation:

> This is a wav file of my wife getting spanked as I fuck her!! She really loves to be spanked hard during sex. She loves it when I slap her face with my cock and slap her cunt with my hand. Then I turn her over and fuck her doggy style and spank her till her white ass is pink. Comments? Trades?

But another man seeking woman wanting discipline took a more fatherly approach:

> Girls, are you in need of a guiding hand from a strong father-figure-uncle?

Do you feel like you really need to be turned over a man's knee and spanked? Do you know deep down that you have been a bad girl and this is the only way to set things right again? E-mail me, and we will discuss it.

And one man in Ohio offered up his woodshed for anyone of either sex who was interested:

Seeking Males or Females 18–26 for a trip to my woodshed... I am a Father or Uncle figure who wants to warm your little ass... 50-year-old white male who is dominate wants your body... E-mail for details.

Meanwhile, a North Carolina man evoked imagery of an old-fashioned whipping by Dad. Or as he described it, in a long two-page fantasy, which was a mix of story and ad:

Do you ever yearn for the days when Daddy would catch you coming in late and promise you a good, old-fashioned butt-whipping as soon as you were ready for bed? Your tummy would twist with dread while you were getting undressed and putting on your pajamas. Then you'd sit there trembling, just waiting for his footsteps... Then you'd find yourself face down over his knee... His big, strong arm would easily hold you down.... Then, naked from your middle to your knees, your bare bottom shamefully exposed, you'd just want to die of humiliation... Finally, he'd give you a final hug, kiss your forehead, and tuck you into bed where you'd sleep the night on your tummy... Well, if you *do* yearn for those days, why don't you e-mail me and let's get to know each other. I'm a safe and sane spanker, a good deal older than you (I'm a healthy 63), know what I'm doing, and will do my best to make your spanking dreams come true.

And yes, there were a number of professional dominants seeking male submissives or slaves who wanted to be spanked or serve, as well as special ads about spanking sites and services, such as an ad for a SPANKING U Web site and an ad for the World's Only All-Spanking Sex Line, featuring "100 percent spanking stories prerecorded for your xxx pleasure," plus there was a "Dominatrix S&M Line." So where was this number that started off with the prefix: 011-592 located? "Oh, that's Guyana," the operator said.

While alt.sex.spanking similarly had a mix of personals and commercial ads, there was also more of a sense of community because of the extended discussions about technique and philosophy, requests for advice, and fantasy stories or accounts of experiences (perhaps true, perhaps fantasies) that were frequently posted with a mix of both female and male dominant or submissive perspectives.

For example, one poster from the United Kingdom posted a three-part story, each about 5 pages long, describing the problem of the hard-working married couple Chris and Carly who had been working too hard. But then Chris wrote up a spanking list of the various things Carly did wrong, like hiding his car keys and tampering with his papers, leading him to give her a spanking with his hairbrush, described in detail by the poster.

And a few other posters asked for advice or opinions, such as these:

> I am curious what everyone's fav position is . . . I like OTK and while my sub is standing, hands tied over his head and lying down and . . . oh hell, I just like spanking his bottom!!!

> Dear ASSville Gang,
> I have a question for you all, so please indulge me: Do you think that those of us who like being on the spanking end of a relationship have a higher/ different pain threshold than the population in general?? I mean for types of pain OTHER THAN SPANKING??? . . . I like an acute injury (like a broken bone) or for the women folk, LABOR!!! What has your experience been like? Is SPANKING PAIN somehow 'DIFFERENT'??? . . . So please respond if you are a 'heavy' player (canes and stuff), medium (whatever the hell that means), or spanko-wuss (hand/light paddle) like me.

To which one poster replied, yes, they are:

> I am not what you'd call a 'heavy' player, but I can take a pretty good spanking (hand/brush/strap). Pain from injury is not at all like pain from a spanking . . . Perhaps it's the erotic element involved with a spanking . . . I enjoy receiving a spanking, but I studiously avoid visiting the dentist . . . I refuse to take injections. I'm a total coward as regards pain . . . except when it comes to spanking. So I would have to say, yes, the 2 types of pain *are* different.

A few posters described the role of spanking or D&S generally in their relationship, and what made it work for them, such as this man and woman who had this to say about their respective relationships:

> My GF and I have a relationship whereby spanking is sex play and not a lifestyle. I never spank her to change 'her behavior but rather to 'raise the temperature of our lovemaking' as she puts it so aptly. The turn-on for me is that she will surrender her bottom to my hand, cane, paddle, riding crop, cat-o'-nine-tails, or yardstick . . . She tells me the turn-on for her is the look on my face, the sound, my reaction . . . .

> My current partner and I play a lot, but all decisions are joint ones, and while I'm happy occasionally playing to be his slave and maybe fetching a beer or something, if he expected it as a matter of course, he'd get his beer outside of the bottle and all over him.

So for the regulars, the newsgroup was a kind of virtual community where they could share their ideas in a kind of ongoing dialogue. In fact, one woman described it as such, explaining why.

> I have been reading these newsgroups for over a year now... Why?... Because I am a member of that unique society that has a spanking fetish... Simply put... spanking 'turns me on'... I have been living with both the fetish, and the guilt of that fetish, for as long as I can remember... And then I discovered alt.sex.spanking... Here I found people from all walks of life... from all over the world... that shared my strange ideas... I felt like I had 'come home'... I found a place where I belonged at long last....
>
> Assville is a community... a very caring and sensitive community... It is made up of people with as many varying ideas as any other community. Each of us has our own personal agenda... our own ideas as to what is acceptable and what is not.

In fact, reinforcing this notion of community, the group even has its own FAQ—or discussion of frequently asked questions, which describes the newsgroup as a "splinter group from alt.sex.bondage" focusing on an interest in spanking, while a.s.b. deals with "the entire breadth of DBSM interests." And besides suggesting what people should post—"just about any test that relates to erotic spanking—fiction, real-life anecdotes, childhood memories, questions, advice, scene information, etc."—there's a detailed discussion about what not to post, including pictures, personal ads, and flames, though there are ads galore.

And finally, I checked out the alt.sex.femdom category. Again, the same mix of commercial and personal ads and "see our Web site" postings. But as in alt.sex.spanking, there was more debate and discussion, even a section FAQ, this time with an emphasis on women being dominant and men being submissive whatever the activity—whether bondage, spanking, or generally playing with power.

For example, in an extended discussion of "How does one find the REAL Female Dommes?," Lady Tanith, who was a frequent participant in the alt.sex.spanking group, too, had this to say:

> I will not date outside the BDSM community. This is a lifetime decision for me, arrived at after several early relationships with vanilla men failed with a lot of pain on both sides... No more of that for me, thanks. If a man has not actively sought out the BDSM community and BDSM activities on his own, showing that his need for BDSM is real... I do not want to be in a relationship with him. It's going to fail. I know it and eventually he will know it too...
>
> So if you date someone for too long before getting honest about your

sexual orientation, that is a hell of a time/energy/emotional investment on your part that might be completely wasted if she turns out to be hard-wired vanilla...So if you are a hard-wired D&S type like me, and the major burning need in your emotional life is to find a dominant or a submissive or to own or to be owned by someone, I think you're a serious schmuck if you lead a straight woman on very far without telling her your hidden agenda.

And in reply, one male submissive, besides recommending others read Lady Tanith's post, had this to say:

Find out who you are, find out what you really want. Chatting, exchanging e-mail or getting turned on by a fantasy story is not always the same as experiencing it in real life...Finding a partner is HARD work and takes some guts. But partners can be found anywhere...Do not give up looking after a couple of bad experiences...If the submissive or dominant part is really inside you, don't settle for a vanilla relationship. It is almost guaranteed that it will fail, or become a quagmire of deceit! However, there is nothing wrong with cultivating a relationship with someone you care for, and if the care is mutual, chances are that she will be open to your desires...(But) do not expect to find a dominant or submissive who is exactly into the things you are into...S&M relationships are the same as any other relationship and involve 'give' and 'take.'

Meanwhile, another ongoing discussion concerned using safe words, reflecting a common paradox of many in the scene—the "paradox of control versus limits." As one woman described this paradox, seeking opinions and advice from others:

He would like to have such complete control that no safe words or anything else are worried about. I don't have a problem with there being no safe word. He stops when he thinks I can't go any further. It's no longer erotic to him if I'm not enjoying it. But it's not completely erotic if he can't just totally let go and disregard me...And it's a problem with hitting the physical limits of the body. We practice a lot of elaborate bondage and there are frequently times where blood flow gets constricted or muscles cramp that just can't be ignored...How do other tops/dom/masters deal with this paradox?

In turn, others replied with their own experiences and advice, such as one man in a permanent relationship with a professional dominatrix with her own 2,000-square-foot dungeon and "every toy imaginable." As he commented:

It's an emotional/mental game between partners that are not formed in concrete, human beings who change and are fluid. Communicate with each other! As a top, I seldom blindfold a sub, because I want to be able to read the eyes, which often say a lot more than the mouth. As a bottom, when things were not going right for me, I would try to give my top a way out.

And then there were the many hopeful ads from mostly submissive men who were hoping to meet a partner online—or at least, describing their fantasy femdom relationship, such as these:

Seattle area male, single... searching for the 'assertive' woman for possible long-term relationship. I'm stubborn but want to learn that serving you is its own reward. Take the time to train me and you'll live in paradise.

I am a 23-year-old-male who lives in New Jersey. I would love to be your virtual slave. My fantasies are of being a little boy turned into a proper young lady and a macho male chauvinist turned into a sissy skirt-wearing male secretary.

In sum, though I only had a chance to skim the surface of these postings, sampling a few of perhaps 20,000 postings in about a two-week period on these seven D&S news groups, they presented a kind of cyberspace version of the range of meetings, classes, newspapers, magazines, and one-on-one get-togethers and sessions that characterized the scene years before and still are a central part of the scene today. But what's different is the global character of these interpersonal communications, and while some may lead to meetings for locals or travelers to an area, (for many posters, some relationships are confined to) e-mail exchanges, including domination with instructions by e-mail, or exchanging or gathering information from the newsgroups or visiting Web sites. Perhaps for some individuals, this has become the '90s safe way to explore in the scene, without any risk of exposure, fully protected by an online code name or an anonymous mail service to do the posting. But for many others, perhaps even most, cyberspace is simply another option for learning about and communicating with others in the scene. It's a way to meet others individually, find out about local meetings, and swap tips and advice to be applied in one's own D&S relationships. And then, for those who want to learn more, it's a way to find out what's out there on the World Wide Web, too—on both personal and commercial sites like home and business addresses in this information age.

VISITING THE D&S CLUB SCENE

Finally, to look at what's new in the scene today, I went to one of the new trendy clubs with a D&S scene. While there were some underground clubs in the 1980s and still are today—clubs like the Hellfire Club in New York, which existed then and now, and has a kind of grungy underground subway atmosphere, what's new is the way some of these clubs have gone mainstream. Such clubs appeal to a typically younger, 20-something audience, and they are in a nightclub setting featuring drinking, dancing, and pop, rock, or house music (generally a mix of industrial, new wave, alternative— sometimes the kind of music you might hear at a rave). This is quite a contrast to the usual D&S party environment, which are typically no-alcohol occasions, since the emphasis is on staying in control in doing a scene. Also, many of these clubs aren't dedicated D&S or S&M style places like the underground clubs; rather they devote a regular night each week or have an occasional D&S event, where attendees are invited to dress up in style—and even participate in scenes if they want.

But instead of a sense of looking in on a private scene as in the underground clubs and typical D&S play parties, there is a sense of observing a D&S performance, with the scene as entertainment, turning the private moment into a kind of theatrical event. While I observed a few of these events from time to time in the 1980s, such as when Kat and several other dominatrixes staged scenes on a stage at my original *Erotic Power* launch party, these were fairly rare then. But now they had become hip and trendy. And with it was gone the kind of guilt I often heard newcomers to the scene express back in the early 1980s about having an interest considered abnormal by many. Instead, now, for many in this younger crowd, an interest in D&S was simply part of the current style or fashionable attitude of the day characterized by a mix of social rebellion and a release of the dark side of the persona, typified in the imagery of many pop and rock stars as well.

This is the kind of atmosphere I found when I went to visit a typical club of this type—the Bondage-a-Go-Go in San Francisco. It's an event held at a club called the Trocadero Transfer. But on Wednesday nights, starting at 9:00 P.M., the club features an evening with a D&S theme, emphasizing bondage and S&M play and dress. And small colored cards promoting the event encouraged attendees to come dressed and ready to play accordingly. For example, one side of the card featured a woman lying on a mattress with a large strap around her arms dangling from a chain, looking a little like a 1920s Jean Harlow-type heroine tied to a railroad track, and on the other side, the invitation went on to announce: "Fetish attire preferrred! Those Dressed to Play Get Front of the Line Privileges." Plus there was "100 Percent Interactive Play Upstairs!," as well as "Exotic Caged Animals"— actually dancers who twisted and writhed in small enclosed areas with bars on the main floor.

As I walked in a few minutes after 9:00 P.M., the evening was just getting started. Like everyone else, I had to show an ID to indicate I was at least 21 ("No exceptions," said the burly bouncer at the door, even though I was clearly well over 21!), and then once inside, I passed by a display of jewelry for sale, and was greeted by two reps for a local weekly newspaper—the *SF Weekly*—which was offering free "Wild Side" ads for men or women who wanted to meet others for erotic relationships. "A headline and 30 words free," one sales rep, a blonde 20-something woman, told me. "And then you can record up to a 3-minute erotic message the caller can hear when he calls." When I looked through the current issue, I saw there were hundreds of such ads divided into categories of Women Seeking Men, Men Seeking Women, and Women and Men Seeking One Another—a category of advertising that was about the same size as a popular section of free romance ads with similar categories. At one time such ads were confined to underground papers, like the *Spectator*, now published by Kat, who had started off in the D&S community as a mistress and occasional teacher of D&S classes about 15 years before. But now they were a growing part of a mainstream weekly paper—still another sign that D&S had gone mainstream.

At first, the crowd was sparse, but upstairs, a small group of people in black leather were gathering behind a roped-off area that would become a kind of ministage for D&S play—a few men in leather pants or jackets and black T-shirts and jeans, a few women in short leather mini-skirts or pants. One of the men had a collection of D&S equipment hanging from his belt—handcuffs, a riding crop, a whip, a hunting knife, handcuffs; another had a couple of bags of equipment, including knives and electrical gadgets; a third was a leather worker who had several masks and cats for sale on display. Meanwhile, a gradually increasing group of onlookers began to gather in front of the rope, waiting for events to begin.

Around 10:30 P.M., they finally did. Perhaps 50 or so people were assembled now, and two of the women now began stepping into the submissive role. One knelt down at one end of the stage in front of the man with the D&S equipment hanging from his belt and he began spanking and then whipping her. Later, he would try out a variety of high-tech techniques on her, including spraying her back with gasoline and running some kind of long-necked device that gave off sparks along her back, creating a kind of buzzing flame—and if it suddenly erupted too much he quickly doused it. Meanwhile, toward the center of the roped area, another woman stripped off her black tights and jersey to her black leather garters and black leather bra, and then raised her arms so her partner, the man with the two bags of equipment, could lock her into a rack on the ceiling with cuffs dangling from it. Then after lightly spanking her, he began running various buzzing electric devices across her body. They looked like various shaped light bulbs and fixtures, and white and blue flashes of electricity snapped through them as he worked. Then, finishing with the electrical play, he rubbed a knife lightly around her body.

Meanwhile, as they continued to play, a few other couples from the audience joined them in the roped area, and began to do scenes as well— again with the male dressed and dominant, the woman submissive—and typically undressed down to a black leather G-string, heels, and top. As for the crowd, here and there a few people wore collars, most of them women, and a few dressed in this same tough dark leather look. But mostly, it was everyday casual dress—T-shirts, jackets, and jeans. And now downstairs in the large dark cavelike room with a few flashing spotlights that swept the room, about 50 couples were dancing while a growing crowd of about 100 people, mostly single males, watched. And in two cages on platforms, a few women and a man in leathers and cape danced.

It was the kind of scene one might see at a punk, rock, or alternative nightclub with a generally 20s something crowd, with a sprinkling of people in their 30s and 40s, except for the addition of the upstairs D&S play space. It also seemed to be a generally, if not exclusively, heterosexual male dominant scene featuring a tough leather and motorcycle look—with the feel of an MTV rock video come to life in a smoky bar setting. Also, the sophisticated high-tech equipment many players used were new, and there seemed to be more of an interest in flirting with danger, such as in the play with gas, electricity, and knives, though it was also clear there was a concern with safety and consensuality, and at the end of the scenes, no one was hurt—no burns, no cuts—though at times, it looked like the potential danger was very real, which perhaps contributed to the excitement of the scene for both the players and the viewers. In any case, the whole look and atmosphere of this scene is very new—and it seems to be part of a growing trend to bring D&S into the clubs with a more mainstream appeal to a younger generation.

When I left around midnight, the club was still going strong—"Until about 1:00 or 2:00 A.M." someone told me as I left, and picked up some small cards announcing other upcoming D&S events on the club circuit—like a SLICK fetish ball, featuring a leather fashion show and S&M and B&D playspace, a "genitorturers" event, and some men-only and women-only events at another local club. Then, as I walked out into the street, I saw a line of about a dozen people, some dressed in leathers, still waiting to get in. It was only midnight, and on the club circuit, the night was still young.

CHECKING OUT THE WORLD WIDE WEB

Finally, to conclude my tour of what's new in the D&S world today, I went to check out the World Wide Web. It was quite different from the news groups, which included some ongoing dialogues along with the personal and commercial ads. By contrast, the Web seemed like more of a collection of commercial billboards, advertising various erotic products and services.

Typically, the sites began with a disclaimer, advising that the site contained explicit—sometimes "very" explicit adult fare. So you should be 18 or older to proceed. Or at least by proceeding, you were stating you were 18 or older. And most of the sites had black backgrounds with white or red printing—perhaps a reminder that this was "dark" side hot stuff.

Then, after offering brief descriptions and sometimes a sampling of photos of scenes of bondage, spanking, or nudity, the sites offered various ways to sign up and pay. One could call an 800 number and join with a credit card, call a 900 number and pay a few dollars a minute for an erotic fantasy call, or sign up as a member online, using a credit card. Only two of the two dozen sites I checked out offered free or noncommercial information—one was a group in New Hampshire that had Fetish Play Parties the fourth Saturday each month, and invited anyone in southern New Hampshire to attend, as well as included a few sample photos from past parties; another was the publisher of an erotic card game *Seduction for 2* that offered a sampling of 50 ways to sexually seduce and excite your lover, such as how to give a sensuous back massage or do intimate slow dancing for two—and then at the end, the publisher also plugged his game.

But the other sites were like cyberspace versions of ads that might appear in a D&S or other erotic newspapers or magazines. For example, one site that called itself "Sunsexxxblvd" offered itself as a kind of "cyberbrothel" with erotic photos and fantasy phone sex. As it explained in its introductory copy:

> **Stop in at the X Mansion**...and play with the girls who call this cyberbrothel home. Sucking, fucking, licking and much much more. These girls do it all...and they'll keep you cuming back time and again!
> **Dial up the Phone Booth**...For the hottest phone fuck of your life, visit the Phone Booth Now. We're HOT, WET and ready for YOU. Nothing is Taboo—we'll talk about anything! So cum on baby, pull down your pants, grab your cock and live out your ultimate sexual fantasy. It's all waiting for you in the phone booth!
> **1-800-**...only $9.95 charged discreetly to your credit card gets you into all the action for 30 days.

Several sites were from other countries, including Kunzmann, a catalog of fetish wear from Germany, and a few porn sites based in Amsterdam, that touted the completely uncensored freedom of the Amsterdam connection. For example, Kunzmann provided a sampling of pages from its catalog, showing small photos of costumes like chain dresses, corsets, boots, and teddies in rubber, plastic, leather, and other materials, along with prices in dollars or deutschmarks and details for ordering. We're "the first on the fetish market," it announced. "Founded in 1950. Here you will get everything your fetish heart can wish for." Meanwhile, the Amsterdam ad pulled no punches, announcing: RED HOT AMSTERDAM...THE HARDEST PORN IN THE WORLD IS DUTCH. IT IS TOTALLY UNCENSORED, TOTALLY UNINHIBITED, TOTALLY UNREGU-LATED...RED HOT AMSTERDAM GIVES YOU FULL-COLOR PIC-TURES AND MOVIES FROM THE HEART OF THE PORNOGRAPHIC WORLD...IF YOU'RE READING THIS PAGE, YOU WANT THE REAL HARDCORE MATERIAL...3 MONTHS OF UNLIMITED ACCESS TO AMSTERDAM AND THE HARDEST PORN NYWHERE, COSTS JUST $10, AND YOU CAN HAVE INSTANT ACCESS."

Another site I contacted was a kind of erotic Web server, which called itself AdultDirect. But now, instead of trying to search for these sites through a more general search engine like Yahoo or Alta Vista, this site had pulled together over 10,000 erotic sites on the Net—from D&S to anything else sexual and erotic. Or to quote from some of the introductory ad copy:

> LINKS TO THOUSANDS OF SEX SITES!...WE NOW HAVE OVER 10,000 Sites! And we are adding more all the time...3 Month Access Special Is Only $39.95!...All membership offers include: Unlimited Access TTime...Use of our Fast and Secure Server...Discrete Billing to your Credit Card...AdultDirect Gives You Adult Entertainment: Adult Internet Sites; Sites with Gifts, Jpegs, AVI, and Quicktime files of adult material...Sites with Erotic stories and text files...IRC Chat Groups listed (the hot channels)...Just press on the HyperText and you are automatically connected to the Adult Sites of YOUR CHOICE! (And then by submitting name, password and credit card information, one could sign up right away).

I also checked out one of the domination sites, sponsored by a publication called *DOMINATION: The Fetish Magazine,* based in Santa Monica, California. It offered hundreds of exclusive photographs, classified by hundreds of categories, and featured a few relatively tame sample photos on its site. Presumably, one could search for just those photos in a particular category, such as:

> nude/pussy/nudity/nudes/porn/sex pictures/oral sex/blowjob/big tits/anal sex/nude celebrities/bestiality/pedophila/cum shots/teen sex/amateur sex/ panties naked men/incest/kinky sex/sadism/nude of the day/watersports/ masochism/doggy style/dildos/x-rated/fellatio/masturbation...etc.

The list went on for 1½ single-spaced pages, with many of the words repeated again and again. The cost? About $20 a month, $90 for a year.

And finally, at the suggestion of numerous mentions on alt.sex.spanking and alt.personals.spanking, I checked out the Spanking-U-Enterprises site (or S.U.E. for short), which like other erotic sites seemed primarily targeted at the male cyberviewer. Its home page featured a group of women bending over to show their bare buts—one bending over a couch, another on an escalater, a third picking up a basket, and then it introduced its main products—several 90-minute spanking tapes, a spanking magazine, a new line of spanking books, and personal ads for spankers. Or as the company explained:

> (We're) a newly formed company that takes the word 'taboo' out of spanking, and reaches the populace with a NEW, FUN approach...that will make it easier for people to talk about their favorite subject, without the normal hesitancy...This will be accomplished through the diversity of products we will offer, not only to spanking enthusiasts, but to EVERYONE!

And then, it described some of its products, featuring both women and men being spanked, such as the following about its 90-minute tapes:

> SUE's Naughty Girl Spanking Fantasies contain 8 arousing stories of SUE's escapades, which always lead her to an over-the-knee, leg kicking, bare bottom spanking that leaves her cheeks crimson red; SUE's Naughty Boy Spanking Fantasies contain 10 tantalizing stories in which SUE finds it very necessary to take naughty boys across her lap, bare their bottoms and give them a very hard, well deserved spanking, leaving their cheeks bright red...These stories are guaraateed to make you want to redden someone's behind!!

And so, with that, I ended my tour of the World Wide Web. It was actually a very slow process, taking several minutes to either load or print most of these pages, even with a 28.8 modem. But then, for those who do browse the Web, there is the opportunity for access sites around the world, as well as sign-up for actually receiving these images, erotic text, or phone calls. And presumably, as the speed and quality of communications on the Web improves, there will be even further developments, such as more quick-time movies and even 3-D images, along with even more privacy and security in accessing these sites. For example, as one new Anonymous Remain Service I found on the Web announced:

> We offer you the chance to send and receive messages with others, or post articles to newsgroups, without others being able to discover your TRUE e-mail address...Speaking of anonymity, how's this?...We don't even ask for your name!

All you need is an e-mail address and a credit card, after trying out the service for free for 3 days.

It seemed a fitting way to end my survey of what the scene is like today. Since I first looked at the scene almost 20 years ago, there has been a continued concern with privacy, and using first names or scene names has been one way to preserve this. And now on the internet and World Wide Web that privacy can be taken even further. Not only is one's identity kept secret by those in the scene, but now one can keep one's identity totally secret from those within it, using a personally created digital persona and anonymous e-mail identity. And then too, one can even create an alternate identity so one can play even more freely in different modes trying out different personas not possible in actual physical encounters (such as becoming a dominant or submissive male or female and experimenting with different fetishes and interests within the scene.

Some individuals in the scene are already trying this, appearing in different guises and under different names when they sign onto the newsgroups or check out various sites on the World Wide Web. And as the Internet and World Wide Web grow, perhaps this is a likely direction for further development of the scene in the 1990s—not only moving into the mainstream nightclubs but becoming more and more a part of virtual reality and cyberspace as well.

22

Conclusion

A s I have tried to illustrate, a vast variety of people with a diverse range of erotic interests participate in D&S. Their backgrounds, activities, and attitudes are quite unlike the social stereotype that depicts D&S as a form of violence, mischief, or mayhem perpetrated by the psychologically unstable who seek to hurt others or to be hurt themselves. In fantasy, D&Sers believe virtually anything may be possible and acceptable. But, in reality, they have a strict code of rules about consensuality, safety, and respect for limits. At times, they may push against these limits, for that is part of the challenge of exploring new forms of sexual expression. But they usually value safety over experimentation—as one practitioner puts it: "You want your partner to be able and willing to play again."

The rare accidents and the tiny minority of psychotic practitioners of S&M seem to attract the attention of the popular press, and such reports may lead the public to judge the whole community to be sick and perverted. But, in fact, at the core of the D&S community are mostly sensible, rational, respectable, otherwise quite ordinary people, for whom D&S is a way of playing with unique, bizarre, unusual, and often taboo forms of fantasy and erotic expression, as a release from the everyday world. Perhaps because these people are otherwise so seemingly normal, D&S exerts a strong compelling power over them—as a fantasy escape from real-life stresses and pressures. They view D&S as a form of adult play and call their equipment "toys"—the very word imbues the objects and devices used in the session, no matter how sinister looking, with a spirit of fun and play.

Thus—quite unlike its public image—the D&S community is a warm, close, and supportive one, and its members avoid truly dangerous or harmful activities. Instead, they emphasize using fantasy, power exchanges, and role playing to create a more intense, and often erotic, experience. The unusualness of these roles and activities are the source of their exciting and erotic effects. But, most importantly, the symbolism and psychological aspects of D&S make these activities pleasurable—for being hit, tied up, humiliated, or disciplined is not enjoyable in and of itself. Rather, the toys, techniques, rituals, costumes, staging, and other accouterments of fantasy give these activities symbolic and psychological meaning.

Furthermore, despite its public image—at least some forms of D&S activity are prevalent among the general public; many couples experiment with D&S to some degree, although they do not call their activities by that name. So there is a continuum between the casual but undefined D&S play of many couples and the conscious and frequent expression of D&S activity among those in the scene.

To sum up some of the major themes we have observed throughout the book, people become involved in the D&S scene for a variety of complex reasons. Most males are attracted to submission as a counterbalance to their overall dominant lifestyle, although some seek sexual submission to complement their overall submissiveness. Similarly, some women are balancers, others are natural dominants. Thus, to understand the dynamics of D&S behavior and preferences, one must look to a given individual's personality and experience; one must look beyond the outward behavior to discover its underlying meaning.

We also noted that although many D&Sers are in higher than average educational, occupational, and income brackets, and tend to be less religious than average Americans, the appeal of D&S cuts across all social categories. No particular social or personality feature appears to account for their involvement in the scene; rather, the determining factors are most often situational. Most usually, the male has had some childhood experiences that provoked submissive fantasies, while the female has been introduced to D&S by a boyfriend, lover, or husband. Both males and females typically first explore D&S privately or in a couple relationship. For most, these explorations go no further.

But a few discover the D&S scene, and in time, some come to identify with a larger D&S community. They take workshops on dominance and submission, meet couples through newspaper and magazine ads, join D&S organizations, go to D&S parties, or get together informally with others involved in D&S. Yet for both those who become extremely active and those who drift in and out of the scene, the couple relationship remains crucial.

Among the issues most couples confront are the individual member's ambivalence about the power exchange—the man's reluctance to yield power and the woman's hesitation to assume it. Of course, each relationship has its particular dynamics, and no two couples follow the same patterns in the importance they attribute to D&S, their preferences, and the ways in which they express D&S. And even in a given relationship, the couple's involvement with D&S may vary sharply over time. Indeed, change and variety are keynotes of the scene, and most D&Sers are excited by new toys, techniques, and approaches to exchanging power and expressing sexuality.

For the most part, D&Sers in the scene have overcome their earlier feelings of guilt, if any, and they are satisfied with their preferred erotic activities. They stress responsible participation that recognizes one's partner's limits, and they adhere to rules, etiquette, and consensuality. But while most D&Sers have come to terms with their activity, they are aware that most members of the general public have not. Accordingly, they are very careful about identifying themselves as D&Sers and reveal themselves only to those they trust will understand or may be prospective participants in the scene.

In contrast to this informal, but close D&S community, we also examined the commercial world of professional dominants and clients. Most males who visit professionals haven't been able to develop satisfying D&S relationships with the women in their lives or are not currently involved with women at all. And although some mistresses truly love being dominant and are active in the noncommercial scene as well, some play dominant strictly for the money. Other aspects of the commercial scene include D&S literature and tapes. These exemplify the pervasiveness of fantasy in the scene, providing readers and viewers with new ideas and entrees to other D&Sers.

Despite the increasing prevalence of both noncommercial and commercial D&S activity, public attitudes toward D&S are extremely negative. Recently, however, news stories and television programs such as *One Foot Out of the Closet* have presented a relatively restrained and neutral view of D&S. Also, a sprinkling of articles have begun to appear in popular magazines, such as one in *Time* in May 1981. Then, too, the imagery of female dominance has gradually entered the world of fashion and advertising. For instance, a fashion spread in *Vogue* in the late summer 1981 featured a series of photos of attractive stylishly dressed women dominating men: one beautiful woman in an evening gown had her foot dramatically poised to kick the rear end of a tuxedoed male crawling on his hands and knees near her bed. Similarly, the punk and New Wave rock scenes express a great deal of D&S imagery, particularly of the tough leather variety.

It also seems possible that the otherwise mainstream, upper-status character of most D&Sers may contribute to D&S's growing acceptability, particularly since many of them are quietly proselytizing interested friends. Although the process of gaining wider public acceptance is a slow one, it seems to be working. The scene itself has grown from a scattering of individuals in the early 1970s to perhaps 10,000 to 20,000 participants who are more or less active in several dozen organized groups.

As more information about D&S becomes public and as more people join the scene, a sense of avant-garde trendiness may become the new public image of D&S.

For a long time, D&S has been an underground movement. But now it seems as if this world is poised at the brink of greater public awareness and activity, much like the hippie movement was in the mid-1960s, and the spiritual cults were in the early-1970s. In both cases, the groups experienced a period of underground expansion, were discovered by the media, and suddenly became trendy. Also, both movements were comprised of mostly middle and upper class members, as are most D&Sers today. Though D&Sers are mostly older, in their 30s and 40s, their focus of interest on the erotic has a broad appeal to youth.

Now it may be D&S's turn to undergo this rapid expansion, particularly if the news media continues to offer informative pieces on D&S and the fashion media continue to glamorize D&S imagery, for this attention will lead the number of people in the scene to increase substantially. This impact can be expected, because beneath the foreboding D&S imagery, the creativity and eroticism involved in D&S activity has potential popular appeal. Ultimately, the heart of the D&S experience will remain within one-to-one relationships. But the desire to experiment and explore will lead many partners in a D&S relationship to link up with the wider D&S scene.

Thus, the following scenario seems likely. Gradually, the media will continue to discover D&S. More and more people will begin to explore D&S because it sounds like something new to do. Many may only explore on their own or within partnerships, as do most members of the current scene. But many will also investigate the organized scene, and as they do, D&S activity will become more acceptable. It will become trendy, the latest fad; and some of its imagery, symbols, and activities will be incorporated into the social mainstream. After a few years, when the scene becomes more sanitized and tamed by its new respectability, the general public will go on to something new. This process has happened repeatedly in the past in American life, and I predict it will happen to D&S, too. In fact, possibly, this book may contribute to this process.